NMS
National Medical Series for Independent Study

Surgery
Casebook

Second Edition

NMS | National Medical Series for Independent Study

Surgery
Casebook

Second Edition

Bruce E. Jarrell, MD

Professor
Department of Surgery
University of Maryland School of Medicine
Baltimore, Maryland

Eric D. Strauch, MD

Associate Professor
Department of Surgery
University of Maryland School of Medicine
Baltimore, Maryland

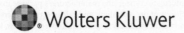

Philadelphia • Baltimore • New York • London
Buenos Aires • Hong Kong • Sydney • Tokyo

Acquisitions Editor: Tari Broderick
Product Development Editor: Amy Weintraub
Editorial Assistant: Joshua Haffner
Marketing Manager: Joy Fisher-Williams
Production Project Manager: Priscilla Crater
Design Coordinator: Terry Mallon
Manufacturing Coordinator: Margie Orzech
Prepress Vendor: Absolute Service, Inc.

Second Edition

9 8 7 6 5 4 3 2 1

Printed in China

Library of Congress Cataloging-in-Publication Data

Jarrell, Bruce E., author.
  NMS surgery casebook / Bruce E. Jarrell, Eric D. Strauch. — Second edition.
    p. ; cm. — (National medical series for independent study)
  Surgery casebook
  National medical series surgery casebook
  Companion to: NMS surgery / [edited by] Bruce E. Jarrell, Stephen M. Kavic. Sixth edition. [2016].
  Includes bibliographical references and index.
  ISBN 978-1-60831-586-4
  I. Strauch, Eric D., author. II. NMS surgery. Complemented by (work): III. Title. IV. Title: Surgery casebook. V. Title: National medical series surgery casebook. VI. Series: National medical series for independent study.
  [DNLM: 1. Surgical Procedures, Operative—Case Reports. 2. General Surgery—Case Reports. WO 18.2]
  RD37
  617—dc23
                                                                                          2015010502

RRS1504

This book is dedicated to several important people that have strongly influenced my ability to pursue a medical student–oriented career.

To Brigadier General Fritz Plugge, MC, USAF (Ret), who has been amazingly kind in his support of this department

To Lazar Greenfield, MD, who has been a wonderful role model for many of us in surgery

To Donald Wilson, MD; James Dalen, MD; Joe Gonella, MD; Frank Calia, MD; Albert Reece, MD; and Jay Perman, MD, my deans, who have each given me the opportunity to be with medical students my entire life

And to my family, Leslie, Noble, Kevin, Gwynneth, Jerry, Dad, and Mom, who have always helped me out

Bruce E. Jarrell, MD

To Stephen Bartlett, MD; Bruce Jarrell, MD; and Roger Voigt, MB, ChB, for being strong role models and their support

To my family, Cecilia, Jacob, Julia, Jessica, Jenna, Dad, and Mom for their love and support

Eric D. Strauch, MD

Preface

During our combined five decades of work with medical students in their clinical years, they have stimulated us to think about how we can do a better job of teaching. The second edition of *Surgery Casebook* is one way of trying to attain that goal. The cases in this book represent how we, as experienced surgeons, think and make decisions about a clinical problem. We have attempted to write it in a way that allows us to talk to you as you read it, so that the book will be the next best thing to teaching in person.

The cases are organized into body systems, and they represent common presentations. The history and physical examination clues help you reach a diagnosis. Illustrations have been added and enhanced with color and are used liberally to help you detect visual clues. Clinical images are also used in abundance. Case variations are also presented to help you consider treatment of patients with various complications and coexisting conditions. An all-new pediatrics chapter has been added that covers common congenital anomalies.

This book is of use to third- and fourth-year medical students in their surgery rotation as well as interns and residents planning to enter the field of surgery. Using this book alone or in combination with *NMS Surgery*, sixth edition, will help you apply your knowledge to decision making in clinical situations and master all of the steps in managing a patient.

Contributors

Emily Bellavance, MD
Assistant Professor of Surgery
Division of Surgical Oncology
University of Maryland School of Medicine
Baltimore, Maryland

Marshall Benjamin, MD
Associate Professor of Surgery
Division of Vascular Surgery
University of Maryland School of Medicine
Director, Maryland Vascular Center
Chairman, Department of Surgical Services
UM Baltimore Washington Medical Center
Baltimore, Maryland

Daniel Bochicchio, MD, FCCP
Assistant Professor
Anesthesiology and Critical Care Medicine
Baltimore VA Medical Center
Baltimore, Maryland

Molly Buzdon, MD, FACS
Chairman
Department of Surgery
Portsmouth Regional Hospital
Portsmouth, New Hampshire

W. Bradford Carter, MD
Medical Director
Alvin & Lois Lapidus Cancer Institute at Sinai and Northwest Hospitals
Baltimore, Maryland

Clint D. Cappiello, MD
Resident in Surgery
University of Maryland School of Medicine
Baltimore, Maryland

John L. Flowers, MD, FACS
Chief of Surgery
Department of General Surgery
Greater Baltimore Medical Center
Towson, Maryland

Joseph S. MacLaughlin, MD
Professor (Retired)
Division of Cardiac Surgery
University of Maryland School of Medicine
Baltimore, Maryland

Thomas Scalea, MD
Physician-in-Chief
R Adams Cowley Shock Trauma Center
Professor of Surgery
Director, Program in Trauma
University of Maryland School of Medicine
Baltimore, Maryland

Katherine Tkaczuk, MD
Professor of Medicine
Director, Breast Evaluation and Treatment Program
Marlene and Stewart Greenebaum Cancer Center
University of Maryland School of Medicine
Baltimore, Maryland

Michelle Townsend-Watts, MD
Assistant Professor of Diagnostic Radiology
University of Maryland School of Medicine
Baltimore, Maryland

Contents

Part I: General Issues

1 Preoperative Care 1
Bruce E. Jarrell, Molly Buzdon, Daniel Bochicchio, Eric D. Strauch

2 Postoperative Care 25
Bruce E. Jarrell, Molly Buzdon, Eric D. Strauch

3 Wound Healing 37
Bruce E. Jarrell, Eric D. Strauch

Part II: Specific Disorders

4 Thoracic and Cardiothoracic Disorders 49
Bruce E. Jarrell, Joseph S. MacLaughlin, Eric D. Strauch

5 Vascular Disorders 96
Bruce E. Jarrell, Marshall Benjamin, Eric D. Strauch

6 Upper Gastrointestinal Tract Disorders 144
Bruce E. Jarrell, John L. Flowers, Molly Buzdon, Eric D. Strauch

7 Pancreatic and Hepatic Disorders 173
Bruce E. Jarrell, Eric D. Strauch

8 Lower Gastrointestinal Disorders 210
Bruce E. Jarrell, Molly Buzdon, Daniel Bochicchio, Eric D. Strauch

9   **Endocrine Disorders** 279
Bruce E. Jarrell, W. Bradford Carter, Eric D. Strauch

10   **Skin and Soft Tissue Disorders and Hernias** 299
Bruce E. Jarrell, Eric D. Strauch

11   **Breast Disorders** 329
Bruce E. Jarrell, Emily Bellavance, Michelle Townsend-Watts,
Katherine Tkaczuk, Eric D. Strauch

Part III: Special Issues

12. **Trauma, Burns, and Sepsis** 360
Bruce E. Jarrell, Thomas Scalea, Molly Buzdon

13. **Congenital Anomalies** 419
Clint D. Cappiello, Eric D. Strauch, Bruce E. Jarrell

Index *439*

*Special thanks to radiologists who assisted
in numerous chapters:*

Barry Daly, MD
Robert Pugatch, MD
Charles White, MD

Chapter 1

Preoperative Care

Bruce E. Jarrell, Molly Buzdon, Daniel Bochicchio, Eric D. Strauch

Key Thoughts

1. The overall goal of a surgery is to make the patient's life better by improving a clinical condition, making a diagnosis, or palliating pain or discomfort.

2. All procedures have a risk/benefit ratio. To make the procedure appropriate and worthwhile, the benefit must outweigh the risk.

3. Risk is difficult to assess but certainly includes understanding: what the surgery intends to correct, how invasive the procedure is, what common complications occur, what pre-existing, cocurrent diseases exist in the patient, and how they are being treated.

4. The most important assessment tool in medicine is the history and physical examination. A good history and physical examination will guide the clinician to what diagnostic laboratory, radiologic, and other interventions are necessary for patient care.

5. Every test that is ordered must be checked and evaluated and the result correlated with the patient's clinical condition. Treat the patient, not the radiographs or laboratory tests.

6. For elective procedures, the patient should be in optimal condition—diabetes, hypertension, and heart disease under control; no infectious processes; not smoking; stable renal function; and no new symptoms or processes. If not, surgery should be postponed until these issues are resolved.

7. For urgent or emergent procedures, managing existing problems to the extent possible is desired.

Case 1.1 Routine Surgery in a Healthy Patient

A 42-year-old fairly active man who can climb stairs and walk for a long distance at a brisk pace has a right inguinal hernia and is planning to undergo elective repair. He has had no other operations. However, his medical history reveals mild hypertension that is currently untreated. His family history is also important; his father died as the result of an acute myocardial infarction (MI) at 68 years of age. In addition, his social history is significant for 20 pack-years of smoking.

Review of systems is negative. His blood pressure (BP) is 140/88 mm Hg. With the exception of an easily reducible right inguinal hernia, examination is otherwise negative.

◆ **How would you assess the patient's operative risk?**

◆ The **American College of Cardiology/American Heart Association (ACC/AHA) has proposed several clinical predictors of increased perioperative cardiovascular risk** (Tables 1-1 and 1-2). This patient has no active cardiac conditions as defined by Table 1-1

Table 1-1: Active Cardiac Conditions for Which the Patient Should Undergo Evaluation and Treatment Before Noncardiac Surgery (Class I, Level of Evidence: B)

Condition	Examples
Unstable coronary syndromes	Unstable or severe angina* (CCS class III or IV)[†] Recent MI[‡]
Decompensated HF (NYHA functional class IV; worsening or new-onset HF)	
Significant arrhythmias	High-grade atrioventricular block Mobitz II atrioventricular block Third-degree atrioventricular heart block Symptomatic ventricular arrhythmias Supraventricular arrhythmias (including atrial fibrillation) with uncontrolled ventricular rate (HR >100 beats per minute at rest)

*Campeau L. The Canadian Cardiovascular Society grading of angina pectoris revisited 30 years later. *Can J Cardiol.* 2002;18(4):371–379. http://reference.medscape.com/medline/abstract/11992130.
[†]May include "stable" angina in patients who are unusually sedentary.
[‡]The American College of Cardiology National Database Library defines recent MI as greater than 7 days but less than or equal to 1 month (within 30 days).
CCS, Canadian Cardiovascular Society; MI, myocardial infarction; HF, heart failure; NYHA, New York Heart Association; HR, heart rate.
From Fleisher LA, Beckman JA, Brown KA, et al. 2009 ACCF/AHA focused update on perioperative beta blockade incorporated into the ACC/AHA 2007 guidelines on perioperative cardiovascular evaluation and care for noncardiac surgery: a report of the American College of Cardiology Foundation/American Heart Association Task Force on Practice Guidelines. *Circulation.* 2009;120(21):e169–e276.

Table 1-2: Cardiac Risk* Stratification for Noncardiac Surgical Procedures

Risk Stratification	Procedure Examples
Vascular (reported cardiac risk often >5%)	Aortic and other major vascular surgery Peripheral vascular surgery
Intermediate (reported cardiac risk generally 1%–5%)	Intraperitoneal and intrathoracic surgery Carotid endarterectomy Head and neck surgery Orthopedic surgery Prostate surgery
Low[†] (reported cardiac risk generally <1%)	Endoscopic procedures Superficial procedure Cataract surgery Breast surgery Ambulatory surgery

*Combined incidence of cardiac death and nonfatal myocardial infarction.
[†]These procedures do not generally require further preoperative cardiac testing.

Table 1-3: Estimated Energy Requirements for Various Activities

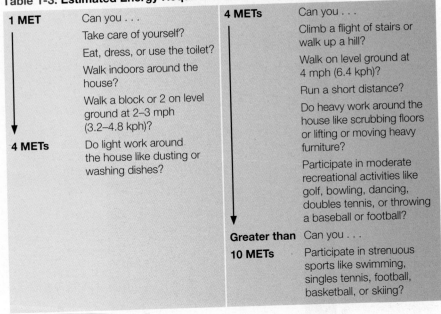

1 MET	Can you . . .	4 METs	Can you . . .
↓	Take care of yourself?	↓	Climb a flight of stairs or walk up a hill?
	Eat, dress, or use the toilet?		Walk on level ground at 4 mph (6.4 kph)?
	Walk indoors around the house?		Run a short distance?
	Walk a block or 2 on level ground at 2–3 mph (3.2–4.8 kph)?		Do heavy work around the house like scrubbing floors or lifting or moving heavy furniture?
4 METs	Do light work around the house like dusting or washing dishes?		Participate in moderate recreational activities like golf, bowling, dancing, doubles tennis, or throwing a baseball or football?
		Greater than 10 METs	Can you . . . Participate in strenuous sports like swimming, singles tennis, football, basketball, or skiing?

MET, metabolic equivalent task.

but does have hypertension, a positive family history, and a significant smoking history. The surgery is a low-risk ambulatory procedure. He needs to be treated for his hypertension and counseled to stop smoking. You can assess his overall functional status using questions that estimate his ability to accomplish physical tasks and then categorizing the level using the metabolic equivalent task (MET) as seen in Table 1-3. This functional status assessment correlates well with maximum oxygen uptake by treadmill testing and can be used to alert you to a higher cardiac risk.

◆ What preoperative tests are necessary?

◆ Standard preoperative testing has not been shown to be of significant value. Testing should be guided by his history and physical examination. Recent guidelines suggest he should have a creatinine level, electrolytes, and an electrocardiogram (ECG) test because of his hypertension and a chest radiograph (CXR) because of his smoking history, although the evidence for value of the CXR to the patient is limited (Table 1-4).

You decide to proceed with the hernia repair.

◆ How would you categorize the patient's anesthesia risk?

◆ All anesthetic techniques are associated with some risk. The American Society of Anesthesiologists (ASA) has attempted to classify anesthetic morbidity and mortality based on physical status (**ASA classes 1–5**) (Table 1-5). This patient presents an ASA 2 risk.

◆ How would you decide whether to use local, spinal, or general anesthesia?

◆ The decision concerning the most appropriate type of anesthesia is multifaceted and should be made in consultation with an anesthesiologist.

Table 1-4: Preoperative Diagnosis-Based Investigations before Elective Surgery

Complete Blood Count	Serum Creatinine and Electrolytes	Blood Glucose	ECG	X-ray Chest	Coagulation Studies
Major surgery	Kidney disease, Hypertension	Diabetes	Cardiac disease	Chronic lung disease	Liver disease
Neonates	Diabetes	Family h/o diabetes	Hypertension	Heavy smoker	Renal dysfunction
Males older than 70 years	Poor nutritional states	Obese	Chronic lung disease	Radiation therapy	Family h/o bleeding disorder
Females older than 45 years	Stroke	Stroke	Diabetes	Aortic aneurysm	On anticoagulant drugs
Chronic renal, liver, lung disease	Medication	Poor nutritional states	Thyroid disease	Cardiomegaly	
Anemia	• Digoxin	Steroids use	Morbid obesity		
Malignancy	• Diuretics	Cushing, Addison	Digoxin therapy		
Poor nutritional states	• Steroids		Males older than 45 years		
Vascular aneurysms	• Chemotherapy		Females older than 55 years		

ECG, electrocardiogram; h/o, history of.

Table 1-5: American Society of Anesthesiologists' Classification of Perioperative Mortality

Class	Definition
1	A normal healthy patient
2	A patient with mild systemic disease and no functional limitations
3	A patient with moderate to severe systemic disease that results in some functional limitation
4	A patient with severe systemic disease that is a constant threat to life and functionally incapacitating
5	A moribund patient who is not expected to survive 24 hours with or without surgery
6	A brain-dead patient whose organs are being harvested
E	If the procedure is an emergency, the physical status is followed by "E" (e.g., "2E").

Class	Mortality Rate
1	0.06%–0.08%
2	0.27%–0.4%
3	1.8%–4.3%
4	7.8%–23%
5	9.4%–51%

From Morgan GE Jr, Mikhail MS. *Clinical Anesthesiology*, 3rd ed. New York: McGraw-Hill; 2002.

 QUICK CUT Most anesthesiologists believe that it is not the technique itself but how well it is used that determines its risk.

Local anesthesia is associated with fewer physiologic consequences than with regional or general anesthetics if a good anesthetic block is achieved. However, with poor local anesthesia, patients experience increased pain, which is stressful and requires large doses of intravenous (IV) sedatives to offset. This significantly increases the risk.

 QUICK CUT Good spinal anesthesia may lead to fewer pulmonary complications than general anesthesia.

However, it may be more dangerous in patients with coronary artery disease, marginal cardiac reserve with low ejection fraction, valvular heart disease, or diabetic peripheral vascular disease with neuropathy. This danger is secondary to either a loss of peripheral vasoconstrictor ability or ability to increase cardiac output when necessary. Thus, hypotension may occur as a result of the vasodilation caused by spinal anesthesia. To restore BP and relieve hemodynamic instability, IV drugs will have to be used, thus increasing the risk. In addition, if a spinal anesthetic fails to provide good anesthesia, patients will require additional IV sedation or even general anesthesia, further increasing the risk.

 QUICK CUT General anesthesia allows excellent analgesia and amnesia while maintaining good physiologic control.

In addition, it provides a secure airway.

QUICK CUT Major drawbacks of general anesthesia are an increased incidence of pulmonary complications and the mild cardiodepression that all anesthetics can cause.

In this particular patient, minimal risk and excellent outcome should be expected regardless of the type of anesthesia used, assuming it is properly administered.

In the following cases, you are faced with making a decision in someone with a pre-existing condition. In each example, your decision making requires balancing the urgency for intervening in an illness requiring surgery with the added risk imposed by the medical condition. In some cases, the pre-existing medical condition may have worsened compared to baseline as a result of the new, acute illness. In other cases, the act of intervening with a surgical procedure will cause or be associated with worsening of the pre-existing condition.

Deep Thoughts

Understanding the urgency of the surgical intervention and thus the time that you have available to optimize the management of the pre-existing condition can make a large difference in the patient's outcome and development of postoperative complications.

A general approach is to consider risk factors in two categories: risks associated with this specific patient and risks associated with the planned procedure. As you go through these cases, try to stratify risks in these two categories as a first step.

For specific patients:

◆ What risks in the patient are pre-existing, and how well are they controlled? (Controlled asthma or controlled diabetes is a much lower risk than uncontrolled.)
◆ What risks are added as a consequence of the new disorder requiring surgical consideration? (An abscess causing generalized sepsis or ischemic bowel incarcerated in a hernia contributes to a much higher perioperative risk than no sepsis or an uncomplicated hernia repair.)
◆ Will treatment of the new disorder return the patient to the pre-existing state or add to the chronic pre-existing problems of the patient? (Removal of a gangrenous appendix should return the patient to the pre-existing state once recovered, whereas amputation of an ischemic foot is an indication of progression of arterial insufficiency as well as a risk for inactivity, postoperative pulmonary embolism, and a prolonged rehabilitation.)

For specific planned procedures:

◆ How invasive and traumatic is the procedure (such as involving vital organs, blood loss, or large fluid shifts vs. none)?
◆ What body cavity or location is invaded (such as thoracic cavity vs. a lower extremity procedure)?

◆ What is the risk of a technical complication occurring, and what new risks arise if the complication occurs (such as what is the risk of a bowel anastomotic leak in a patient with inflammatory bowel disease on steroids vs. someone with a normal immune system)?

◆ What is the risk of failing to correct an abnormality (such as leaving an abscess undrained or leaving necrotic bowel in the abdomen vs. complete drainage or adequate resection)?

The cases and associated tables and figures should be used to assist you in this process, understanding that many risks and mitigation strategies are not always well supported by data or validated.

Case 1.2 Common Risk Factors Associated with Routine Surgery

You evaluate a patient similar to the man in Case 1.1 who is also in need of an inguinal hernia repair.

◆ **How would your preoperative assessment and proposed management change in each of the following situations?**

Case Variation 1.2.1. The patient takes one aspirin per day.

◆ Aspirin and nonsteroidal anti-inflammatory drugs (NSAIDs) can cause platelet dysfunction due to inhibition of cyclooxygenase, preventing prostaglandin synthesis.

 QUICK CUT Aspirin has an irreversible effect on platelet aggregation for at least 7–10 days; NSAIDs have a reversible effect.

In 2 days after cessation of NSAIDS, platelets have recovered normal function. Thus, for an elective procedure, aspirin should be discontinued for 7–10 days prior to the procedure and NSAIDs discontinued for 2 days.

Case Variation 1.2.2. The patient's father and brother both died from acute MIs at 45 years of age.

◆ The man's positive family history should prompt concentrated study of his cardiac history. He should be asked if he has ever experienced anginal symptoms or shortness of breath. An ECG should be performed. An exercise stress test may also be advisable in patients with a strong family history.

Case Variation 1.2.3. The patient's most recent serum cholesterol is 320 mg/dL.

◆ Hypercholesterolemia increases the risk of coronary artery disease, but this factor alone should not postpone surgery. However, he should be treated chronically for his hypercholesterolemia with diet modification, fractionation of his cholesterol, and possibly medical intervention.

Case Variation 1.2.4. The patient's preoperative ECG provides evidence of a previous inferior MI, but he has no knowledge of this MI and is chest pain–free on careful examination.

◆ A previous MI increases the risk of postoperative MI. Appropriate workup includes a **cardiology consultation** and perhaps an exercise stress test to identify stress-induced ischemia.

If signs of ischemia are apparent, cardiac catheterization may be necessary to determine if coronary revascularization is required prior to surgery.

Case Variation 1.2.5. *The patient has diabetes.*

◆ This particular patient, who will be "nothing by mouth" (NPO) after midnight, should be given IV fluids with dextrose.

> **QUICK CUT** Patients who are taking oral hypoglycemic agents should not receive their medication the morning of surgery.

Individuals with insulin-dependent diabetes mellitus (IDDM) should have their glucose levels checked the morning of surgery to ensure that they are not hyper- or hypoglycemic. As a general rule, a slightly elevated glucose level is preferred to a reduced level. If the glucose level is greater than 250 mg/dL, most clinicians would give **two-thirds** of the morning dose of neutral protamine Hagedorn (NPH) and regular insulin. If the glucose level is less than 250 mg/dL, you could administer **one-half** of the morning dose.

Case Variation 1.2.6. *The patient's hematocrit is 34%, and his other laboratory tests are normal.*

◆ **The patient is anemic, and the reason for the anemia must be determined.** The surgery should be postponed. The most common cause of anemia is colorectal cancer, but other causes should be investigated if the workup for gastrointestinal (GI) blood loss is negative.

Case Variation 1.2.7. *The patient's hematocrit is 55%.*

◆ This result suggests that the patient has either hypovolemia or polycythemia due to some other condition.

> **QUICK CUT** Regardless of the cause, the polycythemia should be evaluated and the risk assessed prior to surgery.

If dehydration is present, surgery should be delayed until the patient is well hydrated. Physical signs of dehydration include poor skin turgor and dry mouth.

Important but less common causes of polycythemia such as polycythemia vera, chronic obstructive pulmonary disease (COPD), and erythropoietin-secreting tumors (e.g., renal cell carcinoma, hepatocellular carcinoma) should be diagnosed and treated prior to elective surgery. If patients with polycythemia vera need surgery, the operative risk for thrombotic complications is increased unless the hematocrit is normalized; a combination of hydration and phlebotomy can be used.

Case Variation 1.2.8. *The patient is obese (100 lb overweight) and reports becoming winded easily when climbing stairs.*

> **QUICK CUT** Obese patients have a higher incidence of hypertension and cardiovascular disease. Severe cases result in hypoventilation, hypercapnia, and pulmonary hypertension. These individuals are also at increased risk for adult-onset diabetes mellitus and deep venous thrombosis (DVT).

A complete medical evaluation is necessary, including an evaluation of pulmonary status prior to surgery and optimization of functional capacity with bronchodilators and antibiotics as appropriate. At a minimum, this will involve arterial blood gases (ABGs), as well as pulmonary function studies if ABGs are abnormal. Because the hernia repair is elective, postponing the surgery may be an option if the patient is willing to participate in a weight loss program. Otherwise, **epidural anesthesia and aggressive postoperative pulmonary care** may be used to avoid atelectasis.

 QUICK CUT Sequential compression stockings and/or prophylactic subcutaneous heparin are also important in the prevention of DVT.

Case 1.3 Common Problems in a Patient Waiting to Enter the Operating Room

You plan to repair an inguinal hernia in a male patient. He arrives at the hospital, and you reassess him just before he is moved into the operating room.

◆ **How would your proposed management change in each of the following situations?**

Case Variation 1.3.1. *The patient is known to be diabetic, and this morning his blood glucose is 320 mg/dL.*

◆ Perioperative blood glucose levels should be 100–250 mg/dL, and

 QUICK CUT Surgery should be delayed until the glucose level is brought under control.

The man may need subcutaneous insulin or an insulin drip to lower his glucose level, and he may also require IV drip of a dextrose solution to prevent his blood glucose level from becoming too low. Infection may also be a problem;

 QUICK CUT Patients with poorly controlled diabetes mellitus have a higher incidence of postoperative wound infections.

Case Variation 1.3.2. *The patient has cellulitis from an infected hair follicle in his axilla.*

 QUICK CUT Surgery performed in the presence of an active infection elsewhere in the body is associated with a significant increase in wound infection at the operative site.

◆ Elective surgery should be postponed until the acute infection is resolved, regardless of its location. Unrecognized toe and foot infections are not uncommon in diabetics, who should be examined carefully.

Case Variation 1.3.3. *The patient experiences burning on urination.*

◆ A urinalysis and a urine culture should be performed. If the urinalysis is positive for infection, the surgery should be postponed until the urinary tract infection (UTI) has been successfully treated with antibiotics. A repeat urinalysis and culture indicates resolution of the infection. Urologic consultation may be needed to determine the cause of the UTI.

Case Variation 1.3.4. **His BP, which was 140/88 mm Hg in your office, has risen to 180/110 mm Hg.**

 QUICK CUT Diastolic BP greater than or equal to 110 mm Hg is a risk factor for development of cardiovascular complications such as malignant hypertension, acute MI, and congestive heart failure.

◆ Patients with hypertension have a 25% incidence of perioperative hypotension or hypertension. Significant data suggest that beta-blockers may help reduce the risk of cardiac complications following surgery. This patient should be maintained on antihypertensive medications on the day of surgery. (Beta-blockers, in particular, have a high rate of rebound hypertension if withheld.) Studies have found that postponing surgery for mild hypertension (diastolic BP <110 mm Hg) does not reduce perioperative risk.

Case 1.4   Surgery in a Patient with Pulmonary Symptoms

A 58-year-old man has suffered several bouts of biliary colic in the past 10 days. An ultrasound study 4 days ago showed multiple small gallstones. The man's surgeon says he needs a cholecystectomy.

◆ **How would you interpret the following findings, and how would they affect your proposed management?**

Case Variation 1.4.1. **The patient has daily productive cough and has had this for many years. He smokes two packs per day.**

◆ Questions should be asked about the number of cigarettes smoked daily, the duration of smoking, and any recent change in sputum quality.

 QUICK CUT The relative risk of postoperative complications in smokers is two to six times that of nonsmokers because cigarette smoking is toxic to respiratory epithelium and cilia, resulting in impaired mucous transport and therefore decreased resistance to infection.

Bronchial ciliary function returns to normal after 2 days of smoking cessation, and sputum volume decreases to normal after 2 weeks of smoking cessation.

 QUICK CUT However, studies indicate no improvement in postoperative respiratory morbidity until after 6–8 weeks of abstinence from smoking.

Because the planned cholecystectomy is elective surgery, this patient should be advised that abstaining from cigarettes 6–8 weeks prior to surgery will decrease the risk of postoperative complications. The patient should also be counseled to stop smoking permanently.

Case Variation 1.4.2. **The patient normally has daily sputum production, but his sputum has been green for 3 weeks.**

◆ If this symptom represents **bronchitis limited to the upper airways** as assessed on chest auscultation in the absence of fever, **oral antibiotics** can be given, and the **surgery can be rescheduled after treatment is complete**. Acute or systemic symptoms from pneumonia or other serious diseases warrant further evaluation.

Case Variation 1.4.3. The patient's sputum has been blood-streaked for 3 weeks.

◆ Blood-tinged sputum in patients with a significant smoking history may suggest **active infection or lung carcinoma**. A full workup, including a CXR and most likely a computed tomography (CT) scan of the chest, should be performed prior to surgery to determine the cause of the problem. Bronchoscopy is also necessary to check for endobronchial lesions and obtain samples for cytology.

Case 1.5 Urgent Surgery in a Patient with Severe, Acute Pulmonary Function Problems

You are asked to see a man in the emergency department who is quite ill, with **right upper quadrant (RUQ) pain** and a **temperature of 103°F**. He states that he is a heavy smoker and that he becomes short of breath on mild exertion. He has **scant sputum production**—a thin, white secretion. Examination indicates a barrel chest with decreased breath sounds bilaterally and scattered wheezes, as well as acute tenderness over the RUQ at Murphy's point. CXR findings are typical of **advanced COPD**, and an abdominal ultrasound study shows gallstones and a thickened, inflamed gallbladder. You diagnose his abdominal problem as **acute cholecystitis**.

◆ **How would you manage the patient's pulmonary problem?**

◆ To determine the degree of pulmonary disease, **ABGs**, preferably on room air, are necessary. A Pao_2 of less than 60 mm Hg correlates with pulmonary hypertension, and a $Paco_2$ of more than 45 mm Hg are associated with increased perioperative morbidity. Pulmonary toilet can be given to improve the patient's pulmonary condition including bronchodilators for bronchospasm, anti-inflammatory medications (inhaled or systemic steroids) for inflammation, antibiotics for infection, chest physiotherapy for atelectasis, or mucus plugging. **Knowledge of patients' preoperative pulmonary status helps determine intra- and postoperative management.** If this patient's septic picture worsens, he will need to go to the operating room regardless of his pulmonary function. If his septic picture improves, pulmonary function tests can be used to quantify his pulmonary disease (Table 1-6).

 QUICK CUT Preoperative bronchodilator therapy and other efforts to improve pulmonary status prior to surgery may be appropriate.

It is most likely that the sepsis is secondary to biliary infection from gallstones, **and the patient may respond to antibiotics, hydration, and IV fluids. The surgery can be postponed until the patient is in better condition. However, the course of the disease is unknown at this time, and prompt evaluation is essential.**

The man says that he is normally very short of breath at rest but that his current breathing problems are much worse than usual. **He cannot speak an entire sentence without gasping for air.** On room air, **his Po2 is 49 mm Hg, and his Pco2 is 65 mm Hg**.

◆ **How would your management plans change if the patient has severe COPD in addition to acute cholecystitis?**

◆ This patient is at high risk for **pulmonary failure with surgery**. Further workup should include a CXR to rule out underlying pneumonia. In addition, the man must be asked whether he requires oxygen at home and to determine whether his current respiratory status is at baseline,

Table 1-6: Pulmonary Function Values Suggesting Increased Perioperative Risk of Pulmonary Complications*

Test	Value	Significance
Forced expiratory volume in 1 sec (FEV₁)	<70% of predicted	Moderate risk (major surgery)
	<35% of predicted	High risk (major surgery)
	0.6 L	Pulmonary wedge resection only can be tolerated
	1 L	Major pulmonary resection up to a pulmonary lobectomy can be tolerated
	2 L	Major pulmonary resection up to a pneumonectomy can be tolerated
Forced vital capacity (FVC)	<50%–75% of predicted	Moderate risk
Pulmonary arterial pressure (PAP)	<25 mm Hg	Moderate to high risk
Arterial blood Paco₂	>45 mm Hg	Moderate risk

*Pulmonary risk includes postoperative atelectasis, pneumonia, pneumothorax, inability to wean patient from ventilator, right heart failure, and death.
Adapted from Pett SB, Wernly JA. Respiratory function in surgical patients: perioperative evaluation and management. *Surg Annual*. 1988;20:36.

if he has had any previous pulmonary studies. If the surgery is absolutely necessary, the patient should be taught incentive spirometry before the surgery, and perioperative bronchodilators may be used. Evidence supports the use of incentive spirometry as a risk reduction strategy for pulmonary complications postoperatively. It is also important to minimize the duration of anesthesia. To prevent atelectasis, the patient should be mobilized postoperatively as soon as possible.

Deep Thoughts   The choice of operation may also substantially influence the postoperative course.

For example, **open cholecystectomy** is one option, which may be prudent in this case because of the risk of CO_2 absorption into the blood with laparoscopic cholecystectomy. **Cholecystostomy** is another option. Under local anesthesia, a tube is placed in the gallbladder either under radiologic guidance or via a small incision made in the abdomen. Drainage to the exterior usually resolves the acute sepsis, avoiding the need for cholecystectomy at this time. These examples demonstrate that a high-risk patient's condition influences the choice of surgical procedure. If cholecystostomy is chosen, you are choosing a less definitive procedure. It locally manages the sepsis associated with acute cholecystitis but does not remove the source—the diseased gallbladder—which may need removal at a later date and certainly when the patient is in a lower risk condition.

QUICK CUT Laparoscopy may lead to increased CO_2 absorption into the blood, which then requires excretion through the lungs and increased pulmonary work. This further compromises a patient's pulmonary status and would be contraindicated in this patient.

Case 1.6 Cardiac and Neurologic Risk Associated with Surgery for Peripheral Vascular Disease

A 74-year-old man presents with a recent onset of rest pain in his right foot. He has had non–insulin-dependent diabetes mellitus (NIDDM) for the past 8 years, smokes two packs of cigarettes per day, and has a history of mild hypertension that is well controlled with an angiotensin-converting enzyme (ACE) inhibitor. On physical examination, obvious ischemia of the right foot is evident, with absent popliteal and pedal pulses, dependent rubor, loss of lower leg hair, and shiny skin. The ankle–brachial index is 0.4, indicating severe ischemia of the leg. You recommend a revascularization procedure to salvage the leg. An angiogram indicates that a bypass from the femoral artery to the distal tibial vessels is necessary for adequate revascularization. To proceed safely, you should evaluate the man's medical risk.

A general approach to evaluating cardiac risk for noncardiac surgery has been formulated by the AHA (Fig. 1-1). This algorithm can be used in a stepwise manner as follows:

Step 1: If a patient needs an emergency noncardiac procedure, you would proceed with the procedure and take steps to minimize cardiac stress during the intra- and postoperative period. This is primarily by careful heart rate control and avoiding hypoxia, electrolyte abnormalities, hypotension, and wide fluid shifts.

Step 2: If not an emergency and thus for an elective procedure, evaluate for active cardiac conditions, as seen in Table 1-1. If present, evaluate and treat them by AHA guidelines before proceeding with surgery.

Step 3: For an elective procedure and no active cardiac conditions, look at the surgical procedure planned, as shown in Table 1-2. If a low-risk surgical procedure is planned, then proceed with the surgery.

Step 4: In Step 3, if the surgical procedure is higher risk, then you need to determine the functional status of the patient. For patients who are physically active, this can be estimated using Table 1-3. If the estimate is at or above 4 METS, then proceed with surgery. If physical activity is limited for a variety of reasons, such as with a leg amputation or toe infection, or the METS estimate is below 4, then a more complicated series of steps is recommended based on the number of risk factors present (see Table 1-6).

Noninvasive testing in Step 5 is generally performed if it will change the management of the patient. Cardiac functional assessment helps to establish risk based on cardiac perfusion under conditions of increased oxygen demand as seen in a cardiac stress test.

◆ **How would the following findings alter your plans for evaluation and management?**

*Case Variation 1.6.1. **The man tells you that he has no cardiac problems.***

◆ The patient's cardiac risk should still be evaluated, as the need for vascular surgery makes this patient have a high risk for cardiac complications (reported cardiac risk often >5%). A recommendation algorithm for cardiac evaluation for noncardiac surgery has been formulated by the AHA (see Fig. 1-1).

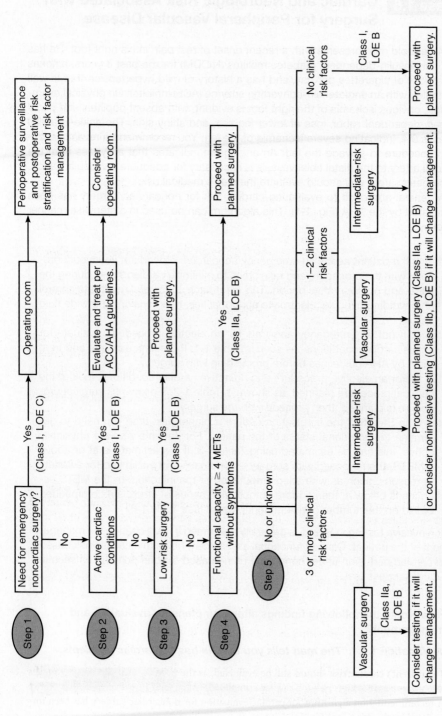

Figure 1-1: Cardiac evaluation and care algorithm for noncardiac surgery based on active clinical conditions, known cardiovascular disease, or cardiac risk for patients 50 years or older. LOE, level of evidence; ACC/AHA, American College of Cardiology/American heart Association; MET, metabolic equivalent task.

QUICK CUT Atherosclerosis is a disease that is not confined to the lower extremities in patients with peripheral vascular disease. Coronary artery disease or carotid artery disease is often present as well.

To determine the degree of disease in other systems, a thorough workup is necessary before any bypass surgery is performed. To achieve a successful outcome, the benefits of peripheral revascularization must exceed the risks underlying the surgery. He should have a rapid cardiac workup prior to surgery. This should include **a comparison of the previous ECG with the current ECG**. Because the man has rest pain, he would not tolerate an exercise stress test, but he should undergo a **Persantine thallium stress test or dobutamine echocardiogram** to assess his current cardiac status.

QUICK CUT If reversible ischemia is present, he may need a cardiac catheterization to determine whether a coronary revascularization procedure is necessary prior to lower extremity bypass.

Case Variation 1.6.2. The man tells you that he had an acute MI 3 years ago.

QUICK CUT The most common cause of early postoperative death following lower extremity revascularization is MI.

◆ Studies have found that the rate of **reinfarction** with **prior history of MI is as high as 15%** in patients undergoing vascular surgery and rises to **37%** in patients who have had a **recent MI**. The risk of cardiac death or recurrent MI decreases as the duration from surgery increases (i.e., the time interval between MI and surgery).

   The patient should undergo a stress test. If reversible ischemia is present, he should undergo cardiac catheterization. If only an irreversible defect is present, no cardiac catheterization is necessary if no other abnormalities are present. The irreversible defect is most likely due to his old MI.

Case Variation 1.6.3. The man tells you that he had an acute MI 3 months ago.

◆ In 2009, the ACC/AHA proposed a set of guidelines to estimate coronary risk related to noncardiac surgery (see Table 1-2). Because he is having a vascular procedure performed, he should have a cardiology evaluation and stress test performed. Occurrence of MI more than 30 days before noncardiac surgery is an intermediate risk factor.

Case Variation 1.6.4. He tells you that he had an acute MI 3 weeks ago.

◆ The ACC/AHA criteria stipulate that MI within 30 days of noncardiac surgery is a major risk factor for perioperative cardiac complications. If possible, the **surgery should be delayed**.

Case Variation 1.6.5. The man tells you that he had a non–Q-wave MI 9 months ago.

◆ Non–Q-wave MIs generally signify a **nontransmural infarct**, which leaves peri-infarct myocardium at risk for further infarction during and after surgery. This patient should have a Persantine thallium stress test to determine whether reversible ischemia is present. If so, coronary revascularization may be necessary before surgery.

Case Variation 1.6.6. The patient's ECG shows left bundle branch block (LBBB).

 QUICK CUT LBBB is never a normal variant and is highly suggestive of underlying ischemic heart disease.

The presence of this conduction disturbance should prompt a **careful evaluation for underlying cardiopulmonary disease**. If invasive intraoperative monitoring is necessary in patients with LBBB, placement of a pulmonary artery catheter increases the risk of concurrent right bundle branch block (RBBB), so transthoracic pacing capabilities should be readily available. **RBBB is a normal variant in up to 10% of the general population, but it is more frequently seen in patients with significant pulmonary disease**.

Case Variation 1.6.7. The patient had a coronary artery bypass graft (CABG) 2 years ago.

◆ There is evidence that **prior coronary artery revascularization may reduce the risk of cardiac complications in patients who are undergoing other surgery**. This situation is most likely in patients who had the cardiac surgery 6 months to 5 years before the noncardiac surgery and who have no symptoms of ischemia with physical activity. In part, this may result from the increased use of internal mammary arterial grafts in the past decade.

Case Variation 1.6.8. The patient had a CABG 10 years ago.

◆ The benefit of CABG is less clear in patients who have had a coronary revascularization procedure more than 5 years prior. **With saphenous vein bypass, the graft occlusion rates** are 12%–20% at 1 year after CABG, 20%–30% at 5 years, and 40%–50% at 10 years. A stress test should be performed to determine whether this patient has reversible ischemia.

Case Variation 1.6.9. The patient had a percutaneous transluminal coronary angioplasty (PTCA) 2 years ago.

◆ The incidence of **coronary restenosis** after PTCA is 25%–35% at 6 months, so a cardiac evaluation with a stress test would be necessary.

Case Variation 1.6.10. The man had a PTCA 2 days ago.

◆ **Noncardiac surgery should probably be delayed for several weeks following coronary angioplasty**, if feasible, because the risk of coronary thrombosis is increased during the first month postsurgery. The recent PTCA may induce a procoagulant state that might be detrimental to a fresh arterial intervention. The presence of a drug-eluding stent may require an antiplatelet drug.

Case Variation 1.6.11. The patient has angina on moderate exertion and uses nitroglycerin.

◆ Because this patient displays evidence of coronary artery disease, **coronary angiography would be appropriate** to determine the extent of disease and whether PTCA or coronary artery revascularization are indicated.

Case Variation 1.6.12. The patient's ECG shows six premature ventricular contractions (PVCs) per minute.

◆ Early studies by Goldman and coworkers in the 1970s showed that preoperative ECGs with more than five PVCs per minute were associated with increased cardiac mortality. Later studies reported that these findings do not necessarily indicate a high likelihood of intraoperative or postoperative ventricular tachycardia. More likely, the cardiac risk of arrhythmia is related to underlying **ventricular dysfunction**. A stress test and an echocardiogram to evaluate left ventricular function and check for underlying cardiac disease would be appropriate. Prophylactic antiarrhythmic therapy has not proved beneficial.

Case Variation 1.6.13. The patient's ECG indicates atrial fibrillation.

◆ If patients have no previous diagnosis of atrial fibrillation, an underlying cause such as **coronary artery disease, congestive heart failure, or valvular heart disease** must be sought. Heart rate must be well controlled, and therapy may involve cardioversion to normal sinus rhythm or beta-blockers to control heart rate. Both cardioversion and chronic atrial fibrillation may require anticoagulation to minimize the risk of embolization. Therapeutic decisions must be made in conjunction with a cardiologist and the surgery planned around them. Oral anticoagulants may also need to be used postoperatively.

Case Variation 1.6.14. The patient has a loud right carotid bruit.

◆ A carotid duplex study should be performed to evaluate for carotid artery disease. Studies have found that one-third of patients with carotid bruits have severe internal carotid stenosis. **For patients with a high-grade stenosis (80%–99%), carotid endarterectomy might be considered** prior to lower extremity revascularization.

 QUICK CUT The primary cause of morbidity and mortality remains myocardial ischemia and infarction.

The risk of neurologic events associated with noncardiac vascular surgery is low (i.e., about 0.4%–0.9%).

Case Variation 1.6.15. The patient had a stroke 2 years ago.

◆ A carotid duplex study should be performed in patients who have had a previous stroke with good neurologic recovery to assess the carotid arteries.

 QUICK CUT Carotid endarterectomy is likely to be beneficial for stroke patients with good recovery of function and 70%–99% stenosis of the carotid artery corresponding to the side of the stroke.

In stroke patients with significant residual neurologic deficit, no further evaluation is necessary.

Case Variation 1.6.16. The man's ankle–brachial index (ABI) is 0.2, and he has a significantly infected large toe.

◆ An infected extremity puts patients at higher risk for gangrene and subsequent amputation because the peripheral circulation does not allow the limb to heal. This particular patient should still have a workup for coronary artery disease, but his need for **peripheral revascularization is more urgent** than in an individual with rest pain and an ABI of 0.4. Thus, it may be necessary to proceed with revascularization despite an incomplete workup of his cardiac disease. If so, the man should be treated as if he were at risk for myocardial ischemia and his anesthesia managed accordingly.

Case 1.7 Surgery in a Patient with Liver Failure

A 47-year-old man with a large umbilical hernia, which has been progressively increasing in size, would like to have it repaired. His history is significant for chronic liver failure secondary to alcohol abuse; he states that currently he is not using alcohol. He is taking a diuretic for control of the ascites. On physical examination, moderate ascites and a 5-cm umbilical hernia are evident. In your assessment, you believe he has alcoholic cirrhosis.

◆ **What factors affect the patient's operative risk, and how are they evaluated?**

◆ The major factors that influence the operative risk relate to the state of compensation and the severity of cirrhosis (Table 1-7). Well-compensated patients can tolerate most surgical procedures, but poorly compensated patients cannot tolerate even mild sedatives. The severity of cirrhosis can be estimated by physical examination and laboratory studies using the Child-Turcotte-Pugh score (Table 1-8) or Model for End-Stage Liver Disease (MELD) score calculated using the serum creatinine, bilirubin (mg/dL), and international normalized ratio (INR) (Table 1-9).

A careful examination and laboratory assessment is necessary to assess the risk fully. In this case, the patient has advanced liver failure and is somewhat decompensated, as evidenced by the ascites. In addition, the ascites is probably part of the cause of the hernia; the constant pressure exerted by the ascitic fluid is certainly making the hernia worse.

Careful examination indicates no evident hepatic encephalopathy and no infections but some mild muscle wasting. Laboratory studies reveal serum albumin, 3.2 g/dL; bilirubin, 2.5 mg/dL; prothrombin time (PT), 15 seconds (reference 1.2 seconds; INR, 1.25); serum creatinine, 2.5 mg/dL; and platelet count, 110,000/mm².

◆ **How does one determine the patient's operative risk?**

◆ **The MELD score is the most common method to assess risk.** The MELD score calculation is 21 points, which indicates a 3-month mortality of approximately 20%, a significant operative risk. Child's classification was originally designed to stratify risk in patients undergoing

Table 1-7: Clinical and Laboratory Evidence of Severe Liver Failure

Clinical Indicators
Jaundice
Ascites
Muscle wasting
Asterixis
Advanced encephalopathy
Caput medusa (dilated periumbilical vessels)
Splenomegaly
History of gastric or esophageal varices
Laboratory Indicators*
Decreased serum albumin
Increased serum bilirubin
Elevated PT
Thrombocytopenia

*Also indicators of marginal hepatic reserve.

Table 1-8: Child's Classification of Liver Failure

	Group		
	A	B	C
Bilirubin (mg/dL)	<2.0	2.0–3.0	>3
Albumin (g/dL)	>3.5	3.0–3.5	<3
Ascites	None	Easily controlled	Poorly controlled
Encephalopathy	None	Minimal	Advanced
Nutrition	Excellent	Good	Poor
Mortality	0%–5%	10%–15%	>25%

From Jarrell BE. *NMS Surgery*, 4th ed. Philadelphia: Lippincott Williams & Wilkins; 2000.

portosystemic shunting procedures, but the risk appears similar in patients undergoing nonhepatic procedures. The system, which combines three laboratory studies with two clinical findings, remains the most accurate measure of hepatic reserve (see Table 1-8). This patient satisfies the majority of the criteria for **group** B and therefore presents an intermediate operative risk.

Deep Thoughts

The benefits of the surgery must outweigh the risks of the surgery; otherwise, the surgery should not be performed.

Table 1-9: Model for End-Stage Liver Disease

MELD uses the patient's values for serum bilirubin, serum creatinine, and the international normalized ratio (INR) for prothrombin time to predict survival. It is calculated according to the following formula:

$$MELD = 3.78[\text{Ln serum bilirubin (mg/dL)}] + 11.2[\text{Ln INR}] + 9.57[\text{Ln serum creatinine (mg/dL)}] + 6.43$$

UNOS has made the following modifications to the score:

- If the patient has been dialyzed twice within the last 7 days, then the value for serum creatinine used should be 4.0.
- Any value <1 is given a value of 1 (i.e., if bilirubin is 0.8, a value of 1.0 is used) to prevent the occurrence of scores below 0 (the natural logarithm of 1 is 0, and any value <1 would yield a negative result).

Patients with a diagnosis of liver cancer will be assigned a MELD score based on how advanced the cancer is.

In interpreting the MELD score in hospitalized patients, the 3-month mortality is:

- ≥40 — 71.3% mortality
- 30–39 — 52.6% mortality
- 20–29 — 19.6% mortality
- 10–19 — 6.0% mortality
- <9 — 1.9% mortality

MELD, Model for End-Stage Liver Disease; UNOS, United Network for Organ Sharing.

◆ **Would you proceed with the surgery?**

◆ As previously stated, patients with chronic liver failure can tolerate most surgical procedures well if they are in a relatively **compensated state preoperatively**. They should **abstain from alcohol** for 6–12 weeks before surgery. If the hernia is repaired but the ascites remains uncontrolled, there is a significant chance of hernia recurrence and bacterial peritonitis. Thus, patients should be **medically optimized** before repair. **Ascites should be controlled** with potassium-sparing diuretics, as well as sodium and water restriction.

In this case, the patient's **serum electrolytes** should be restudied **preoperatively** because diuretic therapy can cause abnormalities. If possible, the patient's **nutrition status should be improved**. In addition, **improvement in the man's liver status** will improve his chance for a successful outcome. Lastly, he has a very **abnormal prothrombin time**, which should be normalized with vitamin K, if possible, prior to surgery.

◆ **What factors might prompt a delay in the patient's surgery?**

◆ A high MELD status, classification in **Child's group C**, and presence of **acute alcoholic hepatitis** make patients generally poor operative candidates. Time and alcohol abstinence allow alcoholic hepatitis to resolve. If surgery can be delayed, efforts to improve a patient's liver status can also be instituted.

You decide to delay the man's surgery and begin efforts to improve his ascites and normalize his prothrombin time.

◆ **How would your proposed management change in each of the following situations?**

Case Variation 1.7.1. The patient has a small ulcerated area on the hernia.

◆ The skin over an umbilical hernia can ulcerate due to pressure necrosis, thus increasing the **risk of rupture**, which has a mortality rate of 11%–43%. This hernia should be repaired in an expedient manner after proper inpatient management of ascites.

Case Variation 1.7.2. The patient returns to the emergency department in a confused, disoriented, and mildly lethargic state.

◆ Evaluation for **mental status change** is necessary. Possible causes include **electrolyte abnormalities, GI bleeding, sepsis, and an intracranial event** (e.g., **subdural hematoma or hepatic encephalopathy**) related to liver failure. Development of **spontaneous bacterial peritonitis** or **peritonitis related to cellulitis** or infection on the umbilical hernia skin is also possible. The ascites should be tapped, and the patient should be treated with antibiotics if the fluid contains more than 250 white blood cells (WBCs)/mm^3.

Case Variation 1.7.3. The patient returns to the emergency department with serous fluid leaking from a small ulcer on the hernia.

◆ Ascitic **fluid leaking** from the umbilical hernia leads to an increased risk of bacterial peritonitis. The mortality rate is high, primarily due to infection. The serous fluid should be sent for cell count and culture, and IV antibiotics should be initiated before culture results return. The hernia should be **repaired urgently**.

Case Variation 1.7.4. You smell alcohol on the patient in the office.

◆ The surgery **should be delayed** until the patient has abstained from alcohol and undergone withdrawal. **Alcohol withdrawal** during the postoperative period is associated with high morbidity and mortality.

Case Variation 1.7.5. The patient tells you that he has severe hemorrhoids he wants removed. Examination confirms several moderate-sized internal hemorrhoids.

◆ Hemorrhoid removal requires **great caution** in patients with cirrhosis and possible **portal hypertension**. Uncontrollable hemorrhage during surgical repair may occur as a result of portal hypertension.

Case 1.8 Surgery in a Patient with Chronic Kidney Problems

A 52-year-old man with aseptic necrosis of his right leg requires hip replacement. His history is significant for chronic renal failure for 10 years secondary to glomerulonephritis. Initial management involved a kidney transplant from a living relative and immunosuppression with cyclosporine and **prednisone**. Recently, he has experienced progressive chronic rejection and has a creatinine of 3.5 mg/dL. On physical examination, multiple stigmata of steroid management, including striae, moon facies, and easy bruisability, are evident. He has mild ankle edema. The patient experiences pain on passive motion of the right hip.

◆ **Would you recommend proceeding with the hip replacement at this time?**

◆ The decision regarding the timing of hip replacement surgery is best made in conjunction with an orthopedist who is experienced in treating patients with renal problems. In patients with progressive deteriorating renal function, repair of the hip should be delayed until the transplant function has stabilized or the necessary dialysis has begun. Once a patient's renal status is stable, the hip can be reassessed and a plan determined. **Repairing the hip during transplant deterioration may complicate or aggravate the rejection process and hasten the need for dialysis.**

◆ **How would you prepare the patient for surgery?**

◆ The major objective is to **resolve any correctable problems** before taking a patient with chronic renal failure to the operating room.

 QUICK CUT Well-dialyzed patients have the most normalized platelet function, hydration state, BP control, and electrolyte status.

Thus, dialysis immediately before surgery is desirable. **Transplant patients** should be adequately hydrated and have well-controlled BP. Infection control is desirable in both types of patients. Many of these patients also have been on steroids in the recent past. If so, there preoperative dosage should be continued, and stress doses of 100–150 mg of hydrocortisone can be given if needed.

Preoperative laboratory tests from 2 days ago reveal a serum potassium of 5.1 mEq/L, and the patient is in the holding area ready for the operating room.

◆ **Is a 2-day-old potassium value an adequate preoperative measurement?**

◆ This measurement is **too old** to rely on for surgery because the potassium can rise to dangerous levels in short periods of time in chronic renal failure. A repeat potassium level needs to be obtained immediately—before the patient proceeds to the operating room.

   You decide to proceed with surgery and encounter intraoperative bleeding due to a "capillary ooze."

◆ **How would you manage the bleeding?**

> **QUICK CUT** Platelet dysfunction due to uremia can contribute to intraop-
> erative bleeding. Transfusion of platelets will not help. Correcting the uremia
> will help.

◆ Several substances can be used to improve platelet function. Desmopressin (ddAVP) may be used acutely. It has a rapid effect of short duration and may induce tachyphylaxis (loss of hemostatic effect with multiple doses); its action is related to release of von Willebrand factor from endothelial cells, and it increases the spreading and aggregation of platelets. Fresh frozen plasma also temporarily corrects the platelet defect. Conjugated estrogens, which have a slow onset of action, may be effective for up to 2 weeks. Finally, postoperative hemodialysis may reduce the uremia and improve platelet function.

The patient becomes hypotensive, with a BP of 80/60 mm Hg, in the operating room. There is no evidence of surgical bleeding.

◆ **In addition to the usual methods to correct hypotension, are there any special measures you might take in this patient?**

◆ The hypotension must be explained; this condition has many causes. Although easy to forget **glucocorticoid deficiency** is one important cause of such low BP in many renal failure patients who have previously taken steroids. The hypotension should be treated with hydrocortisone 25 mg intraoperatively, followed by 100 mg in the next 24 hours.

You successfully replace the man's hip. In the recovery room, his postoperative potassium level returns to 7.1 mEq/L, and he is producing 10 mL/hr of urine.

◆ **How would you manage the patient?**

◆ The patient has oliguria and **hyperkalemia**. He should be adequately hydrated, and his high potassium concentration should be treated. **Peaked T waves** on the ECG suggest that the hyperkalemia is physiologically important and warrants **immediate treatment**. IV **calcium gluconate** should be given to stabilize cardiac membranes. **IV insulin and glucose** should be given to reduce potassium levels, but **hemodialysis** will probably also be necessary.

Case 1.9   Surgery in a Patient with Cardiac Valvular Disease

You are asked to see a female patient who needs an elective cholecystectomy. She has known valvular heart disease.

◆ **How would you manage the following preoperative conditions?**

*Case Variation 1.9.1. **The patient has chronic mitral valve stenosis that is currently well compensated.***

◆ Stenosis of the mitral valve leads to increased left atrial pressure, which may result in passive **pulmonary hypertension and right heart failure**, leading to symptoms of fatigue, dyspnea on exertion, or hemoptysis. The distended atrium is susceptible to **atrial fibrillation or other arrhythmias**. Many surgeons would obtain a cardiology opinion and an echocardiogram to evaluate cardiac function if there is any doubt about the patient's cardiac status. The perioperative mortality for all patients with hemodynamically significant mitral stenosis is as high as 5%.

Because this patient has well-compensated mitral valve stenosis, surgery could proceed. Intravascular volume should be maintained, and hypoxemia, hypercapnia, and acidosis, which all increase pulmonary vascular resistance, should be avoided. Tachycardia should also be avoided because it decreases diastolic filling time. Like all patients with valvular heart disease, this woman should also receive **prophylactic antibiotics** for the prevention of bacterial endocarditis.

Case Variation 1.9.2. *The patient had chronic mitral valve stenosis and an episode of congestive heart failure (CHF) 1 month ago.*

◆ Mitral valve stenosis with underlying CHF increases mortality to as high as 20%. More **extensive cardiac workup** and perioperative monitoring may be necessary, and ECG and echocardiography are indicated to determine the extent of disease. If urgent surgery is needed, **intraoperative monitoring** may include an arterial line and transesophageal echocardiography. The pulmonary artery catheter is of limited usefulness because the pressure gradient across the mitral valve distorts the relationship between the pulmonary capillary wedge pressure and the left ventricular end-diastolic pressure.

Case Variation 1.9.3. *The patient has known aortic stenosis and a grade IV systolic murmur.*

◆ The obstruction to left ventricular outflow leads to left ventricular hypertrophy and increased left ventricular end-diastolic pressure, which may cause angina, dyspnea, syncope, or **sudden death**. The outflow obstruction causes an inability to increase cardiac output. In patients who need **elective surgery, cardiac assessment** and possibly valve replacement would take priority. In patients who need urgent surgery, **perioperative hemodynamic monitoring** with a pulmonary artery catheter, an arterial line, and transesophageal echocardiography should be considered.

Case 1.10 Endocarditis Prophylaxis in a Surgical Patient with Valvular Heart Disease

A 58-year-old woman with mitral valve disease secondary to rheumatic fever is scheduled to undergo a hemicolectomy for diverticular disease.

◆ **When would you consider bacterial endocarditis prophylaxis?**

◆ AMA guidelines recommendations:
Antibiotic prophylaxis is indicated for the following high-risk cardiac conditions:

> Prosthetic cardiac valve
> History of infective endocarditis
> Congenital heart disease (CHD) *(except for the conditions listed, antibiotic prophylaxis is no longer recommended for any other form of CHD)*: (1) unrepaired cyanotic CHD, including palliative shunts and conduits; (2) completely repaired congenital heart defect with prosthetic material or device, whether placed by surgery or by catheter intervention, during the first 6 months after the procedure; and (3) repaired CHD with residual defects at the site or adjacent to the site of a prosthetic patch or prosthetic device (which inhibits endothelialization)
> Cardiac transplantation recipients with cardiac valvular disease

For patients with high cardiac risk, antibiotic prophylaxis is recommended for all dental procedures that involve manipulation of gingival tissue or the periapical region of teeth or perforation of the oral mucosa.

Antibiotic prophylaxis is recommended for invasive respiratory tract procedures that involve incision or biopsy of the respiratory mucosa (e.g., tonsillectomy, adenoidectomy). Antibiotic prophylaxis is not recommended for bronchoscopy unless the procedure involves incision of the respiratory tract mucosa. For invasive respiratory tract procedures to treat an established infection (e.g., drainage of abscess, empyema), administer an antibiotic that is active against *Streptococcus viridans*.

Patients with high cardiac risk who undergo a surgical procedure that involves infected skin, skin structure, or musculoskeletal tissue should receive an agent active against staphylococci and beta-hemolytic streptococci (e.g., antistaphylococcal penicillin, cephalosporin).

If the causative organism of respiratory, skin, skin structure, or musculoskeletal infection is known or suspected to be *Staphylococcus aureus*, administer an antistaphylococcal penicillin or cephalosporin, or vancomycin (if patient is unable to tolerate beta-lactam antibiotics). Vancomycin is recommended for known or suspected methicillin-resistant strains of *S. aureus*.

Antibiotics are **no** longer recommended for endocarditis prophylaxis for patients undergoing genitourinary or GI tract procedures.

Case 1.11   Surgery in a Patient with Cardiomyopathy

You are asked to see a woman with colon cancer who needs a left colectomy. She has a known cardiomyopathy, with mild shortness of breath and fine rales in both lung bases.

◆ **How would you manage the patient perioperatively?**

> **QUICK CUT** Patients with cardiomyopathy are at risk for complications such as arrhythmias, CHF, cardiac outflow obstruction, and sudden death.

◆ Because this patient needs elective surgery, she should be carefully evaluated by a cardiologist. Patients who require urgent surgery should have their fluid status carefully controlled and possible arrhythmias monitored. Pulmonary artery catheterization and/or transesophageal echocardiography may be necessary to manage volume status properly.

Chapter 2

Postoperative Care

Bruce E. Jarrell, Molly Buzdon, Eric D. Strauch

Key Thoughts

1. Ultimately, there is no one formula that best determines postoperative fluid and electrolyte management. Fluid management involves asking several questions.

   Is the patient taking oral fluids?

   - Maintenance fluids should be given on a routine basis for anyone who is on a nothing by mouth (NPO) status.

   What fluid losses and with what electrolyte composition can I measure (i.e., sensible losses) that I need to replace?

   - Nasogastric (NG) tube drainage should be replaced with 1/2 normal saline (NS) with 20 mEq/L KCl milliliter for milliliter.
   - Significant drain output should be replaced with fluid that approximates its composition such as pancreatic drainage with Ringer lactate. The electrolytes of the fluid can be measured to determine the best replacement fluid.

   What nonmeasurable (i.e., insensible) fluid loss sources are present both intraoperatively and postoperatively, and how can I estimate and replace them?

   - High insensible losses (both evaporative losses and leakage into the third space) occur during and after surgical procedures that: involve open body cavities; are invasive and open many tissue planes; are prolonged; are associated with sepsis, inflammatory conditions, and ischemia of organs; result in hypotension; and are done in emergent settings.
   - Fluid losses from the respiratory tree
   - Fever
   - Burns

   What pre-existing disease state and volume or electrolyte deficit abnormalities have to be considered?

   - History of congestive heart failure or pulmonary edema
   - Acute or chronic renal failure and oliguria
   - Hemodynamically significant arrhythmias
   - Low serum protein states, low or high serum potassium

   And then, once a plan has been implemented, continuously reassess the effect of your replacement fluids.

   - Is organ oxygenation and perfusion being maintained? This is not just blood pressure (BP) and pulse—it is also monitoring urine output and renal function; lung auscultation for signs of pulmonary edema, blood oxygenation, chest x-ray for early pulmonary edema; serum electrolyte levels, pH, arrhythmias; mentation; external signs of hydration state, hematocrit, and overall appearance of patient.

- Is the patient improving or at least maintaining status at a sufficient level? If not, are any new processes occurring?

2. A differential diagnosis is always useful when managing patients with clinical problems. This is also true for postoperative patients, particularly those having unexpected problems. For instance, if a patient is oliguric, how many potential reasons can you think of that could cause the oliguria, and which ones are the most likely cause? Once you have that list, you can systematically assess each and arrive at a diagnosis, which leads to a correction plan. Try not to jump to a diagnosis without first going through this process. For example, the usual cause for oliguria in a postoperative patient is hypovolemia and is treated with fluids. However, if the urinary catheter is mechanically blocked, fluids will obviously not solve the problem.

3. When evaluating a patient who is clinically deteriorating, always evaluate the diagnosis in your differential that will lead to the fastest and greatest deterioration. For instance, make sure you rule out a myocardial infarction before aggressively treating gastroesophageal reflux.

4. Management of sick patients requires resuscitation, restoring perfusion, and supporting oxygen delivery. However, your resuscitation will ultimately fail if you do not quickly and accurately find the source of the clinical deterioration and fix that problem.

Case 2.1 | Postoperative Fluid and Electrolyte Management

A 55-year-old diabetic man who has an adenocarcinoma of the sigmoid colon undergoes a colectomy. The operation goes smoothly, and he returns to the recovery room in good condition with an NG tube in place.

◆ **How would you determine whether the intraoperative fluid replacement was adequate?**

◆ Determination of intraoperative fluid replacement requirements involves knowledge of the extent of both measurable, or sensible, and unmeasurable, or insensible, fluid losses. Measurable losses include estimated blood loss (EBL) and urine output. Assuming the patient received no blood in the operating room, replacement of every 1 mL of EBL with 3 mL of isotonic fluid is necessary; approximately two thirds of the intravenous (IV) fluid administered to the patient rapidly leaves the intravascular space (Table 2-1).

Deep Thoughts

Ultimately, adequate fluid replacement is determined by evaluation of the patient, including vital signs, physical exam, ins and outs, and laboratory evaluations.

QUICK CUT Postoperative fluid replacement requires replacement of fluid lost during a procedure; provision of maintenance requirements; and consideration of ongoing losses through drains, NG tubes, and fistulas.

Insensible losses, which occur through evaporation and other processes, are not easily quantifiable. Large amounts of such losses take place in patients who undergo long

Table 2-1: Sample Calculation of Intraoperative Fluid Requirements

Measured Losses	
EBL	500 mL
IV fluids given in OR	1,000 mL
Urine output	200 mL
(EBL × 3 mL isotonic fluid/1 mL blood loss) + 200 − 1000 = 700	
700 mL of isotonic fluid (lactated Ringer or normal saline) should be replaced.	

EBL, estimated blood loss; IV, intravenous; OR, operating room.

procedures, particularly when the peritoneal cavity is open. Insensible losses must be estimated using clinical judgment, based on vital signs, urine output, physical examination, and other physiologic measurements obtained through central venous catheters. A rule of thumb for insensible operative fluid loss is 5–10 mL/kg/hr for large open abdominal procedures, 3–5 mL/kg/hr for smaller open surgical procedures, and 1–2 mL/kg/hr for minor procedures. Obviously, more disruptive procedures are associated with larger insensible losses.

◆ **How would you estimate the patient's routine postoperative fluid and electrolyte requirements?**

◆ Maintenance fluid requirements can be easily calculated using a formula based on body weight (Table 2-2). The combination of $D_5$0.5 NS plus KCl 20 mEq/L satisfies the sodium, potassium, and chloride requirements of the average patient. After a large intraoperative blood loss, lactated Ringer solution or 0.9 NS may be chosen for the first 24 hours. (Because the fluid lost is isotonic, it is replaced by isotonic fluid.) Regardless, the patient's volume and electrolyte status should always be estimated frequently, particularly in the first 24–48 hours after surgery. This involves careful bedside observation, together with analysis of vital signs and laboratory values.

◆ **How would you determine the volume of fluids and electrolytes needed to replace those lost from the patient's NG tube?**

◆ Gastrointestinal (GI) fistulas and tubes placed in certain sites typically drain fluids of a predictable concentration. The amount lost should be replaced milliliter for milliliter (Table 2-3). IV fluids of a known concentration are commonly used for fluid replacement (Table 2-4).

Table 2-2: Estimate of Maintenance Fluid Requirements

Body Weight (kg)	Fluid Requirements (mL/kg/24 hr)
First 10	100
Next 10	50
Beyond 20	20 per kilogram
EXAMPLE: 70-kg patient	
(100 mL/kg × 10 kg) + (50 mL/kg × 10 kg) + (20 mL/kg × 50 kg)	
1,000 mL + 500 mL + 1,000 mL = **2,500 mL/24 hr** (approximately 100 mL/hr)	

Table 2-3: Electrolyte Content of Gastrointestinal Fluids

Gastrointestinal Fluid	Na$^+$ (mEq/L)	K$^+$ (mEq/L)	Cl$^-$ (mEq/L)	HCO$_3^-$ (mEq/L)
Gastric aspirate	100	10	140	0
Pancreatic juice	140	5	75	100
Bile	140	5	100	60
Small bowel drainage	110	5	105	30
Distal ileum and cecum	140	5	70	50
Colon	60	70	15	30

◆ **How do the patient's fluid requirements change during the postoperative course?**

◆ As the man regains GI function and recovers from the surgery, he will begin to mobilize fluid from third-space accumulation. This excess fluid, which must be excreted by the kidneys, represents an additional volume in the intravascular space. Thus, IV fluid requirements decrease during the recovery period. Failure to reduce IV intake may result in fluid overload, edema, and even pulmonary edema.

Case Variation 2.1.1. *The patient has postoperative oliguria, 5 mL/hr for 3 hours with significant tachycardia.*

◆ The patient must be examined, looking for a cause of the decreased urine output and tachycardia. Examination should include the rest of the vital signs, evaluation for jugular venous distention, the presence of rales in the lungs, cardiac rhythm, and evaluation of the abdomen for distention and bleeding or drainage from the wound. The concern is that the patient is hypovolemic. It is important to determine if the hypovolemia is a result of under-resuscitation or bleeding. Hypovolemia is initially treated with bolus isotonic fluid resuscitation. A postoperative hemoglobin and hematocrit (h/h) is obtained. If the patient fails to respond to volume resuscitation, a repeat h/h is obtained. A significant drop in the h/h would be concerning for bleeding most likely from the surgical site.

Table 2-4: Electrolyte Composition of Various Solutions

Solution	Glucose (mg/dL)	Na$^+$ (mEq/L)	K$^+$ (mEq/L)	Ca^{2+} (mEq/L)	Cl$^-$ (mEq/L)	Lactate (mg/dL)
D$_5$W	50	—	—	—	—	—
D$_{10}$W	100	—	—	—	—	—
0.9 NS	—	154	—	—	154	—
0.45 NS	—	77	—	—	77	—
Lactated Ringer solution	—	130	4	3	110	28

W, water; NS, normal saline.

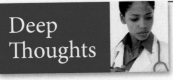

Deep Thoughts

Although uncommon, the h/h can drop from hemodilution. In general, this results in an increase in the intravascular volume, and the hemodynamic parameters of the patient would improve (i.e., the tachycardia would decrease and the urine output would increase). A drop in h/h from bleeding will show all the signs of hypovolemia.

Case 2.2 Postoperative Acute Renal Failure

A 75-year-old man with a history of benign prostatic hypertrophy undergoes a minor ambulatory surgical procedure on his foot. He presents to the emergency department 12 hours later with acute urinary retention. A urinary catheter is placed, and 1,200 mL of clear urine is removed. He is admitted to the hospital.

◆ **How would your evaluation and management change in each of the following situations?**

*Case Variation 2.2.1. **The patient's urine output is 50 mL/hr over the next 4 hours.***

◆ This value represents **normal urine output**, which should be 0.5–1 mL/kg/hr. The patient must remain adequately hydrated; sufficient oral or IV fluids must be given to replace all fluid losses and provide maintenance fluid requirements.

*Case Variation 2.2.2. **The patient diureses 400 mL/hr over the next 4 hours and develops a BP of 80/60 mm Hg.***

◆ This development could be secondary to a number of potential causes, including **pre-existing renal disease with inability to concentrate urine, diabetes insipidus, or a combination of causes. Postobstructive diuresis,** another cause, may account for the increased urine output with resultant dehydration and hypotension. Certain conditions make patients more prone to postobstructive diuresis; these include chronic obstruction, edema, congestive heart failure, hypertension, weight gain, and azotemia.

QUICK CUT The diuresis may be either physiologic—caused by retained urea, sodium, and water—or pathologic—caused by impaired concentrating ability or impaired sodium reabsorption.

The hypotension must be promptly treated with more aggressive hydration and monitoring.

When a patient such as this diureses more than 200 mL/hr for 2 consecutive hours, the urine should be collected over a timed period to determine the cause of diuresis. **Urine with a low osmolality probably indicates a pathologic concentrating defect, whereas urine with a higher osmolality suggests osmotic diuresis.** In most instances, postobstructive diuresis is self-limited, and the blood urea nitrogen (BUN) and creatinine (Cr) return to normal in 1–2 days. In general, urologists believe that it is best to keep the patient's volume expanded during the polyuric phase. The best way to maintain hydration without fluid overloading the patient is to replace some portion of the excess urine volume milliliter for milliliter. The urine electrolytes can be obtained to determine the best fluid for replacement.

Case Variation 2.2.3. The patient's urine output is 10 mL/hr for the next 4 hours.

◆ Most commonly, severe oliguria is caused by either a mechanical problem with the catheter or severe dehydration of the patient. First, catheter patency should be confirmed, either noninvasively using transabdominal ultrasound to detect bladder distension or by irrigating the catheter and demonstrating patency. If no mechanical problem is evident, **volume resuscitation** should be tried. If this fails to increase the patient's urine output, placement of a central venous pressure (CVP) line or pulmonary artery catheter may be necessary to assess the adequacy of the attempts at volume repletion.

Case Variation 2.2.4. The patient's urine output is 10 mL/hr, and his CVP is 12 cm H₂O.

◆ A **pulmonary artery catheter may be indicated** to ensure that preload and cardiac output are adequate. An echocardiogram of the heart can be obtained to look at ventricular function, inferior vena caval filling and diameter, and variation with respiration to help determine intravascular volume status. Other laboratory tests to determine the etiology of oliguria include the fractional excretion of sodium (FeNa), BUN:Cr, urine electrolytes, and osmolality. Obstruction should be ruled out by renal ultrasound (Table 2-5).

Case Variation 2.2.5. The man's first urine sample is cloudy, and he appears confused and disoriented.

◆ This scenario suggests **urosepsis**. The urine should be sent for urinalysis as well as culture, and broad-spectrum antibiotics should be initiated until a specific organism is cultured.

Case Variation 2.2.6. The patient develops gross hematuria as the first 1,000 mL of urine is drained from the bladder.

◆ Hematuria is not uncommon following obstruction due to overdistention of the bladder and bladder wall injury, but a man of this age should also have a urology consult to rule out more serious causes, including malignancy. Infection, kidney stones, trauma, prostatitis, and medications known to cause cystitis (e.g., cyclophosphamide) may also produce hematuria. If the urine output drops, the bladder should be irrigated to dislodge any clots. If clotting occurs and persists, the patient may need constant bladder irrigation with a three-way Foley catheter.

Case Variation 2.2.7. Four hours after insertion of the catheter, the man has a temperature of 104°F and a BP of 80/60 mm Hg. He is confused.

◆ The patient most likely has urosepsis and needs urgent monitoring and fluid resuscitation in the intensive care unit. In addition, he requires a sepsis workup, broad-spectrum antibiotics, and possibly a pulmonary artery catheter.

Table 2-5: Measurements Used in the Evaluation of Oliguria

Cause of Oliguria	Urine Osmolality (mOsm/kg)	Urine [Na⁺] (mEq/L)	FeNa (%)	BUN/Cr Ratio
Prerenal	>500	<20	<1	>20
Postrenal	250–300	>40	>3	<10

FeNa, fractional excretion of sodium.

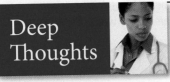

Deep Thoughts

Although this patient needed a catheter, avoiding the catheter in the first place for a situation where it is not required is always a consideration. The simple insertion of a urinary catheter can be sufficient to cause bacteremia and urosepsis, even within hours of inserting the catheter.

Case 2.3 Postoperative Fever

A 45-year-old woman has had a colon resection. You are called to see her on her fifth postoperative day. For the past 24 hours, she has had a temperature of 101°F.

◆ **How would you evaluate this patient?**

◆ A thorough history and physical examination are necessary; they are the most important part of the workup. All sources of fever should be considered. Possible sources of fever in hospitalized or postoperative patients include wound infections, deep space infections, pneumonia, upper respiratory infection, urinary tract infection (UTI), deep venous thrombosis (DVT), infected indwelling catheters, and drug-related fever. The patient should be asked about sputum production, cough, abdominal pain, nausea, vomiting, pain at the wound site, drainage from the wound, bowel function, difficulty urinating, or blood in the urine.

◆ **How would your evaluation and management change in each of the following situations?**

Case Variation 2.3.1. On lung examination, the patient has fine crackles bilaterally.

◆ The **patient probably has atelectasis**, which is collapse of portions of the alveolar structures in the lung.

> **QUICK CUT** A common cause of fever in the immediate postoperative period is atelectasis. It is better to avoid this complication with preoperative training and postoperative use of incentive spirometry. It is diagnosed by physical examination and chest Radiography (CXR). Once atelectasis is present, it is treated with vigorous pulmonary toilet and incentive spirometry. Antibiotics are not used in the treatment of atelectasis.

Atelectasis is one of the most common reasons for a postoperative fever, but several other possibilities should be considered. Pneumonia is diagnosed by the appearance on CXR, as well as sputum suggestive of infection. Antibiotics should be started as soon as the diagnosis of pneumonia is made. Pulmonary edema should also be considered. Although this condition does not typically cause fever, it does occur postoperatively. Pulmonary edema frequently occurs several days into the postoperative period when the patient is beginning to mobilize third-space fluids.

Case Variation 2.3.2. **The man reports burning on urination, and he has noticed some blood in his urine. Urinalysis reveals 10–20 white blood cells (WBCs)/hpf and 3+ leukocyte esterase.**

◆ This patient has a **UTI**, which may be related to the use of a Foley catheter or urinary retention.

> **QUICK CUT** UTI is a common cause of postoperative fever, especially around day 3. Early removal of a urinary catheter can help minimize UTIs, and many hospitals have well-established protocols for early removal or avoidance of catheters.

Retention can be diagnosed by physical examination, bladder ultrasound, or insertion of a catheter. Most infections can be treated with oral trimethoprim–sulfamethoxazole or ciprofloxacin. A urinalysis and urine culture should be performed.

Care should be taken with patients who are elderly or diabetic or show any signs of illness such as nausea, vomiting, or abdominal or flank pain. It may be important to administer the antibiotics intravenously and make certain that patients are well hydrated.

Case Variation 2.3.3. **The man reports some purulent drainage from his wound site with some tenderness. His staples are still in place.**

◆ In this case, **the wound must be evaluated carefully** for signs of cellulitis or fluctuance.

> **QUICK CUT** If the wound exhibits fluctuance, which is suggestive of a fluid collection beneath the skin, sufficient staples should be removed, in consultation with the surgeon, and pus should be drained. The fascial integrity should be determined and local wound care initiated.

The wound should be cultured and treated locally, which often means irrigation and local wound care. If significant cellulitis is present, administration of an appropriate antibiotic is necessary. The most common bacteria found in wound infections are skin flora.

Case Variation 2.3.4. **On examination, you note that the man has an indwelling IV in his right forearm with induration, edema, and tenderness at the site.**

◆ The catheter should be removed. In most cases, after catheter removal, the inflammation will resolve. If significant cellulitis is present, antibiotics should be considered. Most surgeons recommend that all IV insertion sites be rotated every 4 days to prevent this problem.

Case Variation 2.3.5. **You also discover a drop of pus on the skin at the venipuncture exit site.**

◆ This condition is termed **suppurative phlebitis** and is caused by the presence of an infected thrombus in the vein and around the indwelling catheter. Affected patients are apt to have high fevers and positive blood cultures. In addition to removing the catheter, suppurative phlebitis is treated by surgically excising the infected vein.

> **QUICK CUT** In addition to removal of the catheter, excision of the affected vein to the first normal vein segment that is patent and noninfected. IV antibiotics should be administered, and the wound should be left open.

Case 2.4 High Fever in the Immediate
Postoperative Period

A 35-year-old man has received a shotgun wound to the abdomen in which he sustained a blast injury to the abdominal wall and a colon injury. Twelve hours after a right hemicolectomy with ileostomy and mucous fistula, he develops a high fever. You receive a call from a nurse because his temperature is 105°F.

◆ **How would you manage this condition?**

◆ A postoperative fever of this magnitude requires prompt attention because it is a potentially life-threatening problem. It is critical that a wound infection from a gas-forming organism be ruled out. Immediate performance of a careful physical examination must take place. Removal of the abdominal wound bandages and inspection of the wound are necessary. Atelectasis, the most common cause of postoperative fever immediately after surgery, could account for this patient's high temperature. However, for atelectasis to cause such a fever, the patient would have to have massive collapse of an entire lobe or the entire lung. Atelectasis can be evaluated by physical examination and CXR.

The wound appears erythematous, with an advancing edge of brown skin discoloration and bleb formation. There is a thin, watery brown discharge with a foul odor and crepitus near the wound.

◆ **What diagnosis do you suspect?**

◆ A serious wound infection is likely.

 QUICK CUT A gas-forming organism such as Clostridium or group A streptococci can cause a serious wound infection and necrotizing fasciitis. Rapid attention to addressing this infection is critical to its successful treatment and the survival of the patient.

Occasionally, crepitus is a later finding, and its absence should not delay diagnosis because the disease spreads very rapidly along fascial planes.

◆ **How should you treat this infection?**

◆ The wound should be opened and cultured immediately. Clostridial myositis and cellulitis (gas gangrene) is most commonly caused by *Clostridium perfringens*.

 QUICK CUT If gram-positive, spore-producing rods are found, the diagnosis of a clostridial wound infection is made. Debridement of infected tissue is mandatory as the primary therapy.

Administration of high-dose penicillin G should occur, and debridement is necessary. Hyperbaric oxygen therapy may also help stop infection and inhibit the germination of heat-activated spores. Hemolysis is possible from hemagglutinin and hemolysin toxins produced by *Clostridium*. Tetanus immunization is also necessary. Multiorganism infections with *Streptococcus*, *Staphylococcus*, and gram-negative rods can produce similar findings.

Case 2.5 Postoperative Cardiopulmonary Problems

A 47-year-old man has undergone repair of a large ventral hernia. While in the hospital, the man is under your care.

◆ **How would you manage the following situations in the postoperative period?**

Case Variation 2.5.1. The nurses note from the previous night's records a brief episode of shortness of breath. The man, who smokes two packs of cigarettes a day, tells you that he is coughing up yellow sputum.

◆ The man could have dyspnea from atelectasis, bronchitis, or pneumonia. As a smoker, he has a greater risk of developing bronchitis or pneumonia. It is necessary to examine his chest for signs of atelectasis or pneumonia and obtain a CXR and arterial blood gases (ABGs) to evaluate his arterial oxygen saturation. In addition, his sputum should be sent for Gram stain and culture. If he is febrile, empiric antibiotics might be started after the culture is sent based on a CXR finding compatible with pneumonia.

Case Variation 2.5.2. Since yesterday, the patient's oxygen saturation reading on pulse oximetry has dropped from 95% to 85%.

◆ Further evaluation is necessary to determine the cause of the hypoxia.

Case Variation 2.5.3. The man states that he has been coughing up blood-streaked sputum since this morning.

◆ Hemoptysis may be a sign of several conditions.

> **QUICK CUT** Hemoptysis may be secondary to malignancy, bronchitis, pneumonia, tuberculosis, or pulmonary infarction which may be caused by a pulmonary embolism.

If the patient has had hemoptysis prior to hospitalization, malignancy is more likely. If this is the patient's first episode of hemoptysis, it is more likely caused by a pulmonary embolus, especially in the setting of immobilization in the hospital. In either case, further workup is necessary.

Case Variation 2.5.4. The man becomes acutely hypotensive with a BP of 80/60 mm Hg, and his oxygen saturation drops from 95% to 85%.

◆ The man could be having a massive pulmonary embolism (PE) or myocardial infarction (MI). First, his airway should be assessed, which means evaluation of bilateral breath sounds to rule out pneumothorax or another major pulmonary problem. Intubation may also be necessary. Emergent transfer to a monitored setting is required, and CXR and an electrocardiogram (ECG) are necessary. If the patient has ECG changes suggestive of MI, he should be evaluated and treated for this condition. If the man appears to be having a PE, initiation of a heparin infusion may be appropriate; once the patient is stable, the diagnosis can be established usually with a computed tomography (CT) angiogram of the chest with contrast to specifically evaluate the pulmonary arteries.

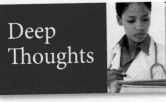

Deep Thoughts

When evaluating an unstable patient, formulate your differential diagnosis. Then evaluate the potential problems in an organized fashion. Look for the diagnosis that will lead rapidly to morbidity and mortality such as an MI or PE quickly. Obtain the diagnostic tests that are simple, quick to obtain, and high yield first such as an ECG, ABGs, or CXR.

Case Variation 2.5.5. *The patient develops cardiopulmonary arrest.*

◆ The advanced cardiac life support (ACLS) protocol, which starts with airway, breathing, and circulation, must be followed. A "code" should be called and the patient intubated emergently. Circulatory arrest may arise from respiratory arrest. Once the patient has been resuscitated, further evaluation is appropriate.

Case 2.6 Management of a Small Bowel Fistula

A 65-year-old woman has had a segment of necrotic bowel resected. On the 10th postoperative day, you notice intestinal contents draining from the wound.

◆ How would you manage this complication?

◆ Enteric contents could originate from a leak at the jejunostomy insertion site, breakdown of the small bowel anastomosis, or a missed enterotomy.

QUICK CUT Although most patients with a small bowel fistula do not need surgical exploration, a patient who shows clinical signs of peritonitis needs operative re-exploration.

Surgical re-exploration may be necessary if the patient has signs of peritonitis. Otherwise, a CT scan is required to rule out an intra-abdominal collection, which can usually be drained percutaneously under CT guidance.

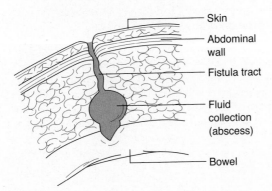

Skin
Abdominal wall
Fistula tract
Fluid collection (abscess)
Bowel

Figure 2-1: A gastrointestinal fistula.

F	Foreign body in the wound
R	Radiation damage to the area
I	Infection or inflammatory bowel disease
E	Epithelialization of the fistulous tract
N	Neoplasm
D	Distal bowel obstruction

Figure 2-2: The *mnemonic* "FRIEND," which can be used to remember the factors associated with failure of a fistula to heal. Some surgeons would add S for steroids.

QUICK CUT If an undrained collection is present in association with a GI fistula, percutaneous or operative drainage should be performed.

If no intra-abdominal fluid collection is evident, and the fistula appears to be draining adequately, this condition can be managed nonoperatively as an enterocutaneous fistula (Fig. 2-1). Treatment involves giving the patient nothing by mouth (making the patient NPO), administering total parenteral nutrition (TPN), and measuring the fistula output daily. Frequent measurement of serum electrolytes is necessary to avoid electrolyte imbalance from a high fistula output. As a result of this management, most fistulas will heal in several weeks. However, in certain circumstances, fistulas will not heal. The mnemonic "FRIEND" can be used to remember these conditions (Fig. 2-2).

Once the GI fistula has become established and is not rapidly closing, a fistulogram or small bowel series may be necessary to examine for explanations of persistent drainage. If the GI fistula persists after 5 or 6 weeks and the patient is free of infection, a definitive repair should be planned.

Chapter 3

Wound Healing

Bruce E. Jarrell, Eric D. Strauch

Key Thoughts

1. Any condition that interferes with the phases of wound healing (hemostasis, inflammation, proliferation, and remodeling) will impair the rate of healing and the final wound strength.

2. Both local and systemic factors have an effect.
   - Local factors:
     a. At closure, wounds should be free of bleeding, hematoma, gross contamination, and necrotic tissue.
     b. Wound edges should be free of tension.
     c. Local tissue should be healthy and well vascularized (irradiated tissue has decreased vascularity).
   - Systemic factors that impair wound healing:
     a. Metabolism: poor nutritional state, zinc and vitamins A and C deficiency, presence of infection elsewhere in the body, hypoxic or low-flow states, smoking, diabetes that is poorly controlled, obesity, diseases such as collagen vascular diseases, and renal and liver failure
     b. Medications: systemic glucocorticoids, some chemotherapeutic and immunosuppressive drugs, and angiogenesis inhibitors

3. For wound infections:
   - If an abscess is present, it must be drained.
   - If there is necrotic tissue, it must be debrided.
   - If a foreign body is present, it must be removed.
   - If there is an enteric leak into the wound, it must be controlled.
   - If crepitus is present, a necrotizing gas-forming infection must be suspected and the wound opened.
   - Systemic antibiotics are not the primary treatment for wound infections.
   - Perioperative antibiotics given to patients with clean-contaminated wounds (which are usually closed) reduce the incidence of wound infections.

Case 3.1 Wound Management and Complications

A 60-year-old man undergoes lysis of adhesions for small bowel obstruction. The wound is closed primarily with staples.

◆ **How would you describe the process of wound healing in this case?**

◆ This is an example of wound healing by **primary intention**. The wound edges are closed with sutures, allowing very rapid coverage by epithelium and rapid wound

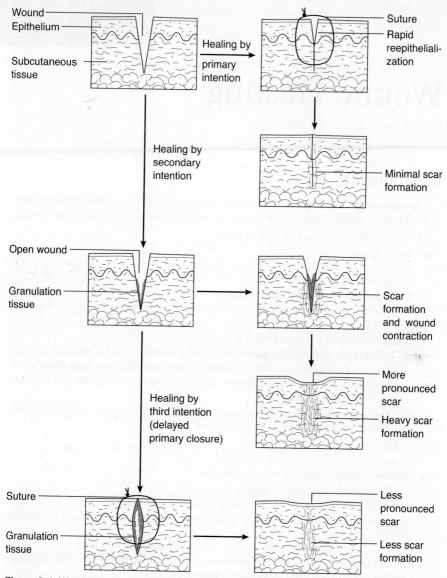

Figure 3-1: Wound healing by primary, secondary, and third intention.

healing. Certain events occur in the wound during the first several weeks of healing (Fig. 3-1).

◆ **What factors are known to delay the process of wound healing?**

◆ **Wound healing is achieved through four programmed phases: hemostasis, inflammation, proliferation, and remodeling. Good nutrition, absence of infection, normal immune function, and adequate oxygenation and blood flow are necessary for normal wound healing.** Several factors are known to delay the process of wound healing (Table 3-1).

Table 3-1: Factors that Slow Wound Healing

Malnutrition
Immunosuppression from any cause
Ischemia; local and systemic
Physiologic stress
Uremia
Obesity
Diabetes
Smoking

Two weeks later, at a return visit, the man asks you when he can return to his job as a loading dock worker.

◆ **What do you tell him?**

◆ You reiterate that the man should not lift significant weight until about the sixth week following surgery.

◆ **What processes are occurring in the patient's wound during the first few weeks postsurgery that support this recommendation?**

◆ Collagen production and cross-linking are still occurring during this phase. Until the collagen matures and reaches a near-final tensile strength, the wound is prone to injury and disruption. Thus, during this phase, the patient should avoid stressing the wound (Fig. 3-2).

The man returns to see you in 3 months. He had no wound complications and his wound has healed. However, he is unhappy with how the wound looks and feels.

◆ **How would you manage the following physical findings at the wound?**

Case Variation 3.1.1. You feel a hard, knot-like structure beneath his skin.

◆ This is most likely a **suture knot**. If absorbable sutures were used in the operation, it may resolve with time. If nonabsorbable sutures were used, you would wait several more months for the wound to completely heal. If the man is still concerned, the knot can be removed under local anesthesia.

Case Variation 3.1.2. The patient has a small, sore, red area that intermittently drains a small amount of pus and then seals over.

◆ A **stitch abscess**, which is an infection of a suture, should be suspected. Usually, this involves the knot and represents a low-grade but persistent infection. Under local anesthesia, the opening can be explored with a hemostat and the suture grasped and removed. This will usually solve the problem.

Case Variation 3.1.3. The man has a 4-cm defect in the fascia that bulges when he coughs.

◆ The man has a postoperative **ventral hernia** due to fascial breakdown (dehiscence). This condition, which may occur as a result of infection, suture failure, or fascial weakness, needs to be repaired surgically to prevent complications of incarceration and pain.

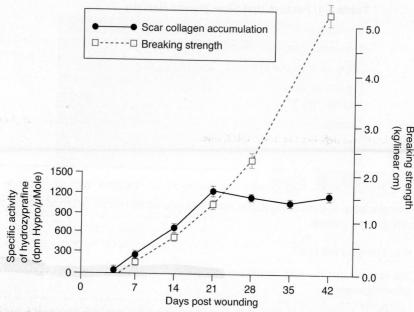

Figure 3-2: Graph of wound strength versus time. Dpm, disintegrations per minute. (Redrawn with permission from Madden JW, Peacock EE Jr. Studies on the biology of collagen during wound healing. III. Dynamic metabolism of scar collagen and remodeling in dermal wounds. *Ann Surg.* 1971;174:511.)

Case Variation 3.1.4. *The man's scar is red and sensitive to touch, and he thinks it is unsightly.*

◆ Some wounds have a prolonged inflammatory process in the later phases of healing.

 QUICK CUT Wound remodeling and maturation continue to occur for at least 6 months.

◆ Assuming no infection is evident, appropriate management involves patient reassurance. The wound should be observed for at least 6 months before considering revision.

Case Variation 3.1.5. *The patient's scar has a raised, hypertrophic appearance.*

◆ This scar, which has remained within the limits of the original incision, is termed hypertrophic. Until the scar stabilizes, it warrants observation. Most hypertrophic scars do not continue to enlarge. Revision may be appropriate, but recurrence is common unless the wound is treated with steroid injections and local pressure dressings, which are inconsistently effective.

Case Variation 3.1.6. *The patient's scar has a raised, hypertrophic appearance, and it is spreading outside the immediate area of the incision.*

◆ This scar, which is similar to a hypertrophic scar, is termed a keloid. It is more pronounced and extends outside the original wound margins. Treatment is the same as that given for hypertrophic scars in Case Variation 3.1.5.

Case 3.2   Wound Infection

You explore a 25-year-old woman for bowel obstruction and perform a lysis of adhesions. When examining the patient on the third postoperative day, you note an area of redness and tenderness in the middle of the wound.

◆ **What should be your next step?**

◆ You should suspect a wound infection. The most important step is to drain the infection completely and **debride any nonviable tissue.**

Deep Thoughts

The mainstay for treating any infection is to control the source. A search for a deeper source such as an abscess or unsuspected intestinal injury is crucial. This can be accomplished with clinical evaluation, imaging of the area and percutaneous drainage, or surgical exploration.

QUICK CUT Many wound infections do not require antibiotics. The key to treatment is drainage, debridement, and creating the environment for healing by secondary intention.

Oral or intravenous (IV) antibiotics are not appropriate. **Antibiotics** are necessary only if the wound cellulitis appears to be spreading despite wound drainage.

You open the wound and drain some purulent material. The wound edges appear viable.

◆ **What treatment is now appropriate?**

◆ Subsequent therapy involves local wound care, which involves debridement of any necrotic tissue surgically, chemically, or mechanically. If there is significant drainage, this is controlled with a negative pressure wound therapy or an absorptive dressing. If it is dry, the wound can be moistened with topical solutions often containing silver ion for its antibacterial properties.

◆ **How would you describe the process involved in the healing of this wound?**

◆ This wound could be described as healing by **secondary intention**. Wounds that heal by secondary intention are typically wounds that were contaminated at the initial surgery and left open by the surgeon or wounds that became infected and required opening in the immediate postoperative period. Leaving the wound open to heal by secondary intention allows bacteria to be removed from the wound rather than accumulate as an abscess. Secondary intention is characterized by the formation of **granulation tissue**, which fills in the cavity that occurs when skin edges are not opposed. **Wound contraction** and re-epithelialization occur following this process (see Fig. 3-1).

Two days later, you examine the wound and find healthy, beefy-red edges, with only a small amount of exudate apparent on the wound surfaces.

◆ **What are the options for wound management at this time?**

Case Variation 3.2.1. You could continue to observe the wound and treat it using local wound care.

◆ This method is perhaps best for wounds in which infection is significant or healing problems develop. However, it is also **slow**, particularly for large or deep wounds, and often results in significant wound contraction.

Case Variation 3.2.2. You could place a split-thickness skin graft.

◆ A split-thickness skin graft is a piece of surgically removed skin from a remote donor site. It is approximately 0.012–0.014 inches thick and contains a layer of epidermis and a part of the dermis. The graft is capable of revascularizing from granulation tissue, a process called inosculation, and causing re-epithelialization of the wound.

 QUICK CUT For a skin graft to attach successfully, the bacterial count on the granulation bed must be less than 10^5 bacteria per gram of tissue.

Once established, split-thickness skin grafts greatly retard the wound contraction process, reducing wound contraction by 60%.

Skin grafts are fragile and easily disrupted in the early stages of attachment and always remain more susceptible to trauma than normal skin. However, they are one of the best ways to resolve wound problems.

Case Variation 3.2.3. You could close the wound using sutures.

◆ This represents wound healing by **third intention**, a method that is commonly performed several days following surgery. Typically, gross wound contamination occurred during the procedure, but with several days of good wound management, the wound has no gross contamination and granulation tissue has taken over. Once the bacterial count has diminished, the wound can be closed with sutures successfully, which allows more rapid healing (see Fig. 3-1).

Your resident asks you what processes are important for regaining strength in the wound.

◆ **How would you respond?**

◆ During the fibrous union phase of wound healing, collagen is generated.

 QUICK CUT In healing wounds, collagen production can be first detected within 10 hours of wounding and peaks in 5–7 days.

Collagen has a low tensile strength until cleavage of procollagen peptides occurs and collagen cross-linking takes place, a process that involves fibroblasts. In wounds that heal by secondary intention, the fibroblasts also contract with smooth muscle elements; these cells are called **myofibroblasts**. This action produces contraction of the wound and may result in contractures, which are distortions of the normal anatomy due to scarring.

Your resident also wants to know which growth factors are most important in the healing process.

◆ **How would you respond?**

◆ Multiple growth factors are involved in wound healing. Platelet-derived growth factor (PDGF), which is chemotactic for fibroblasts, neutrophils, and macrophages, is released early by platelets. Transforming growth factor B (TGF-B), which increases collagen synthesis, follows PDGF. Basic fibroblast growth factor (FGF) hastens wound contraction. Finally, epithelial growth factor (EGF) stimulates epithelial migration and mitosis, speeding wound epithelialization (Fig. 3-3).

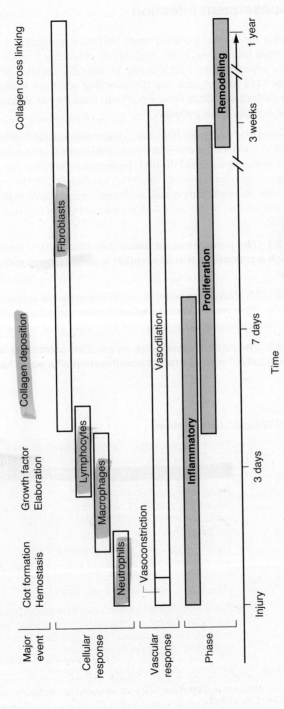

Figure 3-3: Phases and events in wound healing. (Reprinted with permission from Mulholland MW, Lillemoe KD, Doherty GM, et al. *Greenfield's Surgery*, 5th ed. Philadelphia: Lippincott Williams & Wilkins; 2010.)

Case 3.3 Wound Classification Based on Risk of Subsequent Infection

You are planning your day in the operating room. You have an elective ventral hernia repair and an elective colectomy. Both procedures obviously include making an abdominal incision, which carries with it a risk of wound infection. While you are waiting for your first case to start, you also discover that you have to explore a third patient who has a perforated colon. How would you classify the abdominal wound that you will create in these three patients?

◆ Wounds are classified into four categories: clean, clean-contaminated, contaminated, and dirty (Table 3-2). This classification scheme is based on the amount of bacterial contamination present in the operating room and the likely postoperative infection rate if the wound is closed. The rate of postoperative wound infections has dramatically decreased with the advent of better skin decontamination and appropriate prophylactic antibiotics. Thus, wounds can be managed after an operation with some knowledge of expected likelihood of infection (Table 3-3).

Case Variation 3.3.1. The patient has an uncomplicated ventral hernia repair with no mesh. Such a procedure would result in a clean wound with a low risk (<1%) of infection.

◆ The **wound** can be safely **closed primarily**. No antibiotics are given perioperatively, and infection is unlikely. However, if mesh were inserted, most surgeons would administer perioperative antibiotics because of the high morbidity associated with infected mesh.

Case Variation 3.3.2. The patient undergoes an elective colectomy with a preoperative "bowel prep," with operative confirmation of a good "prep."

Table 3-2: Surgical Wound Classifications

Clean	These are uninfected operative wounds in which no inflammation is encountered and the respiratory, alimentary, genital, or urinary tracts are not entered.
Clean/contaminated	These are operative wounds in which the respiratory, alimentary, genital, or urinary tract is entered under controlled conditions and without unusual contamination.
Contaminated	These include open, fresh, accidental wounds; operations with major breaks in sterile technique or gross spillage from the gastrointestinal tract; and incisions in which acute, nonpurulent inflammation is encountered.
Dirty	These include traumatic wounds several days or longer since injury having devitalized tissue and those with retained devitalized tissue and those that involve existing clinical infection or perforated viscera.

Defined by American College of Surgeons National Surgical Quality Improvement Program. *User Guide for the 2008 Participant Use Data File.* Chicago: American College of Surgeons; 2009; Ortega G, Rhee DS, Papandria DJ, et al. An evaluation of surgical site infections by wound classification system using the ACS-NSQIP. *J Surg Res.* 174(1):33–38.

Table 3-3: Comparative Studies of Postoperative Surgical Site Infections Stratified by Wound Classification (Traditional vs. ACS-NSQIP)

	Clean	Clean-contaminated	Contaminated	Dirty
Traditional	1%–5%	3%–11%	10%–17%	>27
ACS-NSQIP SSI	2.58	6.67	8.61	11.80
Superficial SSI	1.76	3.94	4.75	5.16
Deep incisional SSI	0.54	0.86	1.31	2.10
Organ/space SSI	0.28	1.87	2.55	4.54

ACS-NSQIP, American College of Surgeons National Surgical Quality Improvement Program; SSI, surgical site infection.
From Ortega G, Rhee DS, Papandria DJ, et al. An evaluation of surgical site infections by wound classification system using the ACS-NSQIP. *J Surg Res*. 2012;174(1):33–38.

Such a procedure would result in a clean-contaminated wound; there is a low probability of infecting the wound with stool during the operation.

◆ In this situation, most surgeons would close the wound primarily and expect a **less than 10% chance of a wound infection**.

Case Variation 3.3.3. The patient has a perforated colon requiring emergent colectomy and colostomy. Such a procedure would probably result in a contaminated wound—gross wound contamination with stool.

◆ Many surgeons would leave this wound open and treat it with saline-soaked gauze, negative pressure wound therapy, or an absorptive dressing. Once granulation has occurred, some practitioners would close the wound, whereas others would continue to observe wound contraction. Other surgeons might argue that a 50% chance of wound infection with primary wound closure is acceptable. If a wound infection occurs, it can always be managed by opening the wound.

◆ **Several of your clinic patients will be going to the operating room in the next few days. How would you decide which of these patients should receive IV antibiotics preoperatively?**

◆ Prophylactic antibiotics are not necessary in patients who undergo clean surgical procedures or operations that involve implantation of **no permanent foreign body**. In such cases, the rate of wound infection is less than 1% without antibiotics, and the addition of antibiotics does not improve the results. Studies have shown that **perioperative antibiotics** (prophylactic antibiotics), with a preoperative dose and a single, postoperative dose, reduce the wound infection rate in clean-contaminated cases. Prophylactic antibiotics are also usually required in cases involving a brief, predictable exposure to bacteria; implantation of a device or **prosthetic material**; or impaired host defenses such as **immunosuppression** or **poor blood supply** (Tables 3-4 and 3-5).

◆ **How would you administer the antibiotics?**

◆ Surgical Care Improvement Project (SCIP) dictates that prophylactic antibiotics should be received within 1 hour prior to incision. SCIP measures dictate appropriate antibiotics for different procedures (Table 3-6).

Table 3-4: American Heart Association Infective Endocarditis Prophylaxis Recommendations

Cardiac Conditions in Which Prophylaxis Is Reasonable	Procedures* for Which Prophylaxis Is Reasonable (Only in Patients with High-Risk Cardiac Conditions at Left)
Prosthetic cardiac valve or prosthetic material used for cardiac valve repair	All dental procedures that involve manipulation of gingival tissue or the periapical region of teeth or perforation of oral mucosa
Previous infective endocarditis	Invasive procedure of the respiratory tract that involves incision or biopsy of respiratory mucosa
Congenital heart disease (CHD) • Unrepaired cyanotic CHD, including shunts and conduits • Completely repaired congenital heart defect with prosthetic material or device during the first 6 months after the procedure • Repaired CHD with residual defects at or adjacent to site of prosthetic patch or device inhibiting endothelialization	Procedures involving infected skin, skin structures, or musculoskeletal tissue
Post cardiac transplant valvulopathy	

*Antibiotic prophylaxis solely to prevent infective endocarditis is not recommended for gastrointestinal or genitourinary tract procedures.
Reproduced with permission from Wilson W, Taubert KA, Gewitz M, et al. Prevention of infective endocarditis: guidelines from the American Heart Association: a guideline from the American Heart Association Rheumatic Fever, Endocarditis, and Kawasaki Disease Committee, Council on Cardiovascular Disease in the Young, and the Council on Clinical Cardiology, Council on Cardiovascular Surgery and Anesthesia, and the Quality of Care and Outcomes Research Interdisciplinary Working Group. *Circulation*. 2007;116:1736–1754.

◆ **Later in the day, you are asked to see a patient in the emergency department who has been bitten on the face by a dog. How would you manage this wound?**

◆ A dog bite is obviously a contaminated wound and would be left open in most circumstances, except in areas with a particularly rich blood supply. One such area is the face, which has important cosmetic value. Most physicians would close the facial wound and observe it closely. There is evidence that human bites are more likely to result in serious infections than animal bites. Thus, extra precautions should be taken in human bite cases.

Deep Thoughts

All aspects of any potential injury or medical illness must be evaluated. Therefore, a history for potential rabies infection must be evaluated after animal bite and appropriate care given including rabies immune globulin and vaccinations if indicated.

Table 3-5: Dental/Respiratory Procedures

Situation	Agent	Adults	Children
Oral	Amoxicillin	2 g	50 mg/kg
Unable to take oral medication	Ampicillin **OR**	2 g IM or IV	50 mg/kg IM or IV
	Cefazolin or Ceftriaxone	1 g IM or IV	50 mg/kg IM or IV
Allergic to penicillin or ampicillin oral	Cephalexin **OR**	2 g	50 mg/kg
	Clindamycin **OR**	600 mg	20 mg/kg
	Azithromycin or Clarithromycin	500 mg	15 mg/kg
Allergic to penicillin or ampicillin and unable to take oral medication	Cefazolin or Ceftriaxone **OR**	1 g IM or IV	50 mg/kg IM or IV
	Clindamycin	600 mg IM or IV	20 mg/kg IM or IV

Gastrointestinal/Genitourinary Procedures

Use of antibiotics solely for prophylaxis **not** recommended. For procedures involving infected tissue, add enterococcal coverage (e.g., amoxicillin, ampicillin, piperacillin, or vancomycin) to the therapeutic regimen.

Infected Skin and Musculoskeletal Tissue

Include an agent active against staphylococci and beta-hemolytic streptococci (e.g., antistaphylococcal penicillin or cephalosporin; clindamycin or vancomycin in penicillin-allergic patients) in the therapeutic regimen.

Cephalosporins should not be used in an individual with a history of anaphylaxis, angioedema, or urticaria with penicillins or ampicillin.
IM, intramuscular; IV, intravenous.
Modified and adapted with permission from Wilson W, Taubert KA, Gewitz M, et al. Prevention of infective endocarditis: guidelines from the American Heart Association: a guideline from the American Heart Association Rheumatic Fever, Endocarditis, and Kawasaki Disease Committee, Council on Cardiovascular Disease in the Young, and the Council on Clinical Cardiology, Council on Cardiovascular Surgery and Anesthesia, and the Quality of Care and Outcomes Research Interdisciplinary Working Group. *Circulation*. 2007;116:1736–1754.

Table 3-6: Antibiotic Selection Regimen for Surgical Prophylaxis

Surgical Procedure	Approved Antibiotics	
Cardiac or vascular	Cefazolin, cefuroxime, or cefamandole If beta-lactam allergy: vancomycin* or clindamycin*	
Hip/knee arthroplasty	Cefazolin or cefuroxime If beta-lactam allergy: vancomycin or clindamycin	
Colon	**Oral** After effective mechanical bowel preparation, neomycin sulfate + erythromycin base OR neomycin sulfate + metronidazole Administered during 18 hours preoperatively	**Parenteral** Cefotetan, cefoxitin, or cefmetazole OR Cefazolin + metronidazole If beta-lactam allergy: clindamycin + gentamicin or clindamycin + ciprofloxacin** or clindamycin + aztreonam OR Metronidazole with gentamicin or metronidazole + ciprofloxacin**
Hysterectomy	Cefotetan, cefazolin, cefoxitin, or cefuroxime If beta-lactam allergy: clindamycin + gentamicin or clindamycin + ciprofloxacin** or clindamycin + aztreonam OR Metronidazole + gentamicin or metronidazole + ciprofloxacin** OR Clindamycin monotherapy	
Special considerations	*For cardiac, orthopedic, and vascular surgery, if the patient is allergic to beta-lactam antibiotics, vancomycin or clindamycin are acceptable substitutes. **Levofloxacin 750 mg given once may be substituted for ciprofloxacin.	

SCIP uses the combined published recommendations of the American Society of Health System Pharmacists, the Medical Letter, the Infectious Diseases Society of America, the Sanford Guide to Antimicrobial Therapy 2001, and the Surgical Infection Society as the basis for appropriate prophylactic antimicrobial agents. The antibiotic regimens are described in the table.

Chapter 4

Thoracic and Cardiothoracic Disorders

Bruce E. Jarrell, Joseph S. MacLaughlin, Eric D. Strauch

Key Thoughts

1. Lung disease
   - When symptoms or a radiologic abnormality suspicious for a neoplasm or malignancy is detected, then aggressive diagnosis is imperative because a delay in diagnosis can result in significant growth or metastasis and increase mortality. Clinical findings that raise suspicion include a coin lesion on a screening chest radiography, symptoms of dysphagia, and enlarged lymph nodes on physical exam.
   - Small cell carcinoma is considered a systemic disease that begins in the lung and metastasizes early. It is rarely amenable to surgical resection, and chemotherapy is the primary treatment.
   - Non–small cell carcinoma begins as a more local disease that spreads to local and regional lymph nodes before becoming systemic, making surgical resection more likely to be curative.
   - Mesothelioma usually presents in a late stage with low cure rates, but early stages can be cured with extrapleural pneumonectomy.
   - Spontaneous pneumothorax occurs in young, tall, slender adult males due to a rupture of apical blebs. First episodes are treated with a chest tube, but recurrent or bilateral ones undergo thoracoscopic excision of the blebs and pleural abrasion.
   - Empyema is treated with (1) antibiotics, (2) evacuation of pus, and (3) re-expansion of the lung.

2. Cardiac disease

   There are many new technologies and minimally invasive interventions being used to treat coronary artery and valvular disease. Initial treatment of coronary artery disease should consist of lifestyle changes. More aggressive interventions should be used based on the symptoms, extent of disease, and the risk/benefit ratio for the intervention.
   - Patients with left main coronary artery disease have a reduced survival, making it a primary indication for coronary artery revascularization.
   - The internal mammary artery graft, which has a 90% or better patency rate at 10 years, has superior patency over other grafts.
   - Mechanical valves have a long lifetime but require long-term anticoagulation to prevent thromboembolic events. Biologic prosthesis valves have a shorter lifetime but have no need for anticoagulation.

3. Mediastinal masses

- The location of a mediastinal mass accurately formulates the differential diagnosis and focuses the clinical evaluation.
- Anterior: lymphoma, thyroid, teratoma/germ cell tumors, or thymoma. Thymoma can present with myasthenia gravis, diagnosed with anti–acetylcholine receptor antibodies, and be cured with resection.
- Middle: lymphoma, sarcoid, metastatic lung cancer, and cysts
- Posterior: neurogenic tumors

4. Esophageal disorders

- Any patient with dysphagia should undergo esophagogastroduodenoscopy to rule out carcinoma. Squamous cell carcinoma is most common in the upper and middle third and adenocarcinoma in the lower.
- Barrett esophagus is replacement of distal squamous epithelium with columnar epithelium associated with gastroesophageal reflux disease that can undergo malignant transformation. It should be monitored for degree of dysplasia. Severe dysplasia and carcinoma in situ should be resected.
- Carcinoma of the esophagus is treated with multimodal protocols, with surgery reserved for early stages.
- Achalasia is associated with dysphagia and regurgitation. Its findings are dilated esophagus, loss of peristalsis, and increased lower esophageal sphincter (LES) tone showing a bird's beak on barium swallow. It is treated by dilation or transection of the LES (a Heller myotomy).

Case 4.1 Asymptomatic Abnormality Seen on Chest Radiography

A 50-year-old man with an abnormality seen on chest radiography (CXR) seeks a referral before undergoing planned repair of an inguinal hernia. He has no chest-related symptoms.

◆ How would you describe this lesion? (Fig. 4-1)

◆ This lesion is a round, well-circumscribed lesion in the periphery of the lung. It would be called a **"coin"** lesion. For individuals who are 50 years of age, the chance that the lesion is malignant is 50%. Younger than 50 years, the chance decreases progressively, and older than 50 years, the chance increases progressively. Different coin lesions have distinct appearances (Fig. 4-2).

 QUICK CUT Benign lesions usually have a smooth surface, in contrast to malignant lesions, which often have an irregular or spiculated surface.

Granulomas may contain calcium, but cancers rarely do; bull's eye configurations are almost certainly benign; and hamartomas, which are benign, typically have a "popcorn" appearance (see Fig. 4-2).

◆ What history, physical examination, or laboratory studies may help establish a definitive diagnosis?

◆ Information about previous pulmonary illness or previous CXR abnormalities is worth seeking, and review of **previous films**, if possible, is essential. **Coin lesions** are common

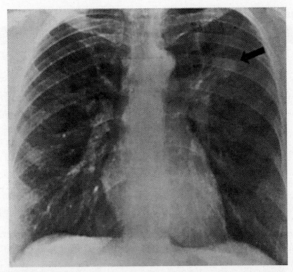

Figure 4-1: CXR of the patient in Case 4.1. *Arrow* is pointing to the coin lesion. (Reprinted with permission from Mulholland MW, Lillemoe KD, Doherty G, et al. *Greenfield's Surgery: Scientific Principles and Practice*, 5th ed. Philadelphia: Lippincott Williams & Wilkins; 2010.)

in the areas in which **fungal disease** is prevalent such as in the southwestern United States, where coccidioidomycosis occurs, as well as in the middle Atlantic region and the Ohio Valley, where histoplasmosis occurs. Physical examination may reveal evidence of a **primary tumor**. Testicular, breast, renal, and colon cancer may manifest as **lung metastases** (Tables 4-1 to 4-3).

◆ **What is the next step in reaching a diagnosis?**

◆ **Computed tomography (CT)** is indicated; it clearly defines the characteristics of the lesion and can evaluate the mediastinum for the presence or absence of enlarged lymph nodes (Fig. 4-3). Using CT guidance, needle aspiration is possible for cytologic examination of the tumor.

QUICK CUT The chances of definitive diagnosis with needle biopsy are 90% or better.

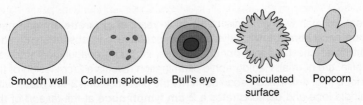

| Smooth wall | Calcium spicules | Bull's eye | Spiculated surface | Popcorn |

Figure 4-2: Radiographic appearances of various types of coin lesions.

Table 4-1: Assessment of Solitary Pulmonary Nodules

Evaluation	Favors Benign Status	Favors Malignant Status
History	Age younger than 40 years	Age older than 40 years
	Nonsmoker	Smoker
	Previous tuberculosis exposure	No previous tuberculosis exposure
	Lives in or frequently travels to endemic, histoplasmosis, or fungal regions	Does not live or travel to endemic, histoplasmosis, or fungal regions
	No previous malignancy	Previous malignancy
Physical examination	No lymphadenopathy	Lymphadenopathy
	No organomegaly	Hepatomegaly; splenomegaly
	OB (−) stools; no hematuria	OB (+) stools; hematuria
Skin test	PPD (+); histoplasmosis (+)	PPD (−); histoplasmosis (−) or (+)
Laboratory workup	Fungal serum titers (+)	Titers may be + or −
	Sputum acid-fast bacilli (+)	Sputum acid-fast bacilli (−)
Radiology	<3 cm on chest radiography	>3 cm on chest radiography
	Distinct margins	Hazy, spiculated, or lobulated margins
	Has not changed in size in 2 years	Has increased in size
	Doubling time <5 weeks or >465 days	Doubling time 5 weeks to 280 days
	Calcification on chest radiography, tomography, or fine-cut CT scans	Noncalcified or rarely eccentrically calcified on chest radiography, tomography, or fine-cut CT scans
	High CT density number (>164)	Low CT density number (<100)

OB, occult bleeding; PPD, purified protein derivative; CT, computed tomography.
From Levine BA, Copeland EM III, Howard RJ, et al. *Current Practice of Surgery*. Vol 2. New York: Churchill Livingstone; 1993:13, with permission.

◆ If the lesion is **malignant or indeterminate** on needle biopsy, **resection** is indicated. The major complication of needle biopsy is pneumothorax. If the pneumothorax is small, it may resolve on its own; however, it may require aspiration.

Case 4.2 Symptomatic Abnormality Seen on Chest Radiography

A 60-year-old man with a history of 40 pack-years of **cigarette smoking** presents with **cough and hemoptysis**. Physical examination reveals absent breath sounds in the right lower chest. Laboratory chemistries, including coagulation studies and a liver profile, are normal. Radiographic examination reveals a 2-cm lesion of the right middle lobe (Fig. 4-4A). A CT scan confirms the presence of a **2-cm mass** within the right middle lobe and demonstrates a **2-cm lymph node** at the *takeoff* of the right mainstem bronchus (see Fig. 4-4B).

Table 4-2: **Masses Simulating Malignancy**

Lesion	Clinical or Radiologic Features Suggesting other than Malignancy
Actinomycosis	Associated dental abscess or sinus
	Chest wall involvement
Histoplasmosis	Concentric or homogeneous calcification
	Endemic area
Coccidiomycosis	Thin-walled cavity often with air-fluid level
	Endemic area
Blastomycosis	Associated chronic skin ulcers
	Endemic area
Cryptococcosis	Superinfection in immunocompromised patient
	Frequent meningeal involvement
Aspergillosis	Mycetoma with "air-crescent" sign (Fungus ball)
Hamartoma	Well-defined border with slight lobulations
Round atelectasis	Adjacent to thickened pleura
	"Comet-tail" vessel pattern

From Levine BA, Copeland EM III, Howard RJ, et al. *Current Practice of Surgery*. Vol 2. New York: Churchill Livingstone; 1993, with permission.

◆ **What are the next steps in patient evaluation?**

QUICK CUT Bronchoscopy is used to obtain a tissue diagnosis and to determine the location of the lesion in the bronchial tree. Mediastinoscopy is used to determine the state of the mediastinal lymph nodes.

Usually, both bronchoscopy and mediastinoscopy are performed using the same general anesthetic. Bronchoscopy involves a flexible fiberoptic scope inserted through the endotracheal tube used for the anesthesia. Mediastinoscopy involves making a small incision above the manubrium; the scope follows the anterior wall of the trachea down to the carina and the origin of the mainstem bronchi (Fig. 4-5).

Table 4-3: **Common Metastatic Pulmonary Tumors**

Primary	5-Year Survival (%)
Colorectal	13–38
Breast	27–50
Renal	24–54

Adapted from Jarrell BD, Carabasi RA, Radomski JS. *NMS Surgery*, 4th ed. Philadelphia: Lippincott Williams & Wilkins; 2000.

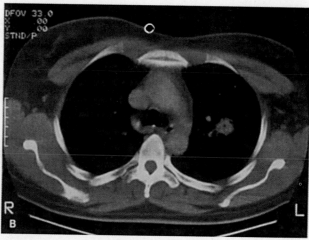

Figure 4-3: CT scan of a coin lesion. (Reprinted with permission from Mulholland MW, Lillemoe KD, Doherty G, et al. *Greenfield's Surgery: Scientific Principles and Practice*, 5th ed. Philadelphia: Lippincott Williams & Wilkins; 2010.)

The bronchoscopy and mediastinoscopy indicate an **adenocarcinoma of the middle lobe bronchus** 2 cm below the origin of the right middle lobe bronchus. The **enlarged lymph node is a result of benign enlargement with inflammation.**

◆ **What is the stage of the tumor?**

◆ Staging is an important modality; it directs treatment and allows comparison of various treatment regimens.

> **QUICK CUT** The tumor-node-metastasis (TNM) system is used to stage lung tumors. T refers to tumor size and characteristics, N to lymph node spread, and M to the presence of metastasis.

By combining T, N, and M, it is possible to determine the stage of the tumor. **Stage I** indicates that the tumor is **localized** to the lung, **stage II** indicates that the tumor involves **lymph nodes** within the lung or is greater than 5 cm without extrapulmonary extension, and **stage III** indicates that the tumor has **spread beyond the lung** (Fig. 4-6). Stage IV disease involves distant metastasis. In this case, T = 1, N = 0, and M = 0. Therefore, this patient's tumor is $T_1N_0M_0$, or **stage I**, and **it is potentially curable by surgical resection.**

◆ **How does cell type affect prognosis?**

◆ Lung cancer is generally categorized as small cell carcinoma or non–small cell carcinoma. **Small cell carcinoma** is considered a **systemic disease** that begins in the lung. Because small cell carcinoma usually has spread beyond the lung by the time it is diagnosed, the disease is rarely amenable to surgical resection. Surgery for small cell carcinoma is used only for early limited-stage disease. **Chemotherapy** is the primary treatment. **Non–small cell carcinoma** begins as a more **local disease that spreads to local and regional lymph nodes** before becoming systemic. Most common non–small cell cancers are **adenocarcinoma and epidermoid (squamous cell) carcinoma**, which occur in about equal proportions.

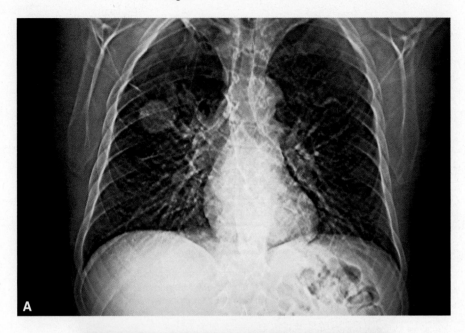

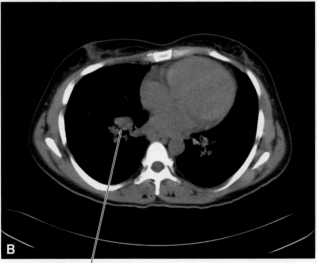

R hilar lymph node

Figure 4-4: A: CXR of the patient in Case 4.2. **B:** CT scan of the same patient confirming the presence of a right hilar lymph node.

 QUICK CUT Surgical resection is the primary mode of therapy for non–small cell cancer, with irradiation and chemotherapy playing adjuvant roles.

Because this patient has a stage I adenocarcinoma of the lung, you proceed to resection, either through a thoracotomy or a thoracoscopy. After exploring the mediastinum, you find no spread outside the lung and can safely perform a right middle lobectomy.

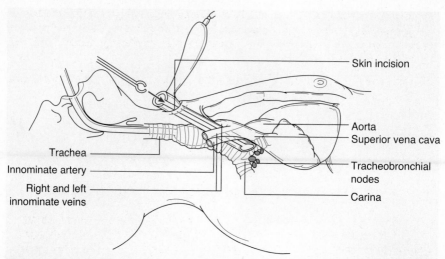

Figure 4-5: Description of mediastinoscopy sampling nodes anterior to the trachea down to the level of the carina. (From McKenney M, Moylan JM, Mangonon P. *Understanding Surgical Disease: The Miami Manual of Surgery*. Philadelphia: Lippincott-Raven Publishers; 1998:250.)

◆ **What are this patient's chances of survival?**

◆ For patients with **stage I** tumors, like this patient, the chance of cure via resection is **50%–70% or better**. For patients with **stage II** tumors, the 5-year survival rate is **30%–50%**. For patients with **stage III** tumors, survival rates are **lower**, depending on how extensively the mediastinal **lymph nodes** are involved and the amount of **distant metastatic disease** present.

Case 4.3 Symptomatic Abnormality Located in the Hilum on Chest Radiography

A 55-year-old man who smokes two packs of cigarettes per day presents with increased cough, hemoptysis, and a 10-lb weight loss. A CXR reveals a **3.5-cm mass adjacent to the right hilum** (Figs. 4-7 and 4-8). **Bronchoscopy demonstrates a tumor growing out of the upper lobe bronchus**, and mediastinoscopy is negative for lymph node metastasis. No peripheral metastasis is evident. Histologic examination reveals undifferentiated squamous cell carcinoma (**non–small cell carcinoma**).

◆ **What cancer stage does this represent?**

◆ This is a stage I tumor because it is not associated with hilar metastasis even though it is a **T2** primary lesion.

◆ **What management procedure would you recommend?**

◆ The patient should still undergo an exploratory thoracotomy, as in Case 2. However, the situation is different here because the mass is **centrally located and involves the right main-stem bronchus**. It will probably require a **pneumonectomy or a sleeve resection** (a surgical procedure that removes a cancerous lobe of the lung along with part of the bronchus, or air passage, that attaches to it; the remaining lobe[s]' bronchus is then anastomosed to the airway—this procedure preserves part of a lung and is an alternative to removing the lung as a whole) for complete removal.

Your assessment of the workup suggests that from a surgical point of view, this patient is a potential candidate for curative resection.

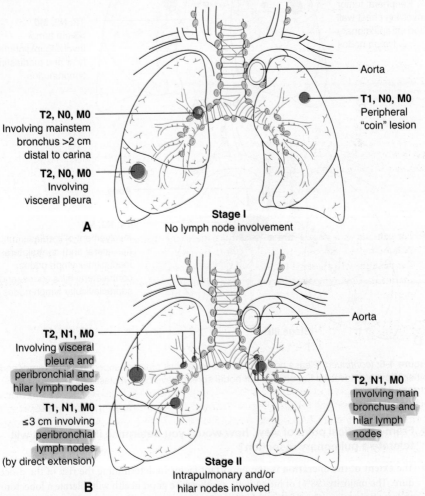

Figure 4-6: Staging diagram for carcinoma of the lung. **A:** Stage IA: A T1 lesion is 3 cm or less; stage IB: A T2 lesion is greater than 3 cm. **B:** Stage IIA: a T1 lesion with a peribronchial lymph node; stage IIB: hilar node involvement or limited extrapulmonary extension. **C:** Stage IIIA: mediastinal or subcarinal node involvement. **D:** Stage IIIB: extensive extrapulmonary tumor invasion of local structures. Stage N1: nodal disease; N2: nodal disease—not pictured. (From McKenney M, Moylan JM, Mangonon P. *Understanding Surgical Disease: The Miami Manual of Surgery*. Philadelphia: Lippincott-Raven Publishers; 1998:261–262. Adapted from Mountain CF, Libshitz HI, Hermes KE. *Lung Cancer: A Handbook for Staging, Imaging, and Lymph Node Classification*. Houston, TX: CF Mountain and HI Libshitz; 1999:28–38.) *(continued)*

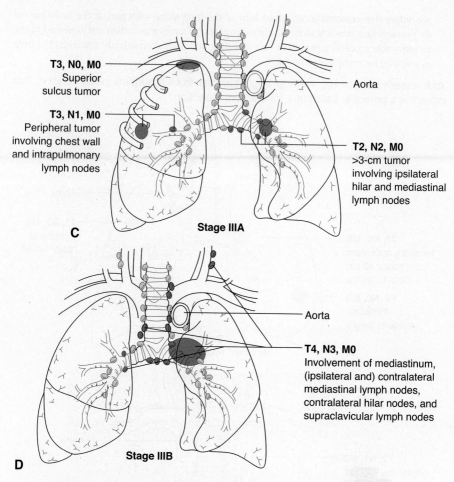

T3, N0, M0
Superior
sulcus tumor

T3, N1, M0
Peripheral tumor
involving chest wall
and intrapulmonary
lymph nodes

Aorta

T2, N2, M0
>3-cm tumor
involving ipsilateral
hilar and mediastinal
lymph nodes

Stage IIIA

C

Aorta

T4, N3, M0
Involvement of mediastinum,
(ipsilateral and) contralateral
mediastinal lymph nodes,
contralateral hilar nodes, and
supraclavicular lymph nodes

Stage IIIB

D

Figure 4-6: (*continued*) Please note: Since this figure was created, superior sulcus tumor and other chest wall invasive tumors without nodal spread have been reclassified as stage IIB.

◆ **From a medical point of view, how would you determine if the patient will tolerate a pulmonary resection?**

◆ The **extent of the operation** is one important factor in determining the risk of the procedure. The majority (98%) of individuals in otherwise good health will tolerate a lobectomy or lesser resection. On the other hand, a pneumonectomy is associated with a far more serious physiologic risk; the risk of perioperative death ranges from 5%–10%, especially in patients older than age 70 years.

QUICK CUT Patients with significant cardiac abnormalities or obstructive airway disease are at particularly high risk, and both cardiac and pulmonary systems require evaluation.

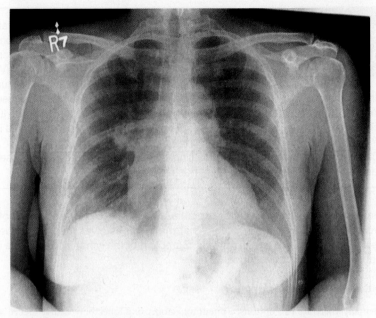

Figure 4-7: CXR of patient in Case 4.3 showing a 3-cm right hilar mass.

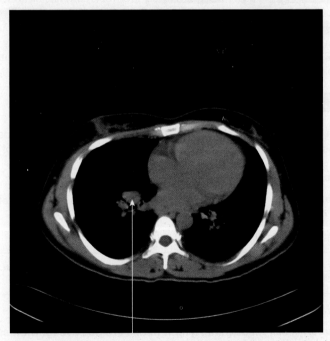

Figure 4-8: A CT scan of the same patient showing a tumor invading a bronchus (*arrow*).

Deep Thoughts

Patients must be able to function adequately postoperatively without the resected pulmonary tissue. To evaluate the lungs, pulmonary function studies are useful. Ventilation-perfusion (V/Q) scans can determine the percentage of functioning lung tissue that remains following resection, and spirometry provides useful information about the mechanics of ventilation. Without sufficient postoperative lung function, life-time mechanical ventilation or living as a pulmonary cripple results in a poor quality of life that can be worse than the cancer.

Cardiac disease is assessed by evaluating evidence of cardiac ischemia, assessing arrhythmias, and evaluating ejection fraction and wall motion.

After determining that the risks are acceptable, you decide to perform a thoracotomy. As a result of this procedure, you learn that the tumor involves the upper lobe with **extension into the mainstem bronchus**. Sampling of the lymph nodes of the hilum and mediastinum is negative for cancer.

◆ **What are the surgical options?**

◆ Essentially, there are two options: a pneumonectomy or a lobectomy with a "sleeve" resection. A **pneumonectomy** involves (1) dividing the right mainstem bronchus just distal to the carina and sewing or stapling it closed and (2) dividing the pulmonary artery and the two main pulmonary veins. A **sleeve lobectomy** involves (1) dividing the mainstem bronchus above and below the origin of the right upper lobe bronchus and (2) reattaching the bronchus by suture technique. The vessels to the right upper lobe are divided, but the blood supply to the middle and lower lobes is left intact. **Although pneumonectomy is easier to perform, it has a higher initial mortality rate. Sleeve lobectomy is safer**, but it may not be feasible because of local invasion of the main pulmonary artery.

Case 4.4 Lung Mass with Possible Metastases

You are evaluating a man with a lung mass. You complete a CT scan, bronchoscopy, and mediastinoscopy of the chest. The patient has a non–small cell carcinoma of the lung.

◆ **How would you manage the following findings?**

Case Variation 4.4.1. Ipsilateral hilar lymph nodes are positive for metastasis and there is no other evidence of disease (see Fig. 4-8).

◆ This represents a stage II lung cancer.

 QUICK CUT The treatment for stage II cancer is similar to that for stage I (surgical resection).

However, the prognosis for stage II carcinoma is worse.

Case Variation 4.4.2. Mediastinal lymph nodes are positive for metastasis on mediastinoscopy (Fig. 4-9).

◆ This represents a stage III lung cancer, which involves a different treatment plan.

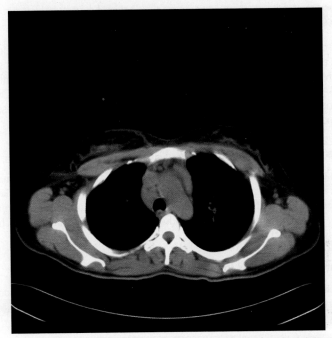

Figure 4-9: CT scan demonstrating mediastinal adenopathy. Adenopathy is seen lateral to each side of the aortic arch. (From Mulholland MW, Lillemoe KD, Doherty G, et al. *Greenfield's Surgery: Scientific Principles and Practice*, 5th ed. Philadelphia: Lippincott Williams & Wilkins; 2010.)

 QUICK CUT Chemotherapy and radiation therapy are appropriate therapy for stage III disease.

If the tumor became smaller and could be downstage, then the patient could undergo resection (Table 4-4).

Case Variation 4.4.3. Positron emission tomography (PET) scan is positive for tumor outside the lung.

◆ It appears that PET scanning is highly reliable and sensitive in detecting lung cancer metastasis. If a lesion is found outside the hilar nodes, then the patient most likely has a stage III or stage IV (distant metastasis) cancer and should receive chemotherapy and radiation.

Table 4-4: Five-Year Survival for Stages II and III Lung Cancer

Stage	Five-Year Survival Rate (%)
II	30–50
IIIa	10–30
IIIb	<10

Case 4.5   Symptomatic Superior Sulcus Tumor

A 45-year-old woman presents with pain in the midback and down the ulnar area of the elbow and wrist. She has little cough or shortness of breath. Cervical spine films are negative. Despite 6 months of treatment with nonsteroidal anti-inflammatory drugs (NSAIDs) and physical therapy, her symptoms have increased. On physical examination, **Horner syndrome** is evident, and on CXR, a vague haziness is visible in the **apex of the lung** (Fig. 4-10A).

◆ **What is the most likely diagnosis?**

◆ This patient most likely has a **Pancoast tumor**, which is a lung cancer originating in the extreme apex of the lung in the groove (superior sulcus) produced by the subclavian artery. It invades the chest wall, the lower cords of the brachial plexus, the subclavian artery, and, at times, the sympathetic ganglia and produces symptoms depending on which structures are involved (Fig. 4-11).

◆ **What are the next steps in making a more definitive diagnosis?**

◆ A **CT scan** would be the next step, and it reveals erosion of the first and second ribs and a superior sulcus mass (see Fig. 4-10B). After CT, **bronchoscopy**, **mediastinoscopy**, and **needle biopsy** of the mass are appropriate.

Bronchoscopy reveals no lesions. Mediastinoscopy reveals no tumor in the mediastinum. Needle biopsy of the mass is positive for adenocarcinoma.

◆ **What is the stage of this tumor?**

◆ In Pancoast tumor, the presence of chest wall invasion makes this a T_3 tumor; this would be a stage IIB if no nodes are present.

◆ **What is the prognosis in this case?**

> **QUICK CUT** Nodal involvement found at surgery is the key to prognosis.

◆ There is little hope for long term patient survival if lymph nodes in the mediastinum contain tumor, but the 5-year survival is 40%–50% without nodal involvement.

◆ **What is the appropriate treatment?**

◆ Treatment of superior sulcus tumors is carried out in **two phases**.

> **QUICK CUT** For patients with no evidence of metastatic disease, concurrent chemoradiotherapy is the recommended initial step in patient management. This is followed by surgical resection if there is no evidence of distant metastases or local progression.

Patients do surprisingly well, considering the extent of tumor involvement and the radical treatment necessary to eradicate it. Before the development of this treatment regimen, patients died in agony because of tumor invasion of bone and nerves.

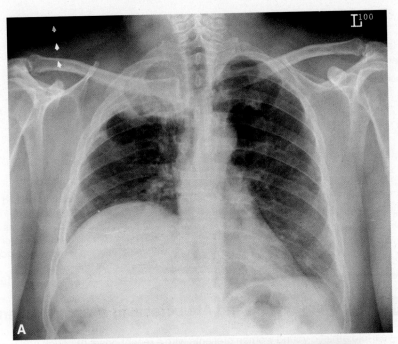

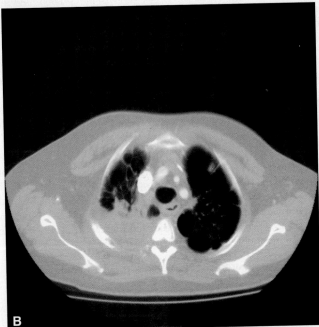

Figure 4-10: A: CXR and **(B)** CT scan of patient in Case 4.5, showing Pancoast tumor in the apex of the right lung.

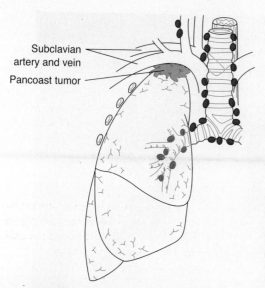

Subclavian artery and vein

Pancoast tumor

Figure 4-11: Pancoast tumor and local structures. (Redrawn from Mountain CF, Libshitz HI, Hermes KE. *Lung Cancer: A Handbook for Staging, Imaging, and Lymph Node Classification*. Houston, TX: CF Mountain and HI Libshitz; 1999:19.)

Case 4.6   Hemoptysis and Atelectasis in a Young Patient

A 25-year-old athletic young woman presents with a recent onset of cough and shortness of breath. Not long ago, she noted that her sputum contained flecks of blood. She does not smoke. A CXR reveals partial collapse of the right upper lobe of the lung.

◆ **What is the differential diagnosis?**

◆ Hemoptysis has many causes, but in an otherwise healthy young woman with atelectasis, an obstructed bronchus is probably present. In such a young person, the most likely diagnosis is **bronchial adenoma**. Cancer would be unusual in a nonsmoker younger than 30 years of age. In addition, although one must always consider tuberculosis, atelectasis is rare with this condition.

◆ **What are bronchial adenomas?**

◆ Bronchial adenomas **arise within bronchi** and often obstruct them. The use of "adenoma" is faulty nomenclature; these tumors have considerable malignant potential. There are two main types: carcinoid tumors and adenocystic carcinomas. Although carcinoid tumors are usually benign when originating in the lung, they may demonstrate significant malignant potential, especially when they develop in the small bowel. Adenocystic carcinomas, which more commonly arise in the upper airway, invade locally.

◆ **What diagnostic measures should be undertaken to establish the diagnosis?**

◆ A CT scan may better delineate the pulmonary anatomy and an obstructed bronchus, but bronchoscopy is required for diagnosis. This is a safe procedure in capable hands. However, **bronchial adenomas are vascular and tend to bleed when biopsied**, and the bronchoscopist must be prepared to coagulate or otherwise control any untoward bleeding.

A bronchial adenoma is visualized by bronchoscopy, and a bronchoscopic biopsy is carried out safely. A diagnosis of carcinoid tumor is made on histopathology.

◆ **What is the next step in treatment?**

> **QUICK CUT** Surgery involves complete resection of the tumor with medi-
> astinal lymph node sampling or dissection. Lobectomy is required in about
> 50% of patients.

◆ This procedure is usually curative, but atypical carcinoid tumors may metastasize widely. Bronchial carcinoids may also produce carcinoid syndrome without the presence of liver metastasis.

Case 4.7 New-Onset Pleural Effusion without Heart Failure

A 65-year-old man, a retired shipyard worker, is admitted with **chest pain and shortness of breath** of 3 months' duration. Physical examination reveals absent breath sounds and dullness to percussion in the right lung base. The CXR reveals an **opacified right lower lung field with pleural effusion** (Fig. 4-12).

◆ **What is the differential diagnosis?**

> **QUICK CUT** Pleural effusion in an older patient signifies cancer until
> proven otherwise.

◆ However, benign effusions as the result of congestive heart failure are more common. The most common cancers are bronchiogenic carcinoma and mesothelioma, particularly considering the patient's history of working in a shipyard and the strong possibility of exposure to asbestos. Benign effusion may be the residual of viral or bacterial pneumonia. Empyema and tuberculosis effusion should also be considered.

◆ **How would you establish a diagnosis (assuming the effusion is not related to congestive heart failure)?**

◆ **Thoracentesis and pleural biopsy** are indicated. Pleural biopsy detects pleural-based cancers (Fig. 4-13). Culture of the pleural fluid for bacteria and tuberculosis is warranted, and examination for the presence of malignant cells is also necessary.

The pleural biopsy reveals mesothelioma.

◆ **What treatment options are available?**

◆ Mesothelioma is an aggressive malignancy that has a low cure rate even with aggressive multimodal therapy including chemotherapy, radiation therapy, and surgery. Mortality is also very high because these tumors are present in a late stage.

> **QUICK CUT** The best results that lead to cure of the rare, early stage
> mesotheliomas have involved extrapleural pneumonectomy.

In this procedure, the entire lung and the parietal and visceral pleura along with, at times, the pericardium and diaphragm are resected en bloc. This exceedingly radical procedure results in high morbidity and mortality but offers the chance for recovery in up to 30% of patients.

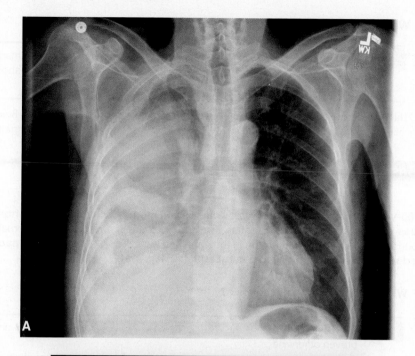

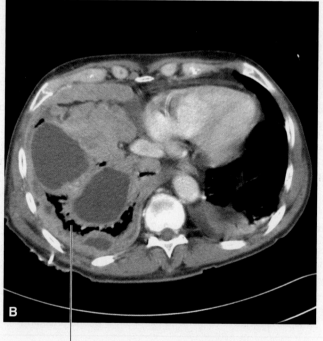

Thick-walled tumor that is pleurally based

Figure 4-12: A: CXR of patient in Case 4.7 showing a right pleural effusion. **B:** CT scan of patient in Case 4.7 confirming the presence of a mesothelioma.

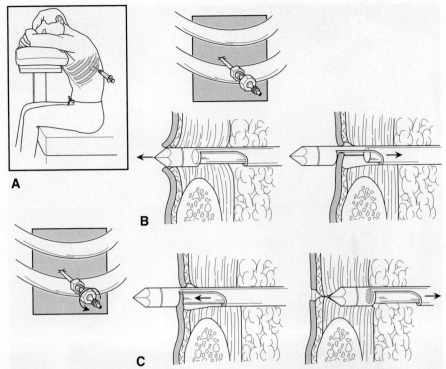

Figure 4-13: A–C: Pleural biopsy procedure. (Redrawn from Urschel HC Jr, Cooper JD. *Atlas of Thoracic Surgery*. New York: Churchill Livingstone; 1995:91.)

Case 4.8 Sudden Chest Pain and Shortness of Breath in a Young Patient

An 18-year-old female college student experiences sharp chest pain followed by shortness of breath while playing tennis. Physical examination reveals an anxious-appearing young woman who is short of breath. The trachea is shifted to the left, **and breath sounds are absent on the right** (Fig. 4-14).

◆ **What is the probable diagnosis?**

◆ **Spontaneous pneumothorax** is a common condition seen in otherwise healthy young people. Its etiology is rupture of **apical blebs**. These typically small clusters of thin-walled, bubble-like structures are formed by the breakdown of the septae in the apex of the lung. Rupture may occur spontaneously or may be related to strenuous activity. **Air escapes into the pleural space, increasing the intrapleural pressure and resulting in lung collapse.** With collapse, the air leak may seal and the lung may re-expand. Continued leakage may lead to a marked increase in pleural pressure. Total lung collapse and mediastinal shift, as seen in this patient, are the hallmarks of tension pneumothorax, which warrants urgent treatment.

◆ **What is the treatment for pneumothorax?**

◆ Air must be removed from the pleural space to allow the lung to expand and the pleural surfaces to coapt and seal the defect. The technique of simple **chest tube drainage (tube thoracostomy)**

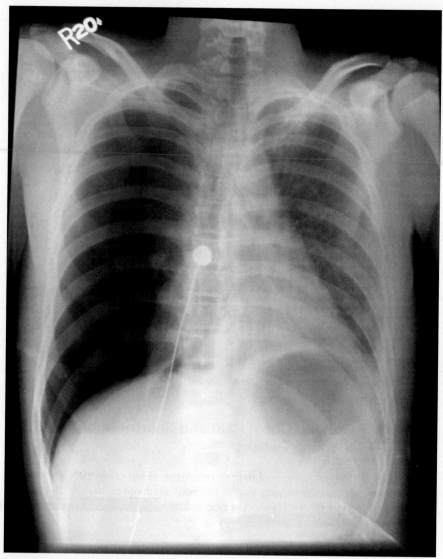

Figure 4-14: CXR of the patient in Case 4.8 showing complete right pneumothorax.

is effective in well over 90% of patients (Fig. 4-15). For a first time pneumothorax, a polyeth-ylene tube with a one-way valve (Heimlich valve) may be sufficient. Most commonly, a small-sized number 24 chest tube is inserted into the chest between the ribs in the lateral chest wall and directed to the apex. The tube is attached to a **water-seal–type** drainage (Fig. 4-16). A pigtail catheter can also be placed into the pleural space using a percutaneous approach.

◆ **How does a water seal function?**

◆ A water seal **maintains a negative pressure in the pleural space and chest tube** such that air and fluids may escape from the chest. The water seal creates a one-way valve mechanism

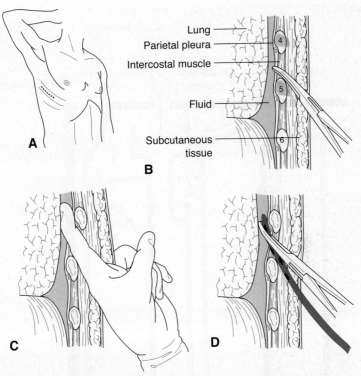

Figure 4-15: **A–D:** Insertion of chest tube. (Redrawn from Hood RM. *Thoracic Surgery*, 2nd ed. Philadelphia: Lea & Febiger; 1993:41–43.)

to prevent air and fluids from re-entering the cavity through the tube. Air that leaks through the injured lung parenchyma traverses through the tube and into the external container (often termed a Pleur-evac). The leaking air may be seen as it bubbles through the water seal, especially when the patient coughs or performs a Valsalva maneuver. Leaking air is termed an air leak. Most air leaks are small and seal in several days.

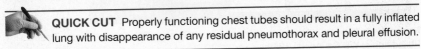

QUICK CUT Properly functioning chest tubes should result in a fully inflated lung with disappearance of any residual pneumothorax and pleural effusion.

◆ **If the lung does not expand, what is the treatment (Fig. 4-17)?**

◆ It is necessary to find the cause of the problem. The most common cause is **an improperly placed chest tube or a leak at the site of entry** into the chest. **Replacement** remedies this problem. Other causes include leaks at tubing connections and large leaks from the lung parenchyma from large blebs or leaks from larger bronchi.

◆ **What is involved in the management of a persistent air leak?**

◆ Initially, it is necessary to eliminate the causes mentioned previously. After ruling them out, the clinician would conclude that there is a parenchymal cause for the leak and surgical intervention is necessary.

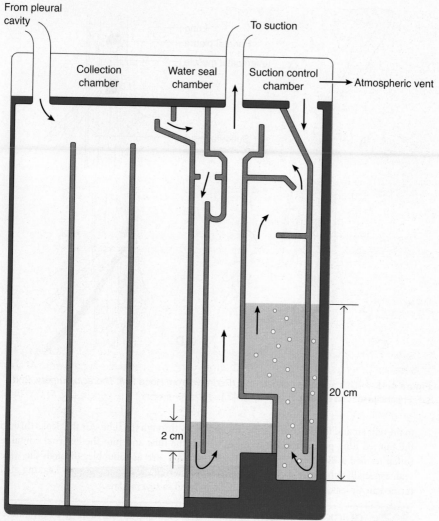

Figure 4-16: Apparatus for chest drainage. (From Symbas PN. *Cardiothoracic Trauma.* Philadelphia: WB Saunders; 1989.)

 QUICK CUT Thoracoscopic excision of the blebs and pleural abrasion (pleurodesis) is highly effective in resolving persistent or recurrent pneumothorax (Fig. 4-18).

Pleurodesis irritates the visceral and parietal pleura, causing them to adhere, thus preventing a future pneumothorax. Pleurodesis is also used in patients with recurrent **spontaneous** pneumothorax as well as in patients **with bilateral spontaneous** pneumothoraces. Obviously, a bilateral pneumothorax is a dangerous event, and the clinician should want to eliminate any possible recurrences.

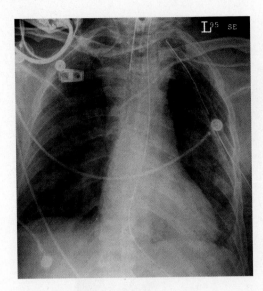

Figure 4-17: CXR of a well-positioned chest tube and a persistent pneumothorax.

Case 4.9   Pleural-Based Chest Pain, Fever, and Pleural Effusion

A 70-year-old woman develops **pneumonia** during a winter influenza outbreak. She receives antibiotics at home, and her condition improves over the next week. At that time, she notes increased pain in her chest, increased cough, and recurrent fever; she is sent to the emergency department. You are asked to evaluate her. A CXR reveals a pleural effusion in the right lung field confirmed on CT (Fig. 4-19).

◆ **What is the most likely diagnosis?**

◆ This patient presents with a classic history of **empyema**. In the community setting, the most common causal bacteria is *Streptococcus pneumoniae*. In the hospital setting, *Staphylococcus*

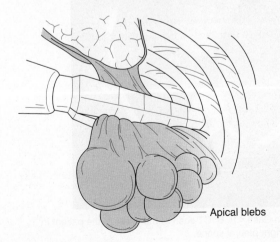

Apical blebs   Figure 4-18: Excision of blebs using a stapler.

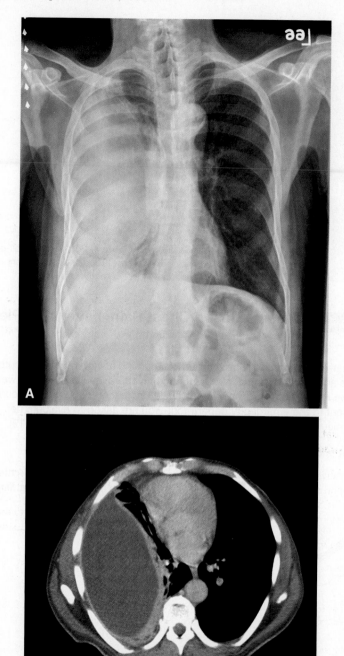

Figure 4-19: A: CXR of the patient in Case 4.9. **B:** CT scan of the chest of the patient in Case 4.9 showing empyema in the right pleural space.

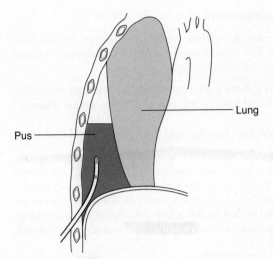

Pus

Lung

Figure 4-20: Empyema drainage. (Redrawn from Hood RM. *Thoracic Surgery*, 2nd ed. Philadelphia: Lea & Febiger; 1993:200.)

and gram-negative bacteria are the usual pathogens. If there is a history of alcoholism, unconsciousness, recent operation, or pulmonary aspiration, the empyema often contains anaerobic organisms. In case series of empyema, up to 35% of cultures are negative because of previous treatment.

◆ **What is the therapeutic approach to management?**

◆ There are three important management principles.

1. **Initiate appropriate antibiotics** as determined by culture and sensitivity.
2. **Evacuate pus.**
3. **Reexpand the lung.**

   Chest tube drainage is the primary mode of therapy and is highly effective in draining the pus and re-expanding the lung (Fig. 4-20). **Failure** to expeditiously accomplish this allows the empyema to become **loculated** by organizing fibrin. If this occurs, **decortication** (removal of the thick inflammatory tissue trapping the lung) is necessary to re-expand the lung. This may be carried out through a mini thoracotomy or by video-assisted thoracoscopic surgery techniques.

Case 4.10 Progressively Increasing Substernal Chest Pain

A 53-year-old man with non–insulin-dependent diabetes (NIDDM) has experienced angina for 3 years. He has been successfully managed medically until recently. In addition to the diabetes, he has a 30-pack-year history of smoking and a history of hypercholesterolemia. He is admitted with a 2-week history of **increasingly frequent and severe chest pain** that appears to be cardiac in nature, and he now has **angina at rest**. The electrocardiogram (ECG) demonstrates an **ischemic pattern**.

◆ **What is the diagnosis?**

◆ The patient suffers from unstable angina, sometimes called **"preinfarction angina."** This is an emergency situation.

◆ **What are the next steps in management?**

◆ Bed rest, sedation, and oxygen are necessary, and the patient should receive beta-blockers. Intravenous nitroglycerine, aspirin, and heparin are warranted. It is important to obtain cardiac enzymes to rule out a myocardial infarction (MI).

As a result of the management, the patient's pain subsides. Cardiac catheterization indicates that the patient has a reduced ejection fraction and "three-vessel disease."

◆ **How would you interpret the ejection fraction and the "three-vessel disease"?**

◆ There are three major coronary arteries, the right, the left anterior descending, and the circumflex; the latter two vessels originate from the left main coronary artery (Fig. 4-21). "Three-vessel disease" is atherosclerotic blockage of all three vessels. Blockage of the left main coronary artery is "left main disease." The ejection fraction is a calculated or estimated reduction of left ventricular chamber size during systole. The normal ejection fraction is 55%–70%, slightly higher in children, and 50%–60% in older persons. **An ejection fraction below 40%–50% is considered abnormal.**

◆ **What is your treatment recommendation?**

◆ The presence of **left main disease**, which indicates significantly reduced survival, is a primary **indication for coronary artery revascularization with coronary artery bypass still the gold standard**. Untreated **high-grade left main disease** is associated with **sudden death**. If not treated, the combination of a reduced ejection fraction and three-vessel disease has a high patient mortality (high risk). Surgery with coronary artery bypass is very effective in improving survival and has been demonstrated to be more effective than with medical treatment alone (Fig. 4-22).

QUICK CUT Patients with three-vessel disease and a reduced ejection fraction benefit more in terms of survival than any other group undergoing coronary artery bypass.

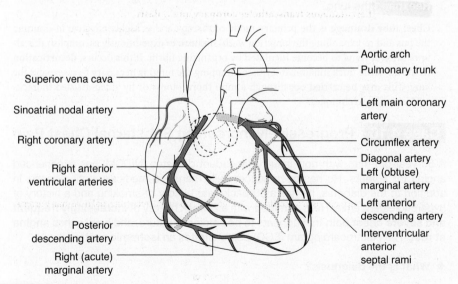

Figure 4-21: Coronary anatomy. (From McKenney M, Moylan JM, Mangonon P. *Understanding Surgical Disease: The Miami Manual of Surgery.* Philadelphia: Lippincott-Raven; 1998:270.)

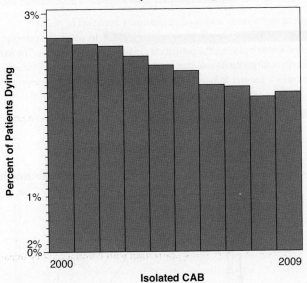

Unadjusted Isolated CAB Operative Mortality
Yearly over last 10 years

Figure 4-22: Unadjusted isolated coronary artery bypass operative mortality: 2000–2009. (Reprinted with permission from Mulholland MW, Lillemoe KD, Doherty G, et al. *Greenfield's Surgery: Scientific Principles and Practice*, 5th ed. Philadelphia: Lippincott Williams & Wilkins; 2010. Society of Thoracic Surgeons.)

◆ **Are viable alternatives to coronary artery bypass available?**

◆ The development of a number of transarterial catheter-based techniques has occurred in recent years. **Percutaneous transcatheter coronary angioplasty**, now frequently used with various **stents** to prolong patency, is capable of dilating an atherosclerotic plaque. Advances in technology including impregnation with antiproliferative drugs have improved outcomes and expanded the indications.

Deep Thoughts

Even with the large number of stents and coronary artery bypass grafts done, the best approaches to treat coronary artery disease still have not been completely elucidated.

◆ **What conduits are used to bypass obstructed coronary arteries?**

◆ Reversed greater saphenous vein grafts and the internal thoracic artery (internal mammary artery) are commonly used, but other veins and arteries have been used with lesser degrees of success.

QUICK CUT The internal mammary artery graft, which has a 90% or better patency rate at 10 years, has the best graft patency by far. The artery is left attached at its origin to the aorta and detached from the chest wall. The distal end is attached to the obstructed coronary vessel.

You decide to proceed with a coronary artery bypass.

There are many ways to perform coronary artery bypass. These include the following:

- Median sternotomy and cardiopulmonary bypass (Fig. 4-23).
- Off-pump coronary artery bypass graft (CABG), in which the coronary arteries are by-passed without placing the patient on cardiopulmonary bypass. The major advantage to off-bypass surgery is its avoidance of the complications of cardiopulmonary bypass, which produces a general inflammatory response and may lead to respiratory, hemorrhagic,

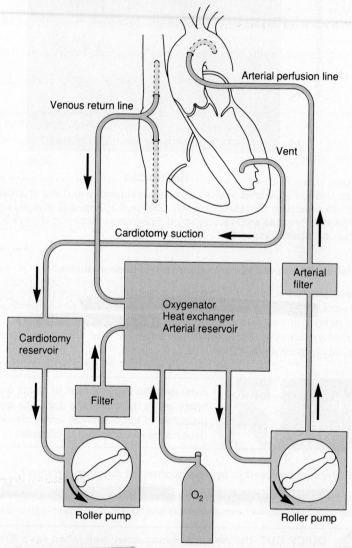

Figure 4-23: Cardiopulmonary bypass circuit. (From Mulholland MW, Lillemoe KD, Doherty G, et al. *Greenfield's Surgery: Scientific Principles and Practice*, 5th ed. Philadelphia: Lippincott Williams & Wilkins; 2010. After Callaghan JC, Wartak J. *Open Heart Surgery: Theory and Practice*. New York: Praeger Press; 1986.)

and myocardial complications in the postoperative period. The postulated benefits of off-pump surgery have not materialized in clinical practice for most patients. For most patients undergoing CABG, today, the use of bilateral internal mammary arteries is far more important than whether surgery is performed on- or off-pump.

- Minimally invasive direct coronary artery bypass grafting (MIDCAB) uses a small anterior left thoracotomy incision and harvesting of the left internal mammary artery with an anastomosis performed to the left anterior descending artery without cardiopulmonary bypass. Procedural success is estimated at 98%. Operative mortality is less than 1% in most series, with low morbidity and good short- and intermediate-term patency rates.
- Robot-assisted, bypass surgery: The major advantage is to avoid the morbidity of the median sternotomy. Because of the added expense and difficulty with learning the technique, robotic bypass is not routine at this time, but this might change with improved technology.
- Multiple arterial CABG procedures: The potential advantage is longer patency rates for the grafts.
- Recently, several studies reported use of a hybrid approach combining minimally invasive left internal mammary artery–left anterior descending artery (LIMA–LAD) bypass procedures with catheter-based interventions on the circumflex or right coronary arteries for the treatment of multivessel disease.

Deep Thoughts

The best approach is dictated by the patient's clinical condition and needs more extensive coronary disease may require more invasive procedures.

QUICK CUT The operative mortality is greater for high-risk patients than for low-risk patients, but high risk patients benefit from bypass surgery the most in terms of survival.

Case 4.11   Mitral Valve Disease that Requires Surgery

A 42-year-old stockbroker with a known heart murmur of 10 years' duration is experiencing increasingly severe shortness of breath and fatigue. An echocardiogram reveals **severe mitral valve regurgitation**.

◆ **What is the likely diagnosis in this case?**

◆ The patient's mitral valve regurgitation most likely is due to **myxomatous degeneration** of the mitral valve. The etiology of this disorder is unknown but is thought to be due to ischemia of the myocardium, particularly the mitral valve apparatus.

◆ **How does this condition differ from prolapse of the mitral valve and mitral stenosis?**

◆ **Prolapse** of the mitral valve (Barlow syndrome) refers to **eccentric closure** of the mitral leaflets, usually without significant mitral valve regurgitation. In young women, this is a common disorder and rarely progresses to mitral valve regurgitation. In men, the presence of prolapse may be a harbinger of severe mitral valve disease. Mitral stenosis is four times as common in young women. Although the disorder is now rare in the United States, it is still common in underdeveloped nations and in immigrants from those countries.

Most commonly, mitral stenosis is caused by rheumatic fever. Inflammation occurs in connective tissues, including those in the heart. The mitral valve leaflets progressively fuse beginning at the commissures, and increasing obstruction occurs. With time, the valve leaflets and annulus undergo calcification. Pressure in the left atrium and pulmonary vessels increases, and right heart enlargement develops. Eventually, the pulmonary arterioles become scarred, and pulmonary hypertension with irreversibility develops.

✦ **What is the treatment for symptomatic mitral valve disease?**

✦ **Repair or replacement of the mitral valve** is warranted. In the early stages, before calcification occurs, correction of mitral stenosis can be performed by percutaneous balloon mitral valvotomy or open mitral commissurotomy. Contraindications to percutaneous balloon mitral valvotomy include left atrial thrombus, moderate to severe mitral regurgitation, calcification of the valve, and severe subvalvular distortion. Open mitral commissurotomy is now rarely performed; procedure consists of splitting the commissures and reconstituting the lumen by mechanical dilators or under direct vision with the use of cardiopulmonary bypass. **It is possible to repair mitral regurgitation** by **excising** the insufficient or redundant portions of the **mitral leaflets** and narrowing and reinforcing the mitral annulus with an **annuloplasty** ring. If repair is not feasible, valve replacement with a prosthetic valve is necessary. The mitral valve can be replaced with a mechanical valve that lasts longer and requires long-term anticoagulation to prevent thromboembolic events or a biologic prosthesis with a shorter lifetime and no need for anticoagulation.

Case 4.12   Aortic Valve Disease that Requires Surgery

An 82-year-old man who experiences **near syncope** is brought to the hospital. History reveals a heart murmur noted at 20 years of age when he was discharged from the army. The man has had progressive shortness of breath for 2 years or more and tightness in his chest when mowing the lawn. Physical examination reveals a bright, healthy-appearing man with a systolic murmur radiating to the neck. An echocardiogram reveals **severe aortic stenosis**. Routine laboratory studies are normal.

✦ **What are the usual causes of aortic valve stenosis?**

✦ Aortic valve stenosis is of three main types: **congenital**, **arteriosclerotic**, and **deteriorative**. Congenital stenosis usually takes the form of a bicuspid valve. Over the years, the leaflets thicken, calcify, and increasingly produce a stenotic opening.

✦ **What are the next steps to be taken in this patient's workup?**

✦ This man has severe aortic stenosis with three major symptoms—**shortness of breath, angina**, and **syncope**. These findings signify an extremely limited life expectancy. **Without surgery, the vast majority of such patients are dead within 2 years.**

Cardiac catheterization is indicated to determine the status of the coronary circulation. The catheterization allows for determination of the **aortic valve lumen size and pressure gradient, ventricular function**, and **presence of coronary artery disease**. Angina is common due to aortic stenosis, but intrinsic coronary artery disease may also be present.

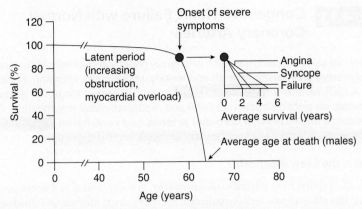

Figure 4-24: Natural history of aortic stenosis. (Mulholland MW, Lillemoe KD, Doherty G, et al. *Greenfield's Surgery: Scientific Principles and Practice*, 5th ed. Philadelphia: Lippincott Williams & Wilkins; 2010. After Ross J Jr, Braunwald E. Aortic stenosis. *Circulation*. 1968;38[Suppl 5]:61.)

Carotid Doppler studies are indicated to rule out internal carotid artery obstruction. Syncope is a common symptom of aortic stenosis and bruits in the neck may be radiated, but identification of carotid artery stenosis is essential. If necessary, it must be corrected to avoid neurologic catastrophe.

◆ **Is this man a candidate for surgery at age 82 years?**

◆ Aortic stenosis is generally well tolerated with good medical management, although, in some instances, congenitally stenotic valves produce symptoms of obstruction early in life (Fig. 4-24).

 QUICK CUT Symptoms do not develop in many patients until their fifth or sixth decade, at which time they are at extreme risk for sudden death. Unfortunately, sudden death may be the first symptom.

A symptomatic patient with **a high-grade stenosis and preserved ventricular function has a good chance** for successful surgery and recovery even at age 82 years. In this case, repair depends on the results of the catheterization, not age.

The results of the catheterization indicate a high-grade aortic valve stenosis and preserved ventricular function. You decide that valve replacement is indicated.

◆ **What operation is performed?**

◆ Aortic valve replacement is usually required. Valve prostheses are of two main varieties, mechanical and tissue. New technology allows the aortic valve to be replaced via a percutaneous approach in some patients.

 QUICK CUT Mechanical valves, which are of metal and plastic construction, are extremely durable and mechanically efficient but require anticoagulation because they are thrombogenic. Tissue valves (human, porcine, or bovine) are nonthrombogenic but deteriorate in the body and require replacement beginning at about 7 years.

Case 4.13 Congestive Heart Failure with Normal Coronary Arteries

A 45-year-old salesman who has been previously healthy and athletically active develops progressive shortness of breath and weakness 3 months following a respiratory illness. A CXR reveals a large heart shadow and congested lungs. An echocardiogram reveals an ejection fraction of 20% and moderate mitral regurgitation. Cardiac catheterization shows **normal coronary arteries** and confirms **an ejection fraction of less than 25% with poor ventricular contraction and dilatation**.

◆ **What is the likely diagnosis?**

◆ This patient suffers from **dilated cardiomyopathy**, probably related to the viral respiratory illness. This association is well documented, but the etiologic mechanism is unclear.

◆ **What is the prognosis?**

◆ Approximately one third of patients recover, one third will stay about the same or slightly improve with medication, and one third will worsen and die.

   Steroids, diuretics, and immunosuppressives were the mainstays of treatment until it was discovered that **beta-blockers markedly improved** heart function in these patients. Still, the **condition of many patients continues to deteriorate. Heart transplantation** may be lifesaving.

◆ **How is heart transplantation performed?**

1. A donor heart must be located from a brain-dead individual.
2. The heart is isolated from the circulation, perfused with cardioplegia solution to protect it, and removed from the donor.
3. The heart is transported in a cold environment.
4. The recipient's heart is removed using cardiopulmonary bypass.
5. The donor heart is sutured to the remnants of the recipient's atria. The aorta and pulmonary arteries are anastomosed and the circulation re-established.

◆ **What is the outlook with a transplant?**

◆ Immediate survival is greater than 90%. A variety of immunosuppressive drugs, often including steroids and cyclosporine or tacrolimus, are useful in the achievement of immunosuppression. Survival at 1 year is 85%–90% and at 3 years is about 75%.

 QUICK CUT Most deaths occur from infection related to immunosuppressive drugs and accelerated coronary artery atherosclerosis, possibly as a form of chronic rejection.

ESOPHAGEAL DISEASE

Case 4.14 Recurrent Regurgitation of Undigested Food

A 55-year-old woman, a department store salesperson, has experienced **regurgitation** of chewed but **not digested** food intermittently during the past 2 years. She has a long history of **dysphagia**. The woman complains of fetid breath, coughing, and choking but denies abdominal symptoms.

◆ **What is the next step?**

◆ A careful head and neck examination is warranted, and it is important to obtain a **barium swallow** (Fig. 4-25) **or upper gastrointestinal (GI) endoscopy**.

The barium swallow reveals a 4- × 3-cm pharyngeal diverticulum.

◆ **What is the etiology of a pharyngeal diverticulum?**

◆ A pharyngeal diverticulum, also called a **Zenker diverticulum**, is a **pulsion diverticulum** that develops in the area between the lower pharyngeal constrictor and the cricopharyngeal muscle.

 QUICK CUT Abnormal uncoordinated constriction of the cricopharyngeal muscle during swallowing increases the pressure in this area of the pharynx and progressively forces out a pouch of mucosa covered by pharyngeal muscle. This action probably results in a pharyngeal diverticulum.

A pulsion diverticulum may also occur at the distal esophageal gastric junction. It is referred to as an epiphrenic diverticulum, which fills with undigested food. The food is regurgitated and may be aspirated, resulting in severe pulmonary infection.

◆ **What is the treatment for a pharyngeal diverticulum?**

 QUICK CUT The most important management principle is transection of cricopharyngeal muscle to relax the esophageal entrance and prevent uncontrolled contraction.

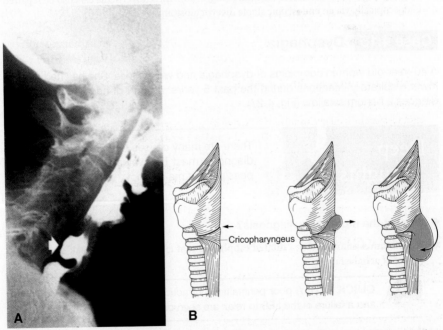

Figure 4-25: A: Barium swallow (*arrow*) of the patient in Case 4.15. **B:** Drawing demonstrating anatomic location.

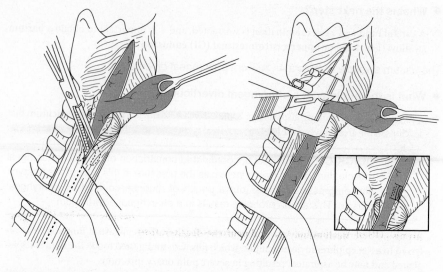

Figure 4-26: Cervical esophagomyotomy and removal of pharyngeal diverticulum. (From Mulholland MW, Lillemoe KD, Doherty G, et al. *Greenfield's Surgery: Scientific Principles and Practice*, 5th ed. Philadelphia: Lippincott Williams & Wilkins; 2010. After Orringer MB. Extended cervical esophagomyotomy for cricopharyngeal dysfunction. *J Thorac Cardiovasc Surg.* 1980;80:669.)

◆ If a pharyngeal diverticulum is large, excision is appropriate at the origin from the posterior pharynx. With an epiphrenic diverticulum, excision and esophageal myotomy at the esophageal gastric junction are necessary (Fig. 4-26). These diverticula can also be repaired endoscopically via an endoscopic staple diverticulostomy.

Case 4.15   Dysphagia

A 40-year-old woman complains of dysphagia and weight loss. She has had several lower respiratory infections during the past 5 years. As part of her workup, she undergoes a barium swallow (Fig. 4-27).

| Deep Thoughts | There are many causes for dysphagia, but the diagnosis must be evaluated because of the possibility of malignancy. |

◆ **What is the most likely diagnosis?**

◆ The barium swallow shows a **dilated esophagus** that ends in a **"bird's beak"** appearance, typical of **achalasia**.

 QUICK CUT A poor peristaltic contraction of the body of the esophagus and a failure of the LES to relax are seen on barium swallow with achalasia.

If this condition is not corrected, the esophagus may greatly **dilate** and essentially become an adynamic sac.

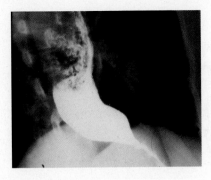

Figure 4-27: Barium swallow of patient in Case 4.15.

◆ **What is the etiology?**

◆ The etiology is not clear, but histopathology usually reveals a **loss of smooth muscle ganglionic cells of Auerbach plexus and neuronal degeneration**. Achalasia is associated with severe emotional stress, physical trauma, weight loss, and Chagas disease (*Trypanosoma cruzi* infection).

◆ **What is the treatment?**

◆ Calcium channel blockers may help, but the classic treatment, which is still most effective, is disruption of the lower esophageal high-pressure zone. Distal esophageal dilation is performed either surgically with a Heller myotomy, which improves approximately 100% of patients, or endoscopically with transesophageal pneumatic dilation, which improves 60% of patients. The Heller myotomy is an incision through the muscular layers of the lower esophagus, which allows the mucosa to bulge out and greatly enlarge the area of previous constriction. It can be performed through either an open thoracotomy or laparotomy or now more commonly via a laparoscopic or thoracoscopic approach (Fig. 4-28). Most surgeons perform a partial esophageal wrap to help prevent reflux postoperatively.

Case 4.16   Dysphagia

A 60-year-old man presents with dysphagia of 3 months' duration. A barium swallow reveals an irregular defect in the esophagus (Fig. 4-29).

◆ **What is the next step in his evaluation?**

◆ Esophagoscopy and biopsy of the abnormality should occur.

◆ **What is the most likely diagnosis?**

◆ This disorder most likely represents cancer of the esophagus. Cancers in the **upper and middle third of the esophagus usually are squamous cell carcinomas**. Tumors in the **lower third** may be **squamous cell carcinomas** but increasingly they represent **adenocarcinomas**.

◆ **What is the etiology of esophageal cancer?**

◆ The exact cause of this cancer is unknown but has been associated with **environmental and dietary conditions, tobacco and alcohol use, and Barrett esophagus**. In Barrett esophagus, **severe reflux esophagitis** leads to ulceration and replacement of lower esophageal squamous mucosa with columnar epithelium (Fig. 4-30). A person with dysplasia of this

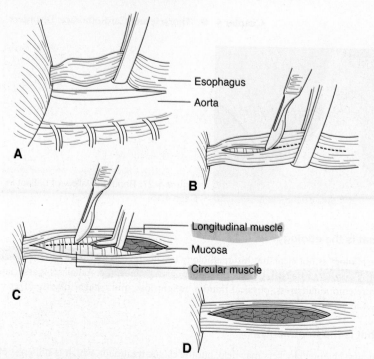

Figure 4-28: A–D: Distal esophagomyotomy procedure for achalasia. (Redrawn from Hood RM. *Thoracic Surgery*, 2nd ed. Philadelphia: Lea & Febiger; 1993:235.)

In figure 4-28 A, labels: Esophagus, Aorta

In figure 4-28 C, labels: Longitudinal muscle, Mucosa, Circular muscle

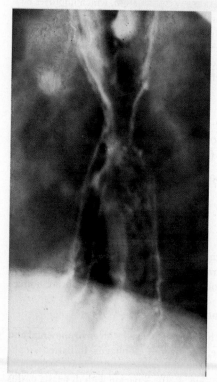

Figure 4-29: Midesophageal cancer.

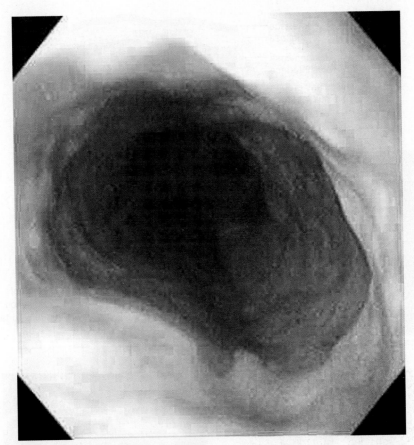

Figure 4-30: Barrett esophagus on endoscopy.

metaplastic epithelium is at high risk of developing adenocarcinoma. **Severe dysplasia is virtually synonymous with carcinoma in situ**; the chance of developing esophageal cancer is 40 times higher in an individual with severe dysplasia than in a normal person.

Esophagoscopy demonstrates a tumor in the middle third of the esophagus that represents squamous cell carcinoma.

◆ **How would you stage this tumor?**

◆ Staging is dependent on **wall penetration and lymph node spread**.

 QUICK CUT Wall penetration is best determined by endoscopic ultrasound examination, which also can identify adjacent node enlargement (Fig. 4-31A–E). Because celiac node involvement in the abdomen is also common, a CT scan of the upper abdomen and chest is indicated.

Local invasion of the tracheobronchial tree and aorta are common in middle third tumors. If studies indicate that there is no evidence of nodal metastases in the mediastinum or the celiac nodes, many centers now perform a thoracoscopic and laparoscopic staging

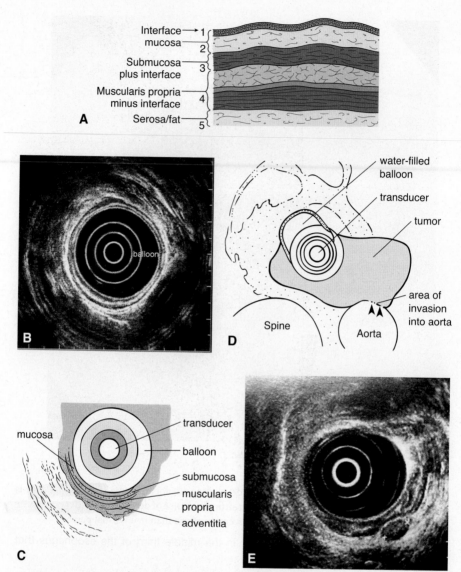

Figure 4-31: Endoscopic ultrasound study (EUS) of an esophageal cancer. **A:** Normal layers of the gastrointestinal wall. **B:** Ultrasound of a normal gastroesophageal junction made with a 12-MHz mechanical sector scanning ultrasound endoscope. **C:** All the anatomic layers, including mucosa, submucosa, muscularis propria, and adventitia with surrounding structures, are seen. **D:** Imaging has been aided by filling a balloon around the radial scanning transducer with water. **E:** EUS of esophagus showing normal wall structure (*left side*) compared to abnormal structure. A mass and local lymph node are seen on *right side*. (Parts **A**, **B**, **C**, and **D** from Yamada T, Alpers DH, LaMe L, et al. *Textbook of Gastroenterology*, 3rd ed. Philadelphia: Lippincott Williams & Wilkins; 1999:3001–3002, 3007.)

procedure to sample nodes and determine the staging more accurately (Fig. 4-32). Unfortunately, most patients have either stage III lesions or distant metastases at the time of diagnosis and are incurable.

The endoscopic ultrasound study, CT scan, and lymph node biopsy all reveal a tumor confined to the esophageal wall and no nodal involvement adjacent to the tumor.

◆ What are the treatment options?

◆ Current protocols for treating carcinoma of the esophagus include **single or combination modality therapy** with irradiation, chemotherapy, and surgical resection. No treatment regimen has demonstrated sufficient superiority in morbidity or survival. The stage of the cancer may be the basis for the selection of treatment methods (Table 4-5). The different therapeutic procedures also are highly dependent on surgeon preference. In addition, the use of videoscopic approaches to perform the thoracic and abdominal parts of the procedure is increasing.

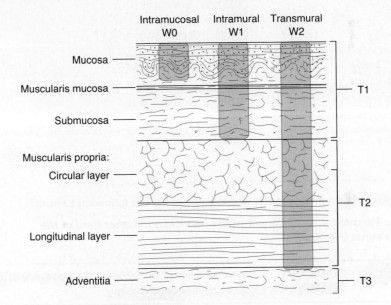

Stage	Classification	Five-Year Survival (%)
0	In situ (intramucosal)	88–100
I	$T_1N_1M_0$	79
IIA	$T_2N_0M_0$	38
	$T_3N_0M_0$	
IIB	$T_1N_1M_0$	27
	$T_2N_1M_0$	
III	$T_3N_1M_0$	13
	$T_4N_1M_0$	
IV	Any T, Any N, M1	0

Figure 4-32: Relationship between the spread of esophageal cancer seen on endoscopic ultrasound and cancer stage.

Table 4-5: American Joint Committee on Cancer Stage Grouping with Recommended Treatment Strategy and Predicted Five-Year Survival

Stage	TNM Designation	Treatment	Five-Year Survival (%)
0	Tis, N0, M0	Surgery alone	95
I	T1, N0, M0	Surgery alone	75
IIA	T2, N0, M0 T3, N0, M0	Surgery alone	30
IIB	T1, N1, M0 T2, N1, M0	Surgery alone or surgery +/− preop chemo/XRT under investigation	20
III	T3, N1, M0 T4, any N, M0	Surgery for T3 lesions with or without preoperative chemo/XRT under investigation Palliation (chemo, XRT, stenting, or combination)	10–15
IVA	Any T, any N, M1a	Palliation (chemo, XRT, stenting, or combination)	5
IVB	Any T, any N, M1b	Palliation (chemo, XRT, stenting, or combination)	1

chemo, chemotherapy; XRT, radiation therapy
From Mulholland MW, Lillemoe KD, Doherty G, et al. *Greenfield's Surgery: Scientific Principles and Practice*, 5th ed. Philadelphia: Lippincott Williams & Wilkins; 2010.

◆ **What treatment approach would you use for the following tumors?**

Case Variation 4.16.1. Cancer of the cervical and upper third of the esophagus (Fig. 4-33)

> **QUICK CUT** The primary treatment of tumors in the cervical and upper third of the esophagus is chemoradiation therapy.

◆ If obstruction persists, resection is appropriate.

Case Variation 4.16.2. Cancer of the middle third of the esophagus

◆ These tumors frequently invade local structures.

> **QUICK CUT** Initial therapy often includes irradiation and chemotherapy to "downstage" or shrink the tumor (neoadjuvant therapy). This may allow surgical resection to remove the entire tumor successfully.

The performance of esophagectomy in this setting represents an attempt to cure the patient. Survival is similar for two procedures: transhiatal esophagectomy and formal esophagectomy. **Transhiatal esophagectomy** allows the stomach to be brought well up into the neck where it is joined with the pharynx (Fig. 4-34). This approach does not require a

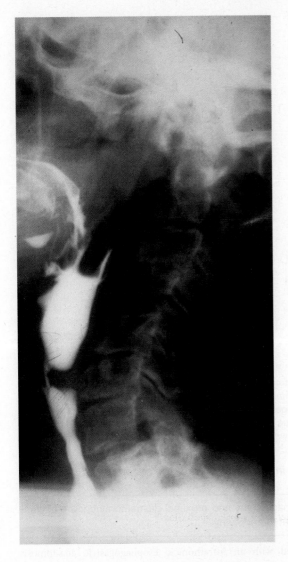

Figure 4-33: Barium swallow showing upper esophageal cancer.

thoracotomy but is performed through simultaneous upper abdominal and cervical incisions. **Formal esophagectomy** (Ivor-Lewis procedure) is accomplished through simultaneous upper abdominal and right thoracotomy incisions, excision of the esophagus, and a gastroesophageal anastomosis in the chest (Fig. 4-35). This approach may be altered to permit anastomosis in the neck. The advantage of a **neck anastomosis** becomes evident if the **anastomosis leaks** postoperatively, which may take place in up to 10% of patients. Because the leak is in the neck, it can be managed with local measures and easily controlled. In contrast, a leak in the chest carries a much higher risk of sepsis and major pulmonary complications. When the stomach is used for reconstruction, a pyloroplasty is usually performed to prevent gastric outlet obstruction.

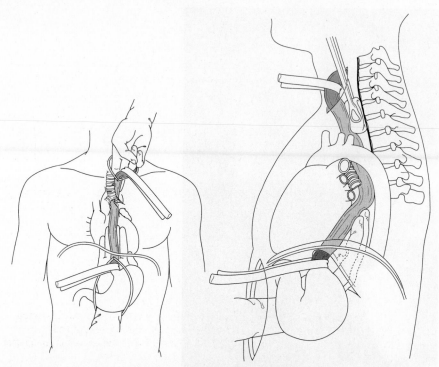

Figure 4-34: Transhiatal esophagectomy. (From Mulholland MW, Lillemoe KD, Doherty G, et al. *Greenfield's Surgery: Scientific Principles and Practice*, 5th ed. Philadelphia: Lippincott Williams & Wilkins; 2010. After Orringer MB. Surgical options for esophageal resection and reconstruction with stomach. In: Baue AE, Geha GL, Hammond GL, eds. *Glenn's Thoracic and Cardiovascular Surgery*, 5th ed. Norwalk, CT: Appleton & Lange; 1990:793.)

Case Variation 4.16.3. Cancer in the lower third of the esophagus (Figure 4-36)

 QUICK CUT Esophagectomy and proximal gastrectomy can be accomplished via left or right thoracotomy.

◆ Reconstruction is accomplished with an intrathoracic esophagogastric anastomosis (Fig. 4-37).

Case 4.17 Dysphagia

A 65-year-old man presents with **severe dysphagia** of 1 year's duration. The dysphagia has been progressive. He now has difficulty swallowing saliva and **coughs** constantly. In addition, he has **lost 50 lb**.

◆ **How would you establish the diagnosis?**

◆ The next steps should include a **barium swallow, esophagoscopy, and biopsy**. The patient most likely has esophageal carcinoma, probably in an advanced state and probably not curable.

A   **B**   **C**

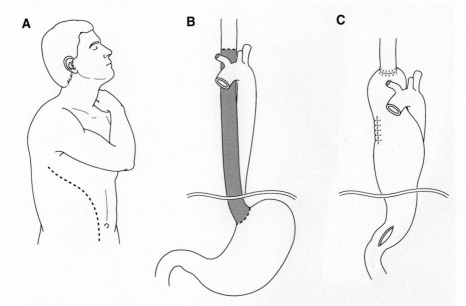

Figure 4-35: A–C: Esophagectomy through the right chest. (From Mulholland MW, Lillemoe KD, Doherty G, et al. *Greenfield's Surgery: Scientific Principles and Practice*, 5th ed. Philadelphia: Lippincott Williams & Wilkins; 2010. After Ellis FH Jr. Treatment of the esophagus and cardia. *Mayo Clin Proc*. 1960;35:653.)

◆ **Why does the man have a constant cough?**

◆ His cough may be secondary to chronic **aspiration from a tracheoesophageal fistula** due to tumor erosion into the trachea.

A barium swallow reveals almost complete obstruction of the midesophagus and a tracheoesophageal fistula. Endoscopic evaluation reveals a tumor constricting the esophageal lumen. Biopsy reveals squamous cell carcinoma.

◆ **What would be your next steps in management?**

> **QUICK CUT** In the vast majority of patients with esophageal cancer, the tumor has either locally invaded a nearby structure or distantly metastasized, precluding cure.

Thus, surgery is inappropriate as a curative procedure. Most **therapy** is therefore aimed at **palliation**; 80% of affected patients will die in the first year after diagnosis despite various treatment regimens involving chemotherapy, radiation, or surgery. Palliative methods include feeding gastrostomy, esophageal stents, radiation, or palliative resection. The incidence of complications and the mortality rate increase progressively with each of these four techniques.

This particular patient is a poor candidate for treatment. He is severely malnourished and probably has pulmonary sepsis, and he certainly will not tolerate a major esophageal operative procedure. Radiation therapy is an option, but the chances of the treatment's

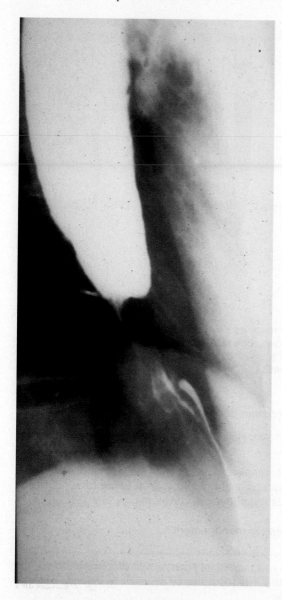

Figure 4-36: Lower esophageal cancer.

worsening a tracheoesophageal fistula and pneumonia are high. Feeding gastrostomy may improve his nutritional status but has not been shown to prolong life. An esophageal stent may help control aspiration from the tracheoesophageal fistula.

Deep Thoughts

In locally advanced or systemically spread esophageal cancer, comfort and palliative care may be this patient's best option.

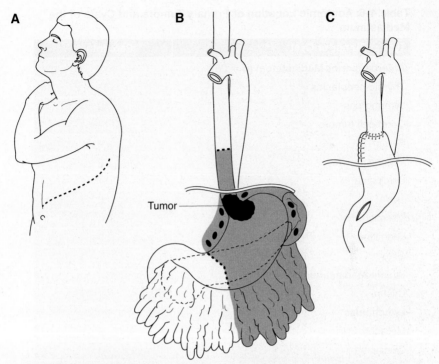

Figure 4-37: A–C: Esophagectomy through left chest and gastric reconstruction. (From Mulholland MW, Lillemoe KD, Doherty G, et al. *Greenfield's Surgery: Scientific Principles and Practice*, 5th ed. Philadelphia: Lippincott Williams & Wilkins; 2010. After Ellis FH Jr. Treatment of the esophagus and cardia. *Mayo Clin Proc*. 1960;35:653.)

Case 4.18 Muscular Weakness and a Mediastinal Mass

A 50-year-old man complains of progressive weakness of the upper and lower extremities and double vision. A radiograph reveals a **mass in the anterior mediastinum**.

◆ **What is the most likely diagnosis (assuming the symptoms are related to the mass) (Table 4-6)?**

◆ This patient has the typical findings of **myasthenia gravis** in association with a **thymus tumor** or hyperplasia. Other tumors in the anterior mediastinum such as **teratomas and lymphomas** and, in younger persons, germ cell tumors, do not produce these symptoms. Calcium deposits in an anterior mediastinal tumor indicate a germ cell tumor, which is often benign but can be malignant. These **teratomas**, predominantly of the epidermal germ layer, may contain **hair and primitive teeth**. Both Hodgkin and non-Hodgkin lymphoma arise commonly occurring in the anterior mediastinum. Hodgkin lymphoma is most common and tends to occur in younger people (Fig. 4-38).

◆ **What is the treatment for these tumor-associated disorders?**

◆ **Radiation and chemotherapy** are indicated for lymphoma. Surgery is unnecessary except in situations where diagnosis cannot be made. **Hodgkin disease** in the cervical and anterior

Table 4-6: Anatomic Location of Primary Tumors and Cysts of the Mediastinum

Type of Tumor or Cyst	Percentage
Anterosuperior Mediastinum (n = 287)	
Thymic neoplasms	33
Lymphomas	19
Germ cell tumors	17
Benign	9
Malignant	8
Carcinoma	11
Cysts	8
Mesenchymal	4
Endocrine	6
Other	2
Middle Mediastinum (n = 98)	
Cysts	61
Lymphomas	21
Mesenchymal	8
Carcinoma	6
Other	4
Posterior Mediastinum (n = 129)	
Neurogenic	53
Benign	41
Malignant	12
Cysts	32
Mesenchymal	9
Endocrine	2
Other	4

From Townsend CM Jr, ed. *Sabiston Textbook of Surgery*, 16th ed. Philadelphia: WB Saunders; 2001:1188.

mediastinum is a highly curable disease. **Surgery** is useful in the treatment of **thymomas and other tumors**; tumor removal can be done through a median sternotomy or a thoracoscopic approach.

◆ **What are the common tumors of the middle mediastinum (see Table 4-6)?**

 QUICK CUT Lymphatic tumors and various cysts are most common in middle mediastinal compartment.

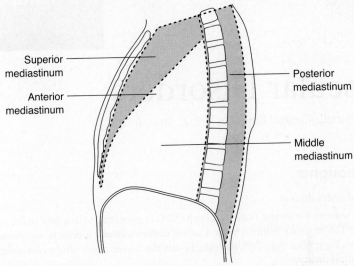

Figure 4-38: Compartments of the mediastinum. (Adapted from Mulholland MW, Lillemoe KD, Doherty G, et al. *Greenfield's Surgery: Scientific Principles and Practice*, 5th ed. Philadelphia: Lippincott Williams & Wilkins; 2010.)

Bronchogenic cysts develop from foregut remnants and may be found in both the lung and the mediastinum. These benign growths are typically lined with columnar epithelium. Pericardial cysts have a typical "water bottle" appearance. Because cysts are symptomatic and have the potential for inflammatory complications such as fistula formation, their removal is usually warranted. Generally, the approach involves resection through a standard posterolateral thoracotomy.

◆ **What are the common tumors of the posterior mediastinum (see Table 4-6)?**

◆ By far, the most common tumors of the mediastinum in most series are **neurogenic tumors**, which occur in the posterior mediastinum adjacent to the vertebral bodies. These neurogenic tumors arise from nerves and nerve sheaths in this area and contain both fibrous and neural elements. The most common type is the neurilemmoma. Most are benign by cell type, but some are malignant by location. They may be dumbbell-shaped within and outside the spinal canal. CT scan is indicated to determine whether tumor is present in the spinal canal. If such is the case, combined thoracic and neurosurgical approach is mandatory. Removal of most posterior mediastinal tumors occurs through a standard posterolateral thoracotomy.

Chapter 5

Vascular Disorders

Bruce E. Jarrell, Marshall Benjamin, Eric D. Strauch

Key Thoughts

1. Carotid artery disease

    - An untreated transient ischemic attack (TIA) is associated with a 40% chance of a second TIA or stroke within 2 years. Carotid endarterectomy, if done in symptomatic patients for greater than 70% stenosis, lowers the 2-year major stroke rate compared to medical therapy.

    - The carotid endarterectomy perioperative risk of a major stroke is 1%–3%.

2. Peripheral arterial disease

    - Acute arterial embolism often is secondary to cardiac thrombi, such as with atrial fibrillation, acute myocardial infarction (MI), and valvular disease.

    - The hallmarks are the 6 P's: pain, pulselessness, paralysis, pallor, paresthesias, and poikilothermia.

    - Revascularization more than 6 hours after ischemia may result in a severely impaired limb or even require amputation time is of the essence.

    - Compartment syndrome may occur following revascularization and is caused by edema increased tissue pressure obstructing capillary blood flow to the tissues. When tissue pressure exceeds capillary pressure($\sim$20–40 mm Hg), muscle ischemia occurs. Because compartment pressure does not exceed arterial pressure, the patient may not present with the signs of arterial occlusion and may have a normal distal pulse.

    - Claudication is reversible ischemia of the leg and is managed by lifestyle modification, including a supervised exercise program, cessation of smoking, control of diabetes, hyperlipidemia and hypertension, and antiplatelet therapy. Revascularization is generally reserved for patients where the claudication interferes with an active lifestyle.

    - Rest pain is constant pain usually across the forefoot and indicates severe ischemia. Tissue loss is imminent and urgent evaluation and revascularization is appropriate.

3. Aortic disease

    - Occlusive disease of the distal aorta, iliac, and femoral arteries (inflow disease) may produce claudication, rest pain, or tissue loss. When it is limb threatening, it should be evaluated and revascularized. Inflow disease should generally be revascularized before outflow disease.

    - Elective repair of abdominal aortic aneurysms that are 5.5 cm in men and 5 cm in women or larger in greatest diameter is appropriate if the patient is likely to tolerate the procedure and has a life expectancy of more than 2 years. Both open and endovascular repairs appear to have excellent long-term durability. Endoleaks are leaks in the space between an endograft and the native vessel and should be repaired.

- Descending thoracic aortic dissection is usually treated with medical therapy to control hypertension. Surgical or endovascular repair is reserved for leaks, rupture, or occlusion of aortic branches. Proximal dissection is a surgical emergency due to risk of coronary occlusion, aortic regurgitation, and tamponade.

4. Arterial bypass grafts

   There are three important facets to a vascular bypass patency.

   - Inflow: If blood flow into the bypass is not strong, the bypass will thrombose.
   - The conduit: If the conduit has a technical problem such as a twist, kink, narrowing, or anything else that impedes flow, the bypass will thrombose.
   - Outflow: If the vessels distal to the bypass are obstructed for any reason, the bypass will thrombose.

5. Venous disease

   - Proven deep venous thrombosis prophylaxis includes intermittent pneumatic compression devices and low-dose anticoagulation. Risk factors are summarized in Virchow triad: stasis, hypercoagulable states, and endothelial injury.
   - Pulmonary embolism is diagnosed with computed tomography (CT) pulmonary angiogram.

6. Upper extremity DVT: usually refers to thrombosis of the axillary or subclavian vein.

   - Secondary UEDVT is increasing in incidence due to increased use of upper extremity catheters. Pulmonary embolus may occur in up to 1/3rd of patients, and post-thrombotic syndrome is common; thus anticoagulation with heparin followed by warfarin is appropriate in most cases.
   - Primary UEDVT (Paget-Schroetter Syndrome) is rare and typically related to extreme arm exercise in sports (effort thrombosis) or thoracic outlet syndrome. It may be amenable to urgent catheter-directed thrombolytic therapy aimed at preventing post-thrombotic syndrome.

PERIPHERAL ARTERIAL DISEASE

Case 5.1 Brief Neurologic Event

A 60-year-old woman presents with a single episode of weakness and numbness in her right arm. The episode lasted for 15 minutes and completely resolved in 1 hour.

◆ **What is the most likely diagnosis?**

◆ A **TIA** is the suspected diagnosis.

 QUICK CUT A TIA is typified by a brief neurologic deficit such as the one described in Case 5.1, which completely resolves within 24 hours.

The neurologic symptoms are most likely vascular in origin because they correspond to an anatomic distribution that receives blood from the appropriate carotid artery.

In this case, the left internal carotid artery is the suspected location of the ischemic event. Current pathophysiologic thinking suggests that atherosclerotic plaques at the

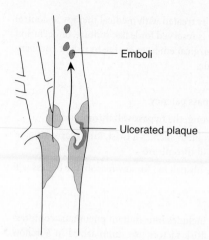

Emboli

Ulcerated plaque

Figure 5-1: Emboli formation in the carotid artery.

carotid bifurcation or internal carotid artery region become ulcerated, allowing cholesterol and platelet debris to break off and **form an embolism in the intracranial circulation
and brain** (Fig. 5-1).

◆ **If this patient is left untreated, what is the risk that she will have a repeat
neurologic event?**

◆ Without treatment, this patient's chance of experiencing another TIA or stroke within
2 years is as high as 40%.

◆ **How would you evaluate this patient?**

◆ An examination for **carotid bruits, residual neurologic deficit,** and **evidence of cardiac
disease,** especially murmurs that might indicate an embolic source, is necessary. If a murmur is present, an echocardiogram would be appropriate. In addition, a **duplex ultrasound
study of the carotid vessels** to check for stenosis or irregular plaque morphology is essential in all patients (Fig. 5-2). Both of these conditions suggest that the carotid artery may be
the source of the neurologic event.

Evaluation indicates a complete resolution of the neurologic symptoms and a left
carotid bruit. No cardiac murmurs are evident. Duplex examination reveals an 80%
stenosis of the left internal carotid artery (Fig. 5-3).

◆ **What treatment option would you select?**

◆ Two therapeutic choices are available: medical treatment with aspirin and, more recently,
the addition of clopidogrel or surgical therapy involving carotid endarterectomy. Recently, a
comparison of the two treatment methods has been the subject of a large number of randomized trials (Table 5-1). Researchers have demonstrated that for a **stenosis of 70% or more
in the internal carotid artery with ipsilateral symptoms** (symptoms that correspond to
the carotid distribution), **surgical treatment results in a significant advantage in stroke
prevention.** In a 2-year period after joining the study, the risk of major strokes was 9% for
surgical patients and 26% for medical patients; this represents a 17% decrease in relative
stroke rate. Table 5-2 gives the indications for carotid endarterectomy. The carotid artery may

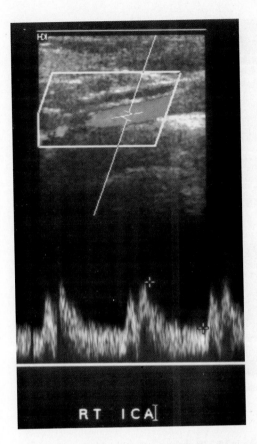

RT ICA

Figure 5-2: Duplex study of a normal carotid artery.

be stented via a percutaneous approach as opposed to the open carotid endarterectomy to prevent stroke from carotid artery stenosis. Current data suggests that carotid artery stenting should be limited to high-risk patients or patients participating in randomized clinical trials.

 QUICK CUT Carotid endarterectomy is three times more effective than aspirin in preventing major strokes over a 2-year period.

You proceed with carotid endarterectomy.

◆ **What additional preoperative evaluation is necessary?**

◆ The recommendation for endarterectomy is dependent on the general medical condition of the patient. However, in most cases, endarterectomy can be safely performed, even with local or regional anesthesia. Blood pressure (BP) should be well controlled preoperatively so wide intraoperative swings in BP can be avoided. An appropriate **cardiac evaluation** is necessary before surgery. In certain settings, a carotid artery angiogram is obtained to describe the anatomy of the lesion in more detail, but this procedure is no longer routine. If coronary artery bypass grafting (CABG) is indicated, it may be safely combined with carotid endarterectomy as one combined procedure in many cases.

The patient wants to know the risk of a stroke during surgery.

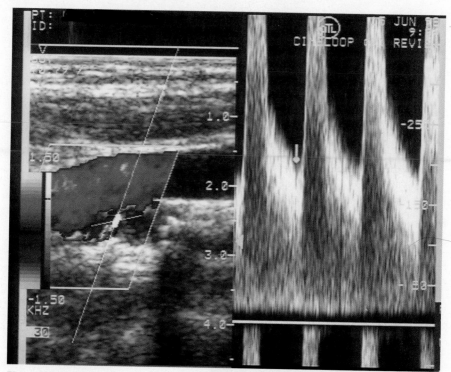

Figure 5-3: Duplex study of an 80% stenosis of the internal carotid artery.

◆ **What do you tell her?**

◆ The **perioperative risk of a major stroke is 1%–3%** during a carotid endarterectomy performed by most experienced vascular surgeons. The operation is technically safe.

◆ **What other surgery-related complications do you discuss with the patient?**

◆ Injury to the hypoglossal nerve, vagus nerve, and the marginal branch of the facial nerve may occur if they are not identified and protected during surgery (Fig. 5-4).

You proceed to the operating room to perform the carotid endarterectomy.

Table 5-1: Risk of Stroke with Medical and Surgical Therapy

Treatment	2-Year Stroke Risk
No treatment (estimated)	~40%
Aspirin	~26%
Carotid endarterectomy	~9%

There was a 65% reduction in relative risk of stroke in the surgical group compared to the aspirin group.
North American Symptomatic Carotid Endarterectomy Trial Collaborators. Beneficial effect of carotid endarterectomy in symptomatic patients with high-grade carotid stenosis. *N Engl J Med*. 1991;325(7):445–453.

Table 5-2: Indications for Carotid Endarterectomy

Ipsilateral hemispheric neurologic symptoms (amaurosis fugax, transient ischemic attack [TIA], completed stroke with major neurologic recovery) AND >70% internal carotid stenosis
Asymptomatic carotid bruit AND >70% internal carotid stenosis

◆ **What are the basic steps in the endarterectomy?**

◆ Patient preparation involves establishment of invasive monitoring with an arterial line to allow careful monitoring of BP during the procedure. Local, regional, or general anesthesia may be used.

The endarterectomy involves the following steps (Fig. 5-5):

- An incision is made along the sternocleidomastoid muscle, and dissection is performed down to the carotid sheath.
- The sheath is opened, the vagus nerve is protected, and the carotid artery is isolated, avoiding denervation of the carotid body.
- The internal carotid artery is exposed to the level of the hypoglossal nerve, which must not be injured.
- The patient is heparinized, and the vessels are clamped.
- The vessels are opened and the plaque is dissected from the underlying vessel media and adventitia, taking care to obtain a smooth distal transition back to normal artery.
- The vessel is then closed with or without a patch, and the neck is closed.

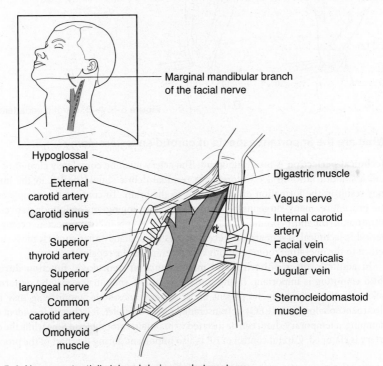

Figure 5-4: Nerves potentially injured during endarterectomy.

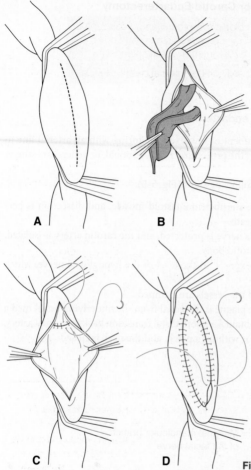

A   B

C   D

Figure 5-5: A–D: Carotid endarterectomy.

◆ **What are the important aspects of carotid endarterectomy?**

◆ **Technical perfection** is most important. The artery must be completely cleared of plaque and a smooth flow surface restored. No residual debris should be left in the lumen; it may result in the formation of an embolus to the brain. To confirm the completeness of the procedure, many surgeons perform an on-table angiogram or intraoperative duplex ultrasound. The most common cause of neurologic events in the immediate postoperative period is technical. If a neurologic event occurs immediately after surgery, most surgeons return to the operating room promptly and re-examine the repair.

In addition, the **monitoring and maintenance of neurologic function during carotid clamping** is important. In the conscious patient, monitoring may be performed by talking to the patient. In the patient under general anesthesia, monitoring may involve electroencephalography (EEG) or transcranial power Doppler. If ischemia is evident during clamping, a temporary shunt can be inserted to maintain carotid blood flow while the carotid artery is clamped. Careful control of BP is also important during this part of the procedure.

The patient recovers from the surgery with no neurologic symptoms.

◆ **What follow-up advice would you give to the patient?**

◆ The patient should be advised that TIA or stroke may result from plaque buildup in the opposite carotid artery or may recur as a consequence of plaque recurrence on the treated side. The risk of recurrent carotid narrowing on the side of the endarterectomy is approximately 13% over 5 years. Most physicians recommend taking **aspirin** after routine endarterectomy.

◆ **What condition is most likely to cause this patient's death?**

> **QUICK CUT** Because atherosclerosis is a systemic disease, any patient who has had a TIA remains at risk for MI in the long term.

◆ Preventive measures in the form of lifestyle modification, including lipid control, smoking cessation, and exercise, are indicated.

Case 5.2 Other Transient Neurologic Events

A 66-year-old woman has had a transient neurologic event. The circumstances are somewhat different from those of the patient in Case 5.1.

◆ **How would you manage the following situations?**

Case Variation 5.2.1. The patient experiences an episode of blindness in the left eye that cleared rapidly, with the occurrence of no other neurologic events.

◆ The ophthalmic artery is the first branch of the internal carotid artery.

> **QUICK CUT** Emboli from the carotid artery bifurcation may travel to the retina, resulting in monocular transient blindness or amaurosis fugax.

Patients may report either painless episodes of monocular blindness or hazy vision described as "a shade being pulled over the eye." Examination of the fundus during the episode may result in observation of a bright shiny spot in a retinal artery, or a **Hollenhorst plaque,** which is presumably a portion of the embolus. Such an episode usually resolves in 15 minutes to several hours and leaves no residua.

In this instance, the left carotid system is the suspected origin of the embolus. Evaluation and treatment are the same as in the first case—duplex scanning of the carotids and carotid endarterectomy would be appropriate if a lesion is present.

Case Variation 5.2.2. The patient, who is right-handed, relates an episode of aphasia, with the occurrence of no other neurologic events.

◆ In most right-handed patients, the speech center is most commonly in the **left hemisphere.** Therefore, the etiology of an aphasic episode most likely involves the left carotid system. An episode of aphasia is a TIA. Evaluation and treatment are the same as in the first case— carotid endarterectomy would be appropriate if a carotid abnormality is present.

Case Variation 5.2.3. The patient experiences marked weakness and numbness in the right arm that is not transient. The condition does not improve in 1 week.

◆ The patient's symptoms do not fit the description of a TIA. Apparently, she has had a fixed neurologic deficit (a stroke). Most physicians would not recommend endarterectomy at this time. A carotid duplex study is appropriate, followed by **observation for improvement.**

Table 5-3: Rate of Major Neurological Events (Stroke and TIA) in the Asymptomatic Carotid Artery Stenosis Study

Treatment	Rate of Neurologic Event (%)
Aspirin	10.6
Carotid endarterectomy	4.8

There was a 55% relative reduction of stroke risk in the surgically treated group.
Walker MD, Marler JR, Goldstein M, et al. Endarterectomy for asymptomatic carotid artery stenosis. Executive Committee for the Asymptomatic Carotid Atherosclerosis study. *JAMA*. 1995;273(18):1421–1428.

When the patient has stabilized, she should be re-evaluated. If recovery is favorable, and neurologic function is good, endarterectomy may be considered based on the duplex findings to prevent future neurologic events. The surgery may occur as early as 2–4 weeks after the diagnosis of stroke or when the patient's neurologic status stabilizes.

Case 5.3   Asymptomatic Carotid Bruit

A 55-year-old man with a bruit in his right neck is referred to you by his primary physician. You review his history and physical examination, which are both normal except for a right carotid bruit. He has no neurologic signs or symptoms.

◆ **How would you evaluate this patient?**

◆ The asymptomatic bruit may originate in the carotid artery. To determine whether an abnormality exists, a carotid **duplex** study is appropriate.

The duplex examination reveals a 65% internal carotid artery stenosis.

◆ **What is the next appropriate step?**

◆ Many surgeons would recommend a carotid endarterectomy in this patient, although this is controversial in asymptomatic patients.
    The most convincing data come from the Asymptomatic Carotid Artery Study (ACAS), in which patients with a 60% or greater stenosis were randomized to medical therapy with aspirin or surgical treatment with endarterectomy.

 QUICK CUT In a 2-year period, major strokes occurred in 2.5% of individuals in the surgical group and 11% of individuals in the aspirin group, a highly significant difference.

One-half of the major strokes in the surgical group appeared preoperatively during the carotid angiogram, indicating the risk of angiography. As in the symptomatic carotid artery trials, the perioperative major stroke rate was about 1%, indicating the high skill of the surgeons. However, performance of endarterectomy is still controversial (Table 5-3).

Case 5.4   Acute Vascular Event in the Leg

A 65-year-old man is brought to the emergency department with a history of sudden onset of pain in his right leg and difficulty moving the leg. He says that the leg has been perfectly normal up until now. On examining his legs, you note the absence of pulses, including the femoral pulse, in the right leg. Pulses are normal in the left leg. The right leg appears cool and cyanotic, with decreased sensation throughout. All muscle groups are weak.

◆ **What is the most likely diagnosis?**

◆ This patient probably has an acute arterial embolus in his right leg. Absence of a right femoral pulse and presence of a left femoral pulse indicate that the embolus is most likely at the right iliofemoral level, a common site of occlusion due to arterial emboli (Fig. 5-6). The common findings in acute arterial occlusion are described by the **"6 P's"**: **p**ain, **p**ulselessness, **p**aralysis, **p**allor, **p**aresthesias, and **p**oikilothermia (Table 5-4).

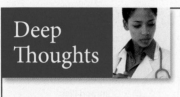

Deep Thoughts	The clinical presentation will give significant clues to the etiology of the disease. If there are no chronic symptoms and the presentation is acute, then an acute occlusion commonly by an embolus is often the etiology of the ischemia.

◆ **What is most important in terms of immediate management?**

◆ **Time is of the essence** with an acute arterial embolus, as some studies strongly indicate. The time interval between the ischemic event and clinical presentation are critical to successful limb salvage.

QUICK CUT The earlier the revascularization after an arterial embolus, the more complete the recovery.

Revascularization more than 6 hours after ischemia may result in a severely impaired limb or even require amputation (Tables 5-5 and 5-6).

◆ **What treatment is appropriate at this time?**

◆ **Administer heparin immediately** and **proceed with surgical or radiological intervention** to allow the earliest revascularization. Arteriography can be performed in the operating room if indicated after removal of the embolus to ensure adequate blood flow and plan any additional interventions.

◆ **What surgical procedure is necessary?**

◆ A **balloon catheter embolectomy** (Fogarty catheter embolectomy) is the procedure of choice and is a quick, safe, and effective method of revascularization after acute ischemia, secondary to arterial embolism.
  The embolectomy involves the following steps (Fig. 5-7):

- The femoral artery is exposed and opened, often under local anesthesia, and the proximal embolus is extracted using a balloon catheter.
- Typically, thrombus is also removed from the distal vessels. An intraoperative arteriogram can then be performed to assess the adequacy of thrombus removal. If necessary, it is possible to lyse thrombus further with intra-arterial thrombolytic therapy if there is residual distal, small arterial thrombus.
- The arteriotomy is closed, and the limb revascularized.

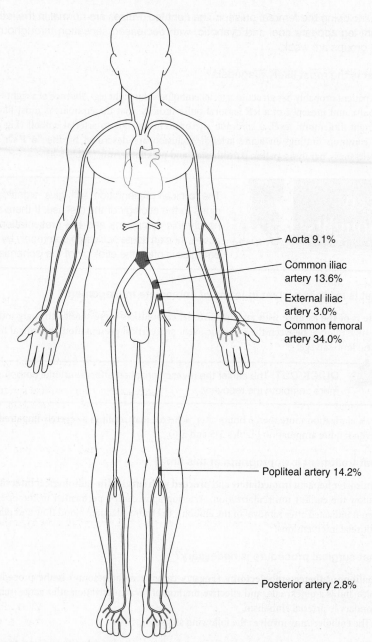

Aorta 9.1%

Common iliac
artery 13.6%

External iliac
artery 3.0%

Common femoral
artery 34.0%

Popliteal artery 14.2%

Posterior artery 2.8%

Figure 5-6: Common sites of lower body arterial occlusion due to arterial emboli
(% represents total body locations).

Table 5-4: The "6 P's": A Mnemonic Device that Can Be Used to Remember the Common Findings in Arterial Occlusion

Pain	Severe, constant ischemic rest pain, usually of sudden onset
Pulselessness	Sudden, unilateral loss of a previously palpable pulse distal to the level of occlusion
Paralysis	The extent reflects the degree of neural and muscle ischemia.
Pallor	Skin is pale or "cadaveric"
Paresthesias	"Pins and needles" feelings. Loss of light touch and proprioception are good clinical indicators of limb viability and degree of peripheral nerve ischemia.
Poikilothermia	The skin is cold below the site of occlusion.

If ischemia is not so severe that the limb is imminently threatened, an acute thromboembolism can be treated with catheter-directed intra-arterial thrombolysis using a thrombolytic such as tissue plasminogen activator (TPA).

Anticoagulants are continued in the postoperative period.

Immediately after surgery, you examine his leg and note good perfusion to the foot and toes but inability to dorsiflex the foot and tenderness in the calf.

◆ **What is the most likely cause of these findings?**

◆ Evidently, this patient has developed a muscular compartment syndrome. Although loss of motor and sensory function may occur in the leg as a consequence of the acute arterial insufficiency, these particular symptoms are most indicative of a **compartment syndrome**. This condition is most common after revascularization of an acutely ischemic limb. However, it should be suspected in any patient who has an ischemic or traumatic injury to a muscle group that causes acute muscular edema.

Compartment syndrome, which can be caused by an **ischemia–reperfusion injury**, occur after reperfusion of an ischemic muscle, resulting in edema of the muscle. Because many muscles are encased in an inelastic, fascial compartment, edema increases the volume, and ultimately the pressure, within the compartment. As the pressure increases, muscle perfusion decreases, resulting in further ischemic injury, which worsens the edema. As the compartment pressure approaches 20–40 mm Hg, **irreversible ischemic injury of muscles and nerves may occur**.

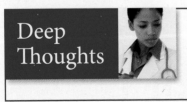

Deep Thoughts

Compartment syndrome can still be present with normal pulses, as the tissue ischemia is a result of obstruction of capillary blood flow from increased tissue pressure, not acute arterial ischemia.

You suspect that this patient has a compartment syndrome.

◆ **How would you manage this patient?**

◆ With a suspected compartment syndrome, the physician **should not wait for advanced symptoms such as motor or sensory loss or loss of the distal arterial pulses**.

Table 5-5: Limb Viability at Presentation (Clinical Categories of Acute Limb Ischemia)

Category	Description	Capillary Return	Muscle Weakness	Sensory Loss	Doppler Signals Arterial	Doppler Signals Venous
Viable	Not immediately threatened	Intact	None	None	Audible (AP >30 mm Hg)	Audible
Threatened	Salvageable if promptly treated	Intact, slow	Mild, partial	Mild, incomplete	Inaudible	Audible
Irreversible	Major tissue loss or amputation, regardless of treatment	Absent (marbling)	Profound, paralysis (rigor)	Profound, anesthetic	Inaudible	Inaudible

AP, ankle pressure.
Modified from Rutherford RB, Flanigan DP, Gupta SK, et al. Suggested standards for reports dealing with lower extremity ischemia. *J Vasc Surg*. 1986;4:80.

Table 5-6: Acute Arterial Embolization

A. Rates of Limb Salvage and Mortality after Catheter Embolectomy	
Limb salvage: perioperative heparin and Fogarty catheter embolectomy	92%
With >12-hour delay in treatment	78%
Mortality of Fogarty catheter thromboembolectomy (worsens to 30%–50% with delay in treatment and presence of arteriosclerotic heart)	10%
B. Common Sources of Arterial Emboli	
Cardiac	75%
Atrial fibrillation	50%–60%
Acute myocardial infarction	20%–25%
Aneurysm or atherosclerotic plaque of aorta	10%–15%
C. Common Sites of Embolization	
Aortic saddle embolus	10%–15%
Iliac	15%–20%
Femoral	40%–45%
Popliteal	15%
Upper extremity	5%–10%
Visceral or renal	5%–10%
Carotid	10%–15%

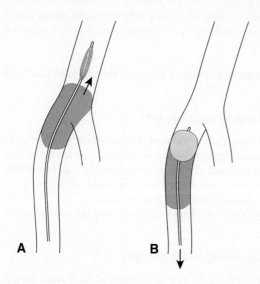

A   **B**

Figure 5-7: A,B: Balloon catheter embolectomy.

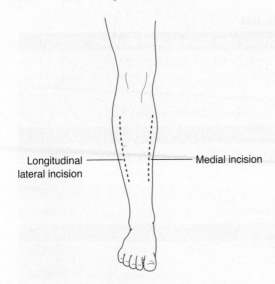

Longitudinal lateral incision ———— Medial incision

Figure 5-8: Fasciotomy of the compartments in the calf will release pressure from edema in the muscles and allow improved perfusion of the muscles. Two compartments are released through each incision.

QUICK CUT Based on a high degree of clinical suspicion, a fasciotomy should be performed. Alternatively, pressure in the compartment can be determined with a needle and pressure-measuring device and fasciotomy based on finding an elevated pressure.

In this case, the fasciotomy should open all four compartments in the calf (Fig. 5-8). Typically, the muscle bulges out at the point of excision, relieving the pressure and improving perfusion. Once the acute episode is resolved, a fasciotomy is typically closed with a split-thickness graft. During recovery, performance of physical therapy is important for maintenance of a full range of leg motion.

The patient recovers from the fasciotomy, receives physical therapy, and retains a functional leg.

♦ **What long-term management plan is appropriate?**

♦ Most surgeons would place this patient on **chronic anticoagulation therapy with warfarin**. Once the patient has recovered, echocardiography and other medical diagnostic techniques such as aortography or CT of the thoracic and abdominal aorta should be used in a **search for an embolic source**. However, in many cases, no definitive diagnosis is made.

  Suppose the presenting physical findings described at the beginning of Case 5.4 occur in an individual who had just undergone a coronary angiogram using the femoral artery approach.

♦ **How would your evaluation and management change?**

♦ Acute arterial ischemia, which is probably caused by a complication of the femoral arterial puncture, is still the diagnosis. **Such punctures can raise intimal flaps, dislodge atherosclerotic plaques, or initiate local thrombotic events.** Because the patient has severe acute ischemia, immediate revascularization is critical. This can be accomplished with open surgery and direct repair or by using endoluminal techniques including angioplasty and stenting (Fig. 5-9).

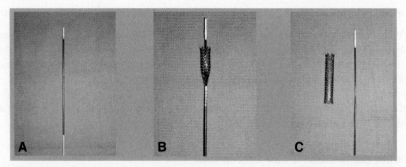

Figure 5-9: These pictures depict a self-expanding stent at various stages of deployment. **A:** The stent ensheathed on the catheter prior to deployment. **B:** The stent partially deployed. Note the expansion of the stent in the unsheathed portion. **C:** The self-expanding stent fully deployed. (From Mulholland MW, Lillemoe KD, Doherty G, et al. *Greenfield's Surgery: Scientific Principles and Practice*, 5th ed. Philadelphia: Lippincott Williams & Wilkins; 2010.)

Acute arterial ischemia may also occasionally be seen in aortic dissection. Here, the false lumen extends to the femoral artery, where it finally impinges enough on the true lumen to cause inadequate blood flow.

Case 5.5   Claudication

A 52-year-old man reports that he develops a cramp in his left calf after walking 100 yards. When he stops walking and sits down, the calf pain slowly resolves in 10 minutes. The man's history is significant for cigarette smoking (two packs/day for 20 years) and mild hypertension.

◆ **What additional history and physical examination findings are important?**

◆ The history findings suggest intermittent claudication, which is exercise-induced ischemic pain of the calf that is relieved by rest.

Examination of the legs is necessary to assess the peripheral arterial system for the presence of pulses, bruits, or thrills; the skin must be examined for ulcerations and the nervous system for intact motor and sensory function (Table 5-7). Other signs such as hair loss; dependent rubor; loss of sensation; or thin, shiny skin suggest the chronic nature of the ischemia. Evidence of other cardiovascular disease related to the cardiac, cerebral, and abdominal vascular systems, as well as diabetes mellitus, may also be apparent.

Table 5-7: Signs of Peripheral Vascular Insufficiency

1. Claudication: **reproducible** muscle pain, cramping, or weakness, typically of the **calf** muscles. It occurs during exercise and is relieved by rest.
2. Rest pain: constant, severe, burning, **forefoot** pain
3. Ischemic ulceration: painful, nonhealing ulceration, typically on the **malleoli and toes** and foot at areas of trauma
4. Gangrene: cyanotic, insensate tissue (pregangrene) progressing to black tissue (dry gangrene) or wet gangrene if infection is present

◆ **What arteries in the legs are typically involved in atherosclerotic occlusions?**

✦ With intermittent claudication, popliteal and pedal pulses are often absent, indicating at least an occlusion of the **superficial femoral artery**, typically at the adductor hiatus. This is the most common location for occlusive disease of the lower extremity. If the femoral pulse is absent, significant aortoiliac disease may also be present.

You examine him and note that pulses are absent in the popliteal, dorsalis pedis, and posterior tibial arteries and present in the femoral arteries.

◆ **What examination is now appropriate?**

✦ The patient should undergo a **noninvasive vascular laboratory examination**, which involves the following steps:

- Calculation of the ankle–brachial index (ABI), which requires measurement of the systolic arterial pressure at the ankle and at the brachial artery with a Doppler device
- Examination of the Doppler tracing of the arterial waveform at various levels to detect stenotic arterial areas, which localizes the level of the occlusion

◆ **What are the typical Doppler findings in peripheral vascular insufficiency?**

✦ Normally, the ABI is greater than 1.0.

> **QUICK CUT** In mild claudication, the ABI is typically about 0.6–0.8. Pressure readings correlate with the severity of ischemia (Table 5-8).

Note that in diabetics, BP measurements may be incorrect. Typically, diabetics may have calcified vessels, preventing arterial occlusion with a BP cuff. As a result, measured BP is often as high as the cuff is inflated (Table 5-9).

Normally, the Doppler waveform is triphasic, with a phase of rapid systolic flow, a brief phase of reverse flow secondary to elastic recoil of the vessel followed by a prolonged phase of diastolic outflow. **As a vessel becomes less compliant due to atherosclerosis**, the Doppler signal changes, and the reverse flow component may be lost. In severe disease, the waveform may be monophasic (Fig. 5-10).

Performance of a Doppler study demonstrates that the ABI = 0.7, and clinical evidence of occlusion of the superficial femoral artery (e.g., absent popliteal and pedal pulses) is present. On the basis of these findings, you decide that the patient has peripheral vascular disease with claudication of the calf.

Table 5-8: Typical Ankle–Brachial Systolic Arterial Pressures Correlate with Severity of Ischemia

Normal	ABI = 0.9–1.1
Mild claudication (single lesion peripheral)	ABI = 0.6–0.8
Severe claudication (multilevel occlusive disease)	ABI <0.5
Rest pain or tissue loss	ABI <0.3

ABI, ankle–brachial index.

Table 5-9: **Five-Year History of Claudication**

Extremity Outcome	
Requires subsequent amputation	10%–15% (1%/yr) of patients
Symptoms remain stable or improve	~70% of patients
Symptoms progress, requiring revascularization	~20% of patients
Survival Outcome: Correlates with Initial Presentation and ABI, Reflecting Associated Cardiovascular Disease	
Mild claudication	97% survival
Claudication, operative	80% survival
Critical limb-threatening ischemia	48% survival

◆ **Would you recommend vascular reconstruction?**

◆ In this case, the principal management decision concerns **the degree to which claudication interferes with the patient's lifestyle**.

 QUICK CUT The management for most patients with claudication alone is to not perform surgery.

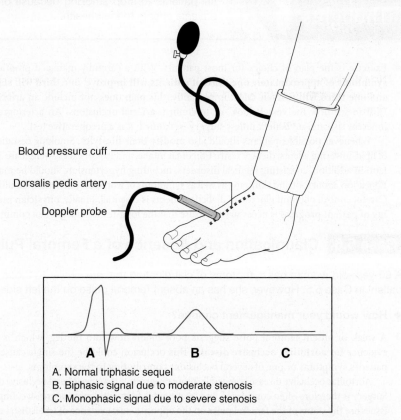

Blood pressure cuff

Dorsalis pedis artery

Doppler probe

A. Normal triphasic sequel
B. Biphasic signal due to moderate stenosis
C. Monophasic signal due to severe stenosis

Figure 5-10: Doppler blood pressure and ankle–brachial indices and Doppler arterial waveform.

The decision regarding surgery is based on a risk–benefit analysis, which compares the risk of an arteriogram and actual operation, including the possibility of thrombosis, infection, and amputation in the poor outcome scenario, with the benefits of increased exercise tolerance in a revascularized limb. A patient and surgeon might consider surgery if the patient's livelihood depends on a higher level of activity than currently tolerated and the patient has an otherwise good medical condition. Even so, there are good nonoperative alternatives, and most patients do not undergo surgery. The presence of an unfavorable medical condition (e.g., concomitant moderate coronary artery disease) or a multivessel disease such as that found in diabetes may detract from surgery. In this particular case, the patient is at no risk for limb loss with this level of perfusion, although the pain is bothersome.

◆ **What nonoperative therapy do you recommend?**

> **QUICK CUT** Nonoperative exercise management and lifestyle changes may prove very successful for these patients with claudication. Cessation of smoking has been shown to reduce the risk of disease progression and can even help diminish claudication symptoms.

Deep Thoughts

A physician always has the obligation to counsel patients to stop smoking because of the adverse effects to their health.

◆ Exercise is the plan of choice for most patients. With a carefully managed program, **the symptoms of approximately one third of patients will improve**, **one third will stabilize**, and **one third will worsen**. Most importantly, this plan does not include an arteriogram "just to see how the vessels look" or to confirm arterial occlusions. An arteriogram has inherent risk and no benefit unless surgery is planned; it is a preoperative test.

Whenever possible, patients should also **modify their lifestyles**. Smoking cessation, use of lipid-lowering agents, dietary restriction of fat intake, and loss of excess weight are important. In addition, coexisting medical disorders, including hypertension, should be managed. Education about foot and skin care, as well as symptoms of worsening ischemia, should occur. Careful control of blood glucose in diabetic patients is essential. Finally, **physician monitoring of patient progress** is necessary to ensure that the long-term management continues.

Case 5.6 Claudication and Absence of a Femoral Pulse

A 60-year-old woman has symptoms of claudication that are similar to those of the patient in Case 5.5. However, she has an absent femoral pulse on the left side.

◆ **How would your management change?**

◆ A weak or absent femoral pulse suggests poor blood flow into the leg, which is strong evidence for **aortoiliac occlusive disease**. This occlusion could be the single cause of the patient's symptoms or one of several occlusions contributing to the symptoms.

Aortoiliac occlusive disease is generally more progressive than peripheral occlusive disease. Surgery is therefore often considered, and treatment is frequently more aggressive. Important issues are the status of the femoral pulse on the opposite side, evidence of small distal emboli,

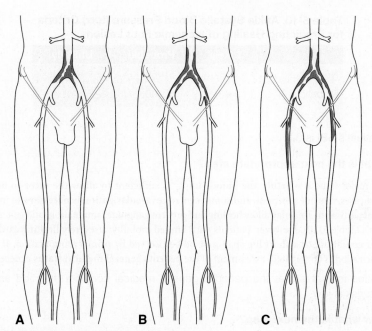

Figure 5-11: Patterns of arterial occlusive disease supplying the lower extremities. **A:** Limited to distal aorta and iliac arteries. **B:** Distal aortoiliac disease combined with proximal extremity disease. **C:** Lower extremity arterial disease combined with disease of the more proximal great vessels.

impotence in males, and claudication in other locations such as the thigh or buttock. **If this patient's disease and symptoms progress, aortoiliac reconstruction with a balloon dilatation and/or stent placement or surgical revascularization will be necessary** (Fig. 5-11).

Case 5.7 Toe Ulceration in Peripheral Vascular Disease

You once recommended an exercise program to a 62-year-old man with claudication who agreed to modify his lifestyle. He is apparently "lost to follow-up" but returns 1 year later complaining of an ulcer on his big toe.

◆ **How would you evaluate this patient?**

◆ An ulceration on the big toe suggests that the **ischemia has worsened**. A vascular laboratory evaluation is appropriate.

 QUICK CUT ABI in a patient with rest pain (constant pain across the forefoot unrelated to exercise) is typically 0.3–0.5.

In addition, the Doppler waveform may show further progression to a monophasic signal. Tissue loss or ulceration may be associated with even lower ABI measurements. Some patients, **especially diabetics**, have predominantly **small vessel disease**, and measuring the BP at the toe level (i.e., a toe BP) may document this condition.

Table 5-10: **Ankle Systolic Blood Pressure (torr) Criteria for Predicting Healing of Ischemic Foot Lesions**

	Likely	Probable	Unlikely
Nondiabetics	>65	55–65	<55
Diabetics	>90	80–90	<80

The patient's ABI is 0.3.

◆ **What is the next appropriate step?**

◆ The major issue is **whether the blood supply is sufficient to allow the ulcer to heal**. In most cases, it is not sufficient, and some form of **revascularization is necessary** to increase distal perfusion. This may allow healing and prevent gangrene, amputation, and generalized sepsis (Table 5-10). However, patients with limited mobility, a severely limiting cardiovascular condition, or a short life span may be best served by primary amputation. If revascularization is anticipated, assessment of the patient's **general medical status** is necessary.

Evaluation indicates that the patient's general medical condition is good and his cardiac risk is low.

◆ **Now what is the next step?**

◆ Assessment of the patient's **vascular anatomy** is necessary to determine whether a vascular reconstruction is likely to be successful. At this point, most surgeons would perform an **arteriogram** to assess the different levels of arterial occlusion to develop a revascularization plan. Generally, results assume two patterns:

1. **Inflow disease**, or inadequate blood flow into the femoral artery, as in iliac artery occlusive disease
2. **Outflow disease**, or single or multiple occlusions of the leg arteries, especially the superficial femoral artery, the popliteal artery, or the distal branches

The surgeon must decide if the occlusion(s) can be bypassed successfully to improve the blood supply to the level of the ulcer. In many cases, **the ulcer will heal with adequate debridement and wound care after revascularization**.

◆ **How would you manage the following findings seen on arteriography?**

Case Variation 5.7.1. The arteriogram shows occlusion of the superficial femoral artery with distal reconstitution.

◆ A **reversed or in situ saphenous vein** graft from the common femoral artery to the popliteal artery is typically used to bypass the obstructions (Fig. 5-12).

Case Variation 5.7.2. The arteriogram shows high-grade stenosis of the iliac artery but patency of the lower extremity vessels (Fig. 5-13).

◆ A **surgical revascularization** using a large-diameter graft from the aorta to the femoral artery or by **balloon dilatation** and/or arterial stent placement is appropriate.

Case Variation 5.7.3. The arteriogram shows high-grade stenosis of the iliac artery and occlusion of the superficial femoral artery.

◆ This case is similar to that in Case Variation 5.7.2, but a **lower extremity revascularization in addition to the aortoiliac reconstruction** may be necessary. The patient has

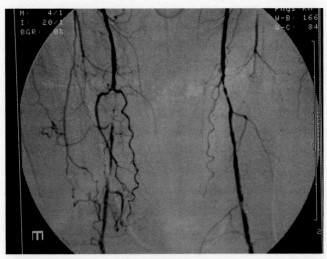

Figure 5-12: High-grade stenosis of superficial femoral artery on left and occlusion on right with distal reconstitution.

multilevel disease. The two procedures may be performed at the same time or sequentially; the inflow (aortoiliac occlusions) can be treated first, and this revascularization may be sufficient to relieve the symptoms (Fig. 5-14).

Case Variation 5.7.4. The arteriogram shows occlusion of the superficial femoral and popliteal arteries with distal reconstitution.

◆ **Femoropopliteal bypass** is indicated for this patient. The best artery continuous with the foot is selected as the outflow tract, with preference given to the popliteal, anterior, and posterior tibial arteries (Fig. 5-15). If the tibial arteries are occluded, the peroneal artery can be chosen for bypass. It is best if it is continuous with one or two of its terminal branches;

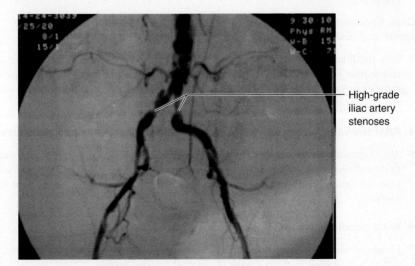

High-grade iliac artery stenoses

Figure 5-13: Aortogram of high-grade iliac artery stenosis.

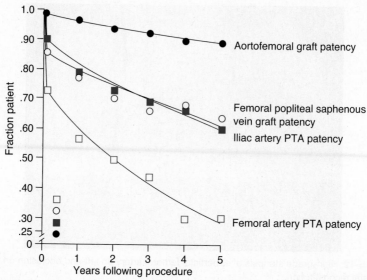

Figure 5-14: Five-year patency of four vascular reconstructions. Aortofemoral reconstruction is a highly successful procedure, whereas percutaneous transluminal angioplasty (PTA) of the femoral artery has poor long-term results. Iliac artery PTA in isolated iliac artery stenosis has a very acceptable long-term result.

however, absence of a plantar arch and vascular calcification is not a contraindication to reconstruction, although it worsens the prognosis. When the length of the vein conduit is limited, a short bypass originating at the popliteal or even tibial artery is useful.

For more distal disease, bypass to the dorsalis pedis, plantar, or tarsal arteries is useful. Typically, diabetics predominantly have tibial disease. The more distal and more diseased the vessels, the more likely the graft is to fail and the patient is to lose his leg (Table 5-11).

Case Variation 5.7.5. *The arteriogram shows multiple obstructions in the upper and distal leg, with only small runoff vessels below the ankle.*

✦ This condition represents severe atherosclerotic occlusive disease, which can be difficult to treat successfully. The decision to reconstruct should be made by an experienced vascular surgeon. **No reconstruction is possible in some cases**, and primary amputation and rehabilitation may be most appropriate in such situations.

◆ After the vascular bypass surgery, what follow-up would you recommend?

✦ After successful reconstruction and healing, clinical follow-up involves frequent **duplex examinations of the graft** to allow early detection of graft stenoses. Most surgeons would place the patient on **aspirin**, advise **control of serum lipids**, and provide **education** about foot care.

◆ What condition is most likely to cause this patient's death?

✦ Peripheral vascular disease is a marker for diffuse atherosclerotic disease. Therefore, this patient is most likely to die as a result of coronary artery disease.

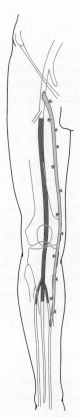

Figure 5-15: A femoral distal bypass procedure for distal popliteal obstruction.

QUICK CUT Although for proximal peripheral arterial bypass, PTFE and saphenous vein have similar long term patency, as the bypass becomes more distal, the patency of PTFE grafts falls off significantly. On the other hand, prosthetic grafts (PTFE and Dacron) in aortic positions perform exceedingly well.

Table 5-11: Four-Year Patency of Femoral-Popliteal Bypass Grafts

Above-Knee Bypass	
Using saphenous vein	69%
Using PTFE	60%
Below-Knee Popliteal Bypass	
Using saphenous vein	77%
Using PTFE	40%
Infrapopliteal Bypass Graft	
Using saphenous vein	62%
Using PTFE	21%

PTFE, polytetrafluoroethylene.

Case 5.8   Aortoiliac Occlusive Disease

A 61-year-old man reports calf and thigh pain on exertion, which is slowly relieved by rest. He also complains of impotence, and he has smoked one and one half packs per day for 30 years. Physical examination reveals absent femoral and lower extremity pulses bilaterally and stigmata of chronic vascular insufficiency in the lower legs.

◆ **How would you evaluate this patient?**

◆ Because the man most likely has aortoiliac occlusive disease secondary to atherosclerosis (Leriche syndrome), ABI measurements and a general medical assessment are appropriate.

> **QUICK CUT** The decision regarding whether to reconstruct his aortoiliac arterial system is based on his operative risk, his discomfort level, and whether or not he has rest pain or ulceration.

Aortoiliac occlusive disease is progressive. Most surgeons would not wait for rest pain or ulceration to develop because these conditions make the procedure more urgent and introduce the added risk of infection from the ulcer to the new vascular graft. An exercise program could be attempted, but few data support its benefit. As with lower extremity disease, an arteriogram should not be performed until a decision to proceed with surgery has been made.

You decide that the patient's symptoms are sufficiently severe that intervention is necessary. The arteriogram shows occlusion of the common and external iliac arteries, with a patent distal aorta and femoral artery.

◆ **How would you manage this patient?**

◆ Several management options are available.

- **Lifestyle modification** is appropriate if the **operative risk for any procedure is prohibitive.** However, without surgery, the patient will most likely progress to amputation or death.
- **Percutaneous transluminal angioplasty (PTA)**, often performed at the time of angiography, is ideal if the patient has **a single, short-segment iliac stenosis.** For common iliac disease, 5-year patency rates approach those of aortobifemoral bypass.
- **Aortobifemoral bypass** is appropriate in this patient, who has **bilateral loss of femoral pulses** and occlusion of the entire iliac system. In a patient who is a poor risk, an alternate procedure that **avoids a large transabdominal maneuver** may be advisable. In such a setting, an axillofemoral bypass graft may be considered. If one femoral artery were patent, a femorofemoral bypass could be performed (Fig. 5-16).

The patient's medical condition is amenable to an aortobifemoral bypass graft, and you decide to perform the procedure.

> **QUICK CUT** Aortobifemoral bypass is still the most durable of all treatment options for aortoiliac disease.

Figure 5-16: A: Aortogram of complete juxtarenal aortic occlusion with retrograde thrombosis to the level of renal artery runoff. (From Mulholland MW, Lillemoe KD, Doherty G, et al. *Greenfield's Surgery: Scientific Principles and Practice*, 5th ed. Philadelphia: Lippincott Williams & Wilkins; 2010.) **B:** drawing of an iliac artery stent, **(C)** drawing of an aortoiliac endoprosthesis, **(D)** drawing of an aortoiliac vascular graft, **(E)** drawing of an axillofemoral vascular graft.

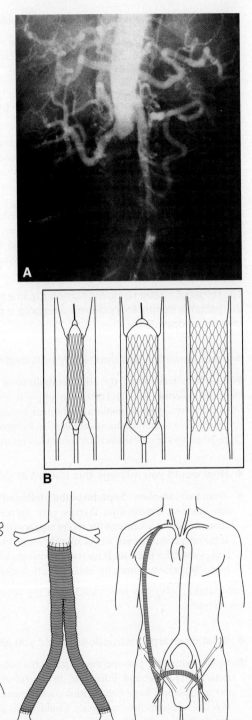

◆ **What are the basic steps in this revascularization operation?**

◆ The abdominal aorta from the level of the renal vein to the distal obstruction is isolated, the vessels are clamped, and a prosthetic graft of Dacron or expanded polytetrafluoroethylene is used to bypass the obstructed segment.

◆ **What part of an aortobifemoral bypass graft operation has the greatest cardiovascular risk?**

◆ As with most operations, **risk is *high* during induction of anesthesia and times of hemorrhage or other stress.** In this particular procedure, the heart is also at increased risk during **aortic clamping and unclamping.** During clamping, the afterload is markedly increased, raising cardiac work. Anticipating clamping and using afterload reduction techniques reduce this stress. During unclamping, there is the risk of bleeding from the graft. The sudden decrease in afterload that occurs due to revascularization of the vasodilated lower torso and extremities and the possible hypotension both demand increased cardiac output. In addition, unclamping flushes blood from the lower body. While this blood is static, it becomes acidotic and hyperkalemic. When released, it may adversely affect cardiac function and rhythm.

The revascularization proceeds smoothly. In a postoperative examination to evaluate the patient's peripheral perfusion, you note a painful, cyanotic big toe that was not present preoperatively.

◆ **What condition has most likely occurred?**

◆ So-called "**trash foot**," the **atheroembolization** of fibrin, platelets, or dislodged atherosclerotic debris, has blocked the small pedal or digital arteries and microvessels during unclamping. Atheroembolization limited to small pedal or digital vessels is generally inaccessible to embolectomy catheters. In the presence of patent tibial vessels and palpable pedal pulses, significant healing commonly results.

◆ **How would you manage this patient at this time?**

◆ Treatment involves **heparinization followed by long-term antiplatelet therapy.** Site-directed thrombolytic therapy may decrease the area of injury but it is usually contraindicated because of the recent surgery (thrombolysis can result in massive bleeding at the operative site even weeks after the surgery). The toe should be protected from injury and assessed for necrosis. If necrosis is present, debridement or minor amputation, which is typically performed once the area has fully demarcated, may be necessary.

The patient, who has recovered from the revascularization procedure, is ready to return home.

◆ **What discharge instructions would you give?**

◆ In the immediate postoperative period, the patient should watch for evidence of infection, including wound infections. In the future, he should seek medical attention for any unexplained fever because this could represent a graft infection, a serious complication. In addition, most surgeons would begin **aspirin therapy** and would recommend **prophylactic antibiotics** similar to bacterial endocarditis guidelines for other procedures that carry a risk of infection.

Case 5.9 Cardiac Risk in Major Vascular Reconstruction

A 68-year-old man with severe stenosis of his distal aorta and iliac arteries needs an aortoiliac graft.

◆ **What is the likelihood that a cardiac event will occur during the patient's surgery?**

◆ In a major vascular reconstruction, **MI, arrhythmia, or heart failure occur perioperatively in up to 10% of patients**, depending on the method of detection and the patient's comorbid conditions. MI rates following infrainguinal bypass are equivalent to those of aortoiliac bypass. Vascular surgery is generally associated with a cardiac mortality of approximately 2%–3%.

◆ **What preoperative evaluation would you perform to assess the patient's ability to tolerate the procedure?**

◆ A careful history, physical examination, and laboratory examination to check his cardiac, neurologic, pulmonary, and renal status are necessary. This patient, like most others, should undergo a carotid duplex study, a screening procedure for carotid artery disease.

The patient's **cardiac status** is the most important medical consideration prior to major abdominal revascularization. Most vascular patients have underlying coronary artery disease to varying degrees, and they should undergo cardiac risk assessment with some form of stress test or cardiac catheterization. As many as 70% of perioperative and late fatalities after peripheral vascular surgery are due to cardiac events.

◆ **What constitutes the patient's cardiac evaluation?**

◆ Cardiac risk assessment in vascular patients remains controversial, despite extensive studies based on numerous cardiac risk indices (e.g., Goldman Risk Assessment) and diagnostic modalities to identify a subgroup of patients who would most benefit from aggressive cardiac testing.

> **QUICK CUT** Although there is general agreement that severe, unstable, or post-MI angina requires coronary catheterization and that truly asymptomatic patients can often proceed with vascular surgery, considerable debate regarding appropriate workup for those with chronic stable angina continues.

Some experts routinely recommend coronary angiography, and others believe that essentially no preoperative testing is necessary. When significant coronary artery disease is found, prophylactic CABG may be recommended. In general, patients whose coronary artery disease is severe enough to warrant prophylactic CABG have a higher mortality rate than those patients with vascular disease who do not need CABG.

Most surgeons promote selective use of noninvasive testing and coronary revascularization. Stress echocardiography, ambulatory Holter monitoring, and in particular, **dipyridamole-thallium scintigraphy (DTS)** are the most useful procedures (Fig. 5-17). When DTS is used to rule out cardiac ischemia, it has an excellent negative predictive value (96%–99%) but a poor positive predictive value (1%–20%), resulting in a high rate of coronary angiograms. Although standard electrocardiography (ECG) may suggest coronary artery disease, a normal ECG does not exclude significant disease. The usefulness of stress ECG is limited; due to claudication, a large number of patients are unable to complete the protocol.

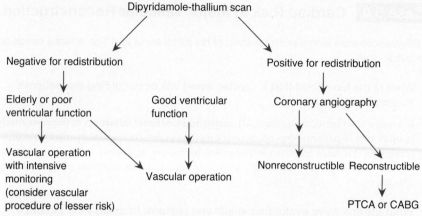

Figure 5-17: Decision-making algorithm for management of heart disease in patients undergoing vascular surgery. PTCA, percutaneous transluminal coronary angioplasty; CABG, coronary artery bypass graft.

 QUICK CUT A left ventricular ejection fraction of less than 30% is a reliable indicator of postoperative heart failure but does not adequately predict myocardium at risk for ischemia (i.e., MI).

◆ **What are your management options?**

◆ Once clinically significant coronary artery disease is identified, treatment options are varied.

- Cancellation or delay of surgery for intensive medical optimization
- Selection of a less invasive vascular procedure such as an extra-anatomic bypass or endovascular option
- Performance of a preoperative CABG or percutaneous transluminal coronary angioplasty to reduce the patient's cardiac risk
- Performance of the vascular surgery as scheduled, using intensive cardiac monitoring such as pulmonary artery catheters and/or transesophageal echocardiography, and accepting an increased cardiac risk

◆ **How would the presence of an MI 3 weeks prior influence the preoperative evaluation and/or the operative procedure?**

◆ At present, the patient is not at risk for immediate limb loss, and the vascular surgery remains an elective procedure. To reduce the intra- and postoperative risk of recurrent MI, the **vascular procedure should be delayed for at least 3 months**. During that time, the patient should be thoroughly evaluated to determine whether the patient should undergo coronary artery revascularization to improve blood flow in coronary lesions. If the patient has been revascularized, the cardiac risk approaches normal.

Case 5.10   Pulsatile Mass in the Abdomen

A 59-year-old man complains of a prominent bulge in his upper abdomen that seems to pulsate with every heartbeat. Physical examination confirms the finding of a non-tender, pulsatile, epigastric mass.

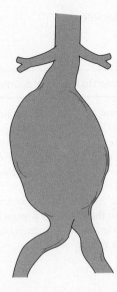

Figure 5-18: Drawing of an AAA.

◆ **How would you evaluate this patient?**

◆ An abdominal aortic aneurysm (AAA) is the suspected diagnosis in a patient with a pulsatile mass. The patient is pain-free and does not have symptoms suggestive of a ruptured AAA. Evaluation should begin with **ultrasound or CT examination** of the abdomen, which allows for reliable diagnosis, determination of the level of the aorta involved, and accurate measurement of the size of the AAA (Figs. 5-18 and 5-19).

◆ **What other aneurysms are associated with AAAs?**

◆ In general, aneurysms are more common in males, but in certain families, the male-to-female ratio is 4:1, and the incidence is increased 11 times in first-degree relatives. In persons with AAAs, the incidence of iliofemoral and popliteal aneurysms is increased. Fifty percent of patients with popliteal aneurysms have AAAs, and 50%–75% of popliteal aneurysms are bilateral.

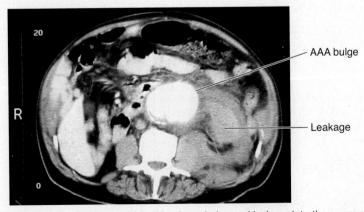

Figure 5-19: CT scan showing an AAA with a huge bulge and leakage into the surrounding tissue. This AAA was found, at operation, to be ruptured.

The CT scan reveals that the AAA is 7.0 cm in diameter.

◆ **What is the next appropriate step?**

QUICK CUT The size of an AAA is related to the risk of spontaneous rupture.

◆ Repair of the AAA may be necessary to prevent rupture, an occurrence that may lead to death.
Elective repair of AAAs that is 5.5 cm in men and 5 cm in woman or larger in greatest diameter is appropriate if the patient is likely to tolerate the procedure and has a life expectancy of more than 2 years. In asymptomatic patients with small AAA, most surgeons would follow the patient for development of enlargement as seen on ultrasound or development of symptoms. AAAs of this size can rupture, even though on average they enlarge at about 4 mm/year.

In addition, the operative risk is less when the AAA is smaller because most people are healthier when first seen for the condition than they are several years later. Certainly, patients with known or symptomatic cardiac disease should be appropriately assessed for operative risk and revascularized first prior to AAA repair.

◆ **What are the steps in the repair of an AAA?**

◆ An AAA can be repaired via an open approach or an endovascular approach. The endovascular repair can be done with a high success rate and low conversion to open rate. The best long-term approach has not been worked out, but most patients seem to prefer an endovascular approach if technically feasible. Whether done via an open technique (Fig. 5-20) or an endovascular technique, it is important to exclude the aneurysmal vessels to prevent future rupture while maintaining blood flow through the important vessels such as the iliac, femoral, and mesenteric arteries.

◆ **What postoperative problems are common following open AAA repair?**

◆ All patients who undergo repair of an AAA suffer postoperatively from major fluid shifts. In the initial 1–2 days after surgery, this patient will have large third-space losses and extra fluid requirements. By the third day, this patient, like most others, will be mobilizing this fluid; he may require diuresis and restriction of intravenous (IV) fluids. If these needs are

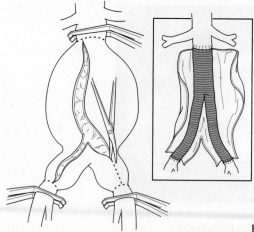

Figure 5-20: Operative repair of an AAA.

not anticipated, he may develop respiratory difficulties from pulmonary edema, resulting in unplanned reintubation.

This patient should also be carefully monitored for cardiac problems, including arrhythmias from the fluid and electrolyte shifts and MI from both the stress of the procedure and the effects of aortic clamping and unclamping.

◆ **What postoperative problems are common following endovascular AAA repair?**

◆ The endovascular approach is still a major operation with exposure of a major blood vessel such as the femoral artery for access to the vascular system. There is less operative dissection and potentially less fluid shifts and third-space losses. Still, there are significant complications specific to the endovascular approach. These include those associated with intravascular dye necessary for the procedure, particularly renal injury and allergy. Endovascular repair is associated with endoleak, where the aneurysm sac is perfused outside the lumen of the endograft. Endotension is the presence of pressure within the excluded aneurysm sac. The concern regarding endoleaks and endotension is that the pressure transmitted to the aneurysm wall may result in rupture of the aneurysm. Aneurysms repaired endovascularly need long-term follow-up for the presence of endoleaks.

The patient recovers from the surgery but returns to the office complaining of impotence.

◆ **What is your recommendation?**

◆ Any complaints of erectile dysfunction should be noted preoperatively because the incidence of this condition is high, and this knowledge would mean that this is not a postoperative complication. Erectile dysfunction may occur as a result of aortic dissection and interruption of the hypogastric circulation or autonomic nerves on the anterior surface of the aorta near the inferior mesenteric artery, which course over the aortic bifurcation. The patient should see a urologist for a more complete evaluation.

Case 5.11 Ruptured Abdominal Aortic Aneurysm

A 68-year-old man is brought to the emergency department appearing pale and in acute distress, with a BP of 105/60 mm Hg and a pulse rate of 120 beats per minute. Although he is obese, he has been in good health, but he passed out this morning in the bathroom. He complains of abdominal pain and weakness. His abdomen reveals tenderness in the epigastrium and suggestion of a pulsatile mass.

◆ **What is the likely diagnosis?**

◆ The syncope, hypotension, and a pulsatile abdominal mass are considered evidence of a ruptured AAA until proven otherwise. The **pulsatile mass** is a telltale sign but often is not present. In addition, the patient's history of syncope and abdominal pain is typical for a ruptured AAA, although other abdominal catastrophes can present in a similar fashion. It is **important to suspect a ruptured AAA because a delay in diagnosis is often fatal**. More than 50% of patients with this condition die before arriving at the emergency department (Table 5-12).

◆ **How would you evaluate and manage this patient?**

◆ Most surgeons would **proceed straight to the operating room** after a sample of the patient's blood is sent for typing, cross-matching, and routine laboratory studies and an ECG is obtained.

Table 5-12: **Risk of Rupture Data for AAA**

Size	Yearly Rate of Rupture (%)	5-Year Rupture Rate
<5 cm	~4%	~20%
5–7 cm	~7%	~33%
>7 cm	~19%	~95%

It is also known in autopsy series that up to 20% of ruptured AAA are 4–5 cm in diameter and 10% that are <4 cm rupture over time.

Active resuscitation in the emergency department may be counterproductive; an increase in volume and BP could convert a contained rupture into a free intraperitoneal rupture, resulting in death. Resuscitation can be better performed once the aorta is controlled either by cross clamp via the open approach or by balloon placed endovascularly in the operating room.

Suppose no hypotension or pulsatile abdominal mass is evident, but an AAA is suspected because of a history of syncope and abdominal pain.

◆ **How would your management change in this situation?**

◆ If the patient is hemodynamically stable, most surgeons would obtain a **CT scan or ultrasound of the abdomen** to visualize the aorta. If an AAA is present, especially with evidence of a nearby hematoma, the patient should go to the operating room.

◆ **How would you describe the surgical procedure?**

◆ This operation is similar to elective repair of an AAA and can be done open or through an endovascular approach depending on the anatomy of the aneurysm and the technical experience and facility resources. **The important first step is controlling the proximal aorta either by clamping via the open technique or with a balloon via the endovascular technique.**

◆ **What are the major perioperative risks in this patient?**

◆ Patients with ruptured AAAs have a higher risk of **exsanguination** in the operating room, leading to death. Perioperative mortality is around 50% and may be less if the procedure can be done through an endovascular approach. Postoperative complications include acute renal failure, MI, and multiorgan system failure.

Case 5.12   Complications of Abdominal Aortic Replacement

A 72-year-old man undergoes repair of a ruptured AAA. The surgery is difficult, but the bleeding is controlled and the aorta is repaired.

◆ **How would you manage the following findings?**

Case Variation 5.12.1. The patient develops fever and a small amount of bloody diarrhea on the third postoperative day.

◆ An **ischemic injury to colon,** which occurs in about 2%–3% of aortic reconstructions, is the suspected cause of the patient's symptoms. The ischemic colitis usually involves the rectosigmoid segment and is due to interruption of a patent inferior mesenteric artery in the setting of compromised collateral flow from the superior mesenteric and hypogastric arteries.

Postoperative symptoms include liquid brown or bloody diarrhea, abdominal pain or tenderness, prolonged ileus or increasing abdominal distention, and signs of sepsis or peritonitis.

Immediate sigmoidoscopy is necessary to diagnose ischemic bowel following AAA repair.

1. Treatment of ischemia (edema or hemorrhage) limited to the mucosa:
   ◆ Bowel rest, NG drainage, antibiotics
   ◆ Maintenance of adequate hydration, hematocrit, oxygenation and perfusion
   ◆ Frequent re-examination, including repeat endoscopy

2. Treatment for full-thickness necrosis of the bowel wall (50% mortality):
   ◆ resection of nonviable bowel, end colostomy and Hartman pouch

Case Variation 5.12.2. Two months later, the patient returns with a fever and an inflamed femoral incision.

◆ **Vascular graft infection**, one of the most serious complications of aortic surgery, is a concern. Graft infection most commonly results from contamination by skin flora, most often *Staphylococcus epidermidis* or *Staphylococcus aureus*, at the implantation site. Methicillin-resistant *Staphylococcus aureus* (MRSA) must always be considered as the pathogen until cultures and sensitivities are obtained. Clinical manifestations may not be evident for months to years postoperatively, particularly infection with *S. epidermidis*, which evades host defenses by production of glycocalyx slime. Presenting signs include systemic sepsis, wound abscess, pseudoaneurysm, sinus tract, GI hemorrhage, and abdominal or back pain. CT confirms the diagnosis.

 QUICK CUT Therapy usually involves complete removal of the graft, debridement of all infected tissues, revascularization by extra-anatomic bypass, and long-term antibiotics.

However, management is complex, and treatment is individualized.

Case Variation 5.12.3. One year later, the patient returns with an upper GI bleed.

◆ Any patient who has had aortic surgery and implantation of a vascular graft and develops upper GI bleeding should be carefully evaluated for an **aortoenteric fistula**. This lesion develops as the result of erosion of the graft into the third or fourth part of the duodenum. The diagnosis is confirmed by endoscopy, CT of the abdomen, or angiography. However, endoscopy may miss this lesion because the fistula is in the distal duodenum and is often difficult to visualize. Clinicians should persist with the workup even if the bleeding has stopped because many affected patients have a small, or sentinel, bleed followed 1 or 2 days later by a massive bleed. **Treatment usually requires removal of the graft, repair of the GI tract, and extra-anatomic bypass** (Figs. 5-21 and 5-22). Mortality or limb loss approaches 50%.

Case 5.13 Chronic Postprandial Abdominal Pain and Weight Loss

A 49-year-old woman presents with a 6-month history of postprandial abdominal pain, a 20-lb weight loss, and intermittent diarrhea. On physical examination, multiple abdominal bruits are evident.

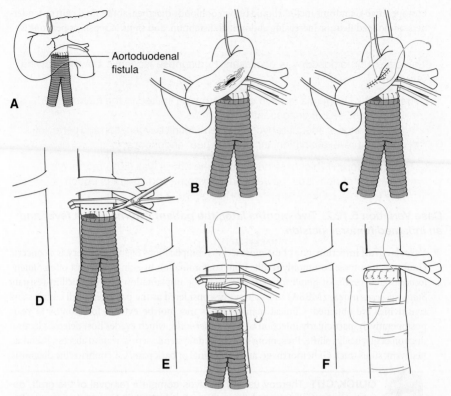

Figure 5-21: Anatomy and repair of aortoenteric fistula. If the aorta is grossly infected, it may require excision, closure of the proximal stump, and creation of an extra-anatomic bypass to perfuse the lower extremities. **A:** Anatomy. **B:** Separation of the duodenum from the aorta. **C:** Closure of the duodenum. **D:** Removal of the vascular graft. **E:** Closure of the proximal aortic stump. **F:** Reinforcement of the closure.

◆ **What is the suspected diagnosis?**

◆ The history and physical examination are typical of **chronic mesenteric ischemia**, which is usually secondary to atherosclerotic occlusion of the celiac and superior mesenteric arteries. Postprandial pain due to ischemia of the intestines causes fear of food, leading to weight loss. Heme-positive stools are usually not present. Signs and symptoms of atherosclerosis elsewhere in the body are also not unusual.

◆ **How would you evaluate and manage this patient?**

◆ If ischemia is suspected, the patient should first undergo a **mesenteric arteriogram** to establish a diagnosis and then planned revascularization, when appropriate to avoid later bowel infarction presenting urgently. **Revascularization can be** performed using a bypass graft from the aorta, which is reconnected to the superior mesenteric artery and celiac axis distal to the obstructions or via endovascular approach with angioplasty and stenting. Both prosthetic and saphenous vein grafts are used for this procedure (Fig. 5-23). The endovascular approach is becoming more commonplace; however, long-term data comparing endovascular repair versus open repair are lacking.

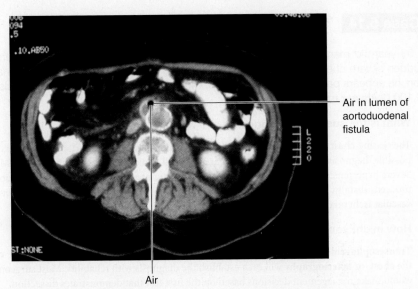

Air in lumen of
aortoduodenal
fistula

Air

Figure 5-22: CT scan showing aorta at area of aortoduodenal fistula. Dye can be seen extravasating into the duodenum, which has a small bubble of air within its lumen.

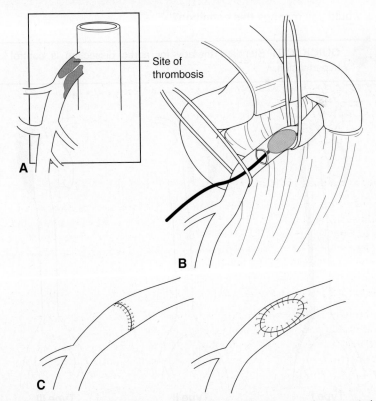

Site of
thrombosis

A

B

C

Figure 5-23: Revascularization of stenosis **(A)** or embolus **(B)** of the superior mesenteric artery. **C:** The arteriotomy can be repaired by end-to-end anastomosis with or without prosthetic graft or with a patch.

Case 5.14   Tearing Chest and Back Pain

A 58-year-old man is brought to the emergency department with diaphoresis and sudden severe chest and back pain that is tearing in nature. On physical examination, he appears pale and in acute distress, with a BP of 200/140 mm Hg and a pulse of 100 beats per minute.

◆ **What is the suspected diagnosis?**

◆ The tearing chest or back pain should make you quite suspicious of aortic dissection as a possible diagnosis. Affected patients appear acutely ill and diaphoretic, just as in acute MI. Severe hypertension is characteristic. The pain may migrate to other areas as the dissection proceeds distally. Stroke, paraplegia, mesenteric ischemia, renal ischemia, and peripheral vascular ischemia may also occur.

◆ **How might you evaluate this patient?**

◆ **Transesophageal echocardiography, magnetic resonance imaging (MRI), spiral CT of the chest, or arteriography** will each establish the diagnosis with reliability. Most surgeons would make management decisions based on the first test that demonstrates dissection.

You establish that the patient has a type III aortic dissection (Fig. 5-24).

◆ **How would you manage this condition?**

 QUICK CUT Standard therapy for aortic dissection is control of the hypertension.

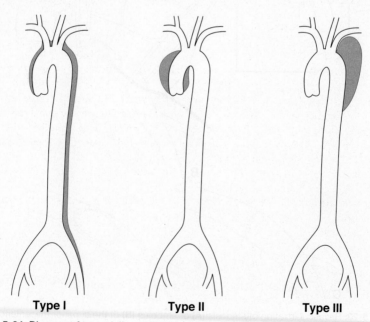

Type I   **Type II**   **Type III**

Figure 5-24: Diagram of types I, II, and III thoracic aortic dissections.

◆ Beta-blockers and other potent antihypertensive agents are effective. Conditions such as dissection of the ascending aorta, which are usually surgically repaired either open or endovascularly, are exceptions to medical management. Although aortic dissections are usually treated medically, if they are leaking, there is rupture, or there is compromise of a major aortic branch, surgery will be required. Endovascular or open surgery can be performed depending on patient anatomy and technical factors.

VENOUS DISEASE

Case 5.15 Postoperative Leg Swelling

A 67-year-old woman undergoes a colectomy for a colon polyp that cannot be removed by colonoscopy. She develops some mild swelling in the left leg postoperatively, and you become concerned that this might represent deep venous thrombosis (DVT).

◆ **How reliable is physical examination for diagnosing DVT?**

◆ Findings from history and physical examination are accurate only 50% of the time as diagnostic signs of DVT. Up to 50% of patients have occult DVT (i.e., with no signs or symptoms). The most common symptom is unilateral, dull leg pain that increases with movement. The **most reliable clinical sign of DVT is new-onset, unilateral leg swelling**, which is evaluated by comparing the circumference of the calf and thigh of the affected leg with that in the contralateral limb. Calf pain on dorsiflexion of the ankle (Homans sign), a palpable cord (often indicative of a thrombosed superficial vein), and thigh and/or calf tenderness, when they occur, are not reliable indicators for DVT (Fig. 5-25).

◆ **How would you verify the diagnosis?**

    QUICK CUT Duplex ultrasound is used to confirm the diagnosis of DVT.

◆ Duplex ultrasound combines B-mode ultrasound, which can visualize tissue structures, with Doppler ultrasound, which can detect flow in vessels. The sensitivity and specificity of this technique is more than 90% for the diagnosis of thrombi between the iliac vein and the knee (Fig. 5-26). Venous duplex ultrasound is considered the test of choice for the detection of DVT. Contrast venography, formerly the gold standard for the diagnosis of DVT, is now used only rarely.

Duplex examination of the common femoral vein reveals that it contains a thrombus, confirming the diagnosis of DVT. There is extension into the proximal thigh but no other abnormalities.

◆ **How would you treat the patient?**

◆ **Systemic anticoagulation is achieved with IV heparin or low-molecular-weight heparin.** A 70–100 U/kg bolus is given initially, followed by a maintenance infusion of 15–25 U/kg/hr administered for 4–6 days. It should be noted that heparin has an anti-inflammatory component that dramatically reduces the discomfort associated with DVT.

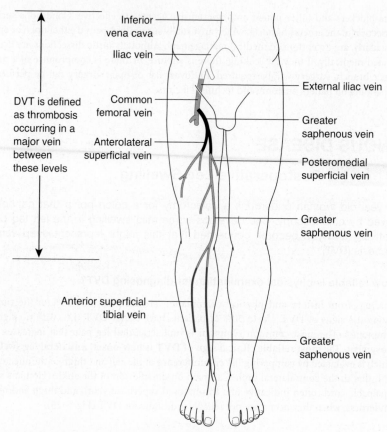

Inferior vena cava

Iliac vein

DVT is defined as thrombosis occurring in a major vein between these levels

Common femoral vein

Anterolateral superficial vein

External iliac vein

Greater saphenous vein

Posteromedial superficial vein

Greater saphenous vein

Anterior superficial tibial vein

Greater saphenous vein

Figure 5-25: Drawing showing the anatomic definition of DVT.

Both **standard heparin and low-molecular-weight heparin** (LMWH) are effective in anticoagulation. LMWH, which is produced by the fractionation of heparin and possesses significant antifactor-Xa activity, does not anticoagulate to the same extent as unfractionated heparin as measured by the partial thromboplastin time (PTT), but it has a strong therapeutic effect.

◆ **How would you monitor the patient's treatment?**

◆ The patient's **PTT should be followed and maintained 1.5–2 times the normal value** if the heparin administration is to remain therapeutic. The half-life of heparin is approximately 90 minutes, so the PTT should be evaluated 6 hours after the initial dose, every 8 hours for the next 24 hours, and once a day thereafter. Because approximately 5% of patients taking heparin develop **thrombocytopenia**, the patient's platelet counts must be followed. Paradoxic arterial thrombosis associated with heparin-induced thrombocytopenia may also develop. If this condition develops, the heparin should be discontinued. Newer methods using LMWH in home settings to treat DVT are under study; these approaches may be as effective as inpatient treatment and reduce costs dramatically.

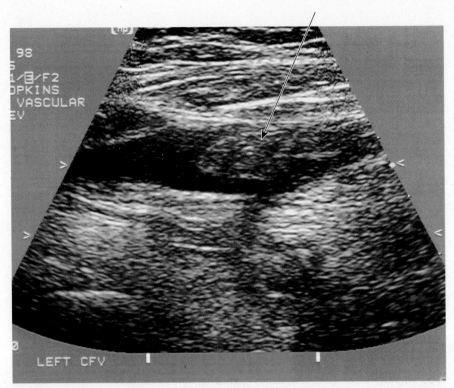

Figure 5-26: Duplex study demonstrating thrombus (*arrow*) within the common femoral vein.

◆ **What long-term treatment plan is appropriate?**

◆ **After the diagnosis of DVT is made, anticoagulation therapy must be continued for 3–6 months.** Warfarin (Coumadin) may be started within the first few days of heparin administration, although the patient should receive 5–7 days of heparin therapy. Warfarin is an anticoagulant that inhibits hepatic synthesis of vitamin K–dependent clotting factors II, VII, IX, and X; it also decreases production of protein C and S. The inhibitory effect lasts 1–10 days, depending on coagulation factor. Goals of therapy are to achieve and maintain an international normalized ratio (INR) of 2.0–3.0 (1.3–1.5 times control prothrombin time) for 3–6 months. Warfarin can induce a protein C deficiency (a relative hypercoagulable state) early after treatment is begun, so patients must remain on heparin for several days after warfarin is started.

◆ **What do you tell the patient about the long-term morbidity of DVT?**

◆ **Recurrence and post-thrombotic syndrome** are the two principal complications of DVT that are likely to develop. Recurrence is most common in the first several months following the initial episode (Fig. 5-27). Therapy involves admission and IV heparin. Long-term treatment with warfarin should also be considered following discharge. At all future admissions, patients with a history of DVT should be considered at high risk for the development of DVT and should receive DVT prophylaxis. Chronic venous insufficiency occurs about 25% of the time after appropriate anticoagulation for DVT. This disease can be very debilitating; therefore, the uses of thrombolytic agents are becoming more commonplace in an attempt to clear the clot rapidly and prevent long-term chronic venous insufficiency. All patients

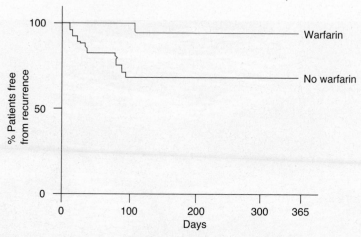

Figure 5-27: Graph of the incidence of recurrent DVT versus time after DVT.

who have DVT are likely to demonstrate venous valvular insufficiency and a tendency to develop edema in the involved extremity. Chronic use of support hose will lessen the edema and easy fatigability in the leg.

Case 5.16 Prevention of Deep Venous Thrombosis

A 55-year-old man has a substantial hernia, which is occasionally painful and has been enlarging. His past history is significant for a right colectomy 4 years ago for carcinoma of the colon. Physical examination reveals a moderately obese patient with a large, easily reducible, ventral hernia. No other significant physical findings are present. Your attending physician asks the following.

◆ **Does the patient have any risk factors for DVT or pulmonary embolism (PE)?**

◆ DVT is defined as thrombosis of the larger veins that may affect either an upper or lower extremity. **In the leg, DVT may involve thrombosis of the popliteal vein, femoral venous system, iliac veins, or the inferior vena cava (IVC).** In the arm, DVT may involve thrombosis of the axillary, subclavian, innominate, or internal jugular veins. DVT develops following 20% of general surgical procedures and in as many as 70% of major orthopedic procedures that involve the leg (Fig. 5-28).

Risk factors for DVT and PE are the same: static blood flow, hypercoagulable states, and endothelial or intimal injury, which are generally known as the Virchow triad. Many conditions may lead to DVT (Table 5-13). In this patient, obesity, increased age, and a history of carcinoma each may contribute to an increased risk. Of these conditions, certain ones have lower or higher risks for DVT and PE (Table 5-14).

Because the patient is at increased risk for DVT, you would like to use **DVT prophylactic therapy.**

> **QUICK CUT** Two preventive measures whose effectiveness has been clearly demonstrated are intermittent pneumatic compression devices and low-dose anticoagulation.

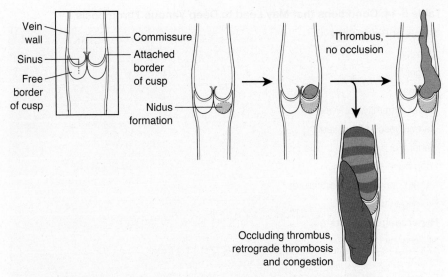

Figure 5-28: Drawing of the relationship between DVT and venous incompetence.

Table 5-13: Risk Factors for Deep Venous Thrombosis

Low Risk
Healthy patient younger than age 40 years
Short-duration surgery
Bleeding disorders, such as chronic renal or hepatic failure
Moderate Risk
Patients older than age 40 years
Moderate-length procedure (2–3 hours)
Upper abdominal and chest surgery
Minor risk factors such as obesity, smoking
High Risk
Older patients
Previous DVT or PE
Long-duration surgery
Pelvic or orthopedic surgery
Major surgery for cancer
Procoagulant states, such as polycythemia vera
Hyperviscosity syndromes, such as multiple myeloma
History of MI, congestive heart failure, or COPD

DVT, deep venous thrombosis; PE, pulmonary embolism; MI, myocardial infarction; COPD, chronic obstructive pulmonary disease.

Table 5-14: Conditions that May Lead to Deep Venous Thrombosis

Stasis of Blood Flow

Obesity

Surgery

Trauma

Lower extremity paralysis

Cerebrovascular accident

General or spinal anesthesia

Long bone fractures

MI with congestive heart failure

Prolonged bed rest

Hypercoagulable States

Malignancy

Pregnancy

Puerperium (first 42 days postpartum)

Oral contraceptive use

Polycythemia vera

Connective tissue disease

Antithrombin III deficiency

Protein C or S deficiency

Disseminated intravascular coagulation

Heparin-associated thrombocytopenia

Thrombosis

Inflammatory bowel disease

Nephrotic syndrome

Myeloproliferative disorders

Homocystinemia

Lupus with anticardiolipin antibodies

Paroxysmal nocturnal hemoglobinuria

Intimal Injury

Surgical injury

Trauma

Indwelling catheters

Varicose veins

Advanced age

Pacemaker wires

History of DVT

Operative manipulation

The terms in boldface type are often referred to as Virchow triad.
MI, myocardial infarction; DVT, deep venous thrombosis.

Intermittent pneumatic compression devices are thought to increase venous velocity as well as increase blood fibrinolytic activity. LMWH or low-dose unfractionated heparin can be used for DVT prophylaxis, although data shows that LMWH is more efficacious. Intermittent compression and low-dose anticoagulation have comparable prevention efficacy and may enhance prophylaxis even further when used concurrently.

You decide to use LMWH.

Case 5.17   Postoperative Shortness of Breath

A 50-year-old man, who is otherwise healthy, undergoes a laparotomy for small bowel obstruction due to adhesions. He has been doing well postoperatively. On the morning of the fourth postoperative day, he relates a brief episode of shortness of breath that occurred the previous night. No new findings are apparent on examination. The man's vital signs are all within normal limits, his lungs are clear and heart sounds are normal, his wound looks fine, and his abdomen is flat and not distended.

◆ **What potential problems could explain this episode?**

◆ The long list of potential causes includes asthma, bronchospasm, aspiration, chronic obstructive pulmonary disease (COPD), paroxysmal nocturnal dyspnea, anxiety, PE, MI, pneumothorax, and infection. The etiology of the episode is more likely to be acute because there is no history of chronic pulmonary or cardiac problems. Because of the brief episodic nature of the incident and the absence of physical findings, **PE is suspected** and an effort should be made to rule it out.

◆ **What would be your initial steps to establish a diagnosis?**

◆ An appropriate history and physical examination should be performed. Common practice involves obtaining an ECG to investigate for MI as well as an arterial blood gas (ABG) measurement and pulse oximetry. The most common ABG abnormality is a **decreased Pco_2 due to hyperventilation**; a decreased Po_2 is less likely. A chest x-ray (CXR) should be performed to examine for pneumonia, atelectasis, and pneumothorax. If no diagnosis is evident at this time, a CT pulmonary angiogram should be performed.

A PE is seen on the CT scan (Fig. 5-29).

◆ **What would be your next step?**

◆ Confirmation of the diagnosis of PE is necessary, although some clinicians might treat the patient for PE at this point. This most commonly involves the performance of a CT pulmonary angiogram. If IV contrast cannot be used secondary to an allergy or renal insufficiency, then a pulmonary ventilation-perfusion scan can be performed.

A diagnosis of PE has been established.

◆ **How would you treat the patient?**

◆ **Treatment of PE, which is identical to treatment of DVT** (see Case 5.16), involves IV heparin. An initial bolus of 5,000–10,000 U of heparin IV followed by an IV heparin drip of 1,000 U/hr is appropriate. This dose would be adjusted to maintain PTT ~2 times the control. The patient would then be started on warfarin (Coumadin) and treated similarly to a patient with DVT.

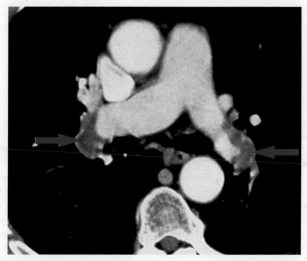

Figure 5-29: CT demonstrates filling defect in the right and left PAs diagnostic of pulmonary embolism (*arrows*). (From Brant WE, Helms C. *Fundamentals of Diagnostic Radiology*, 4th ed. Philadelphia: Lippincott Williams & Wilkins; 2012.)

◆ **What are the long-term complications of PE?**

◆ Most patients recover fully after anticoagulation therapy and demonstrate no evidence of pulmonary insufficiency, pulmonary hypertension, or recurrent embolism. Perfusion scans performed 1 month later have usually returned to baseline. Elderly individuals and patients with pre-existing cardiopulmonary disease are exceptions.

Case 5.18 Confounding Findings in Pulmonary Embolism

A 48-year-old man recently underwent a colectomy. On the third postoperative day, he develops acute shortness of breath. After examination, you suspect PE, and you initiate an evaluation.

◆ **How would you manage the patient with these findings?**

Case Variation 5.18.1. Normal ECG

◆ A normal ECG does not rule out either MI or PE, although MI is unlikely. Evaluation should continue.

Case Variation 5.18.2. Normal CXR

◆ A normal CXR rules out pathologic processes such as pneumothorax, pneumonia, and larger areas of atelectasis but not PE or areas of microatelectasis. Pre-existing pulmonary disease such as COPD, bronchitis, and restrictive disease can complicate interpretation of the CXR, particularly if a pre-existing CXR is not available for comparison to separate old disease from new-onset disease. Evaluation should continue.

Case Variation 5.18.3. Small right pneumothorax on CXR

◆ The pneumothorax is the likely cause of the shortness of breath. This patient is symptomatic with shortness of breath and should have a tube thoracostomy chest tube inserted.

Case Variation 5.18.4. *Right basilar atelectasis on CXR*

◆ If this is a new finding, it may explain the patient's symptoms. If not, CT pulmonary angiogram is the next step.

Case 5.19 Recurrent Pulmonary Embolism on Anticoagulation Therapy

A 24-year-old man who was in an automobile crash and required a chest tube for a pneumothorax has developed shortness of breath. After an evaluation, you diagnosed a PE and began standard therapy with IV heparin. The patient has been fully heparinized for 3 days and doing well, with a PTT consistently maintained at twice controls level. Bowel function has returned to normal, and he has had no recurrent episodes of dyspnea, chest pain, or complications from the heparin treatment.

A nurse reports an acute episode in which the patient was extremely short of breath. His BP was 90/60 mm Hg for several minutes, and he appeared ashen and cyanotic. The nurse administered nasal oxygen, "turned up" his IV fluids, and is now calling you. The patient's vital signs have returned to normal, and he is feeling better. On examination, you note a heart rate of 120 beats per minute, a respiratory rate of 28 breaths per minute, and a normal BP. The lungs are clear and heart sounds are normal. The abdomen is flat with no pain or tenderness, and the wound is healing normally.

◆ **How would you establish the correct diagnosis?**

◆ The patient, who most likely has either a recurrent PE or an acute MI, should be transferred to the intensive care unit. A rapid evaluation, including a brief history and physical examination, pulse oximetry, ECG, ABG, and CXR, is necessary. He should undergo a repeat CT pulmonary angiogram and have a workup for MI, including evaluation of cardiac isoenzymes, serial ECGs, and cardiology consultation. In addition, his PTT should be checked again to determine the degree to which he is anticoagulated.

The CT pulmonary angiogram reveals a new segmental perfusion defect in the lung opposite to the side of the first PE. There is no evidence of an acute MI. The patient continues to be fully anticoagulated.

◆ **How would you manage this patient?**

◆ He most likely has a **recurrent PE**. Let us assume that he has remained therapeutically anticoagulated with no lapses in treatment.

 QUICK CUT A PE on heparin therapy represents a failure of anticoagulant therapy.

Because this lung scan confirms the diagnosis of recurrent PE with reasonable certainty, a second-line method of PE prevention is necessary. The most acceptable form of additional protection is **IVC interruption** using an IVC filter, a metal device placed in the infrarenal IVC using a percutaneous technique (Fig. 5-30). The device is safe and prevents recurrent PE in more than 95% of patients. The knowledge that more than 90% of pulmonary emboli originate from the lower extremities is the basis of the infrarenal location. The most common indications for the Greenfield filter are heparin failure to prevent PE and heparin

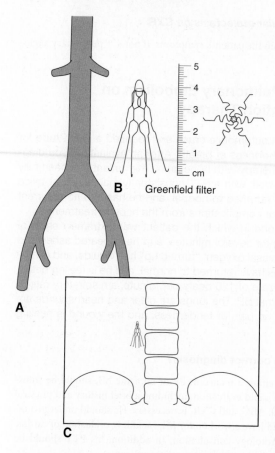

B   Greenfield filter

A

C

Figure 5-30: A–C: Drawing of a Greenfield filter in the inferior vena cava.

complications such as bleeding. If no anticoagulation contraindication exists, most surgeons would maintain therapeutic anticoagulation for 3–6 months.

Case 5.20   Gastrointestinal Bleeding as a Complication of Anticoagulation Therapy

A 60-year-old woman with chronic rheumatoid arthritis that has been treated with nonsteroidal anti-inflammatory drugs (NSAIDs) undergoes an elective left knee joint replacement. She develops evidence of DVT postoperatively, and duplex examination confirms the diagnosis of DVT of the left femoral vein. Accordingly, she receives an IV heparin bolus of 5,000 U followed by a heparin drip infusion of 1,000 U/hr, which maintains her PTT at 2 times control. On the third day of heparin therapy, she vomits 100 mL of bright red blood but otherwise feels fine and has stable vital signs.

◆ **How would you evaluate and manage this patient?**

◆ Because upper GI bleeding represents a life-threatening condition, **systemic anticoagulation should be discontinued immediately. Alternate PE protection with IVC interruption** using a device such as the IVC filter should be provided. Appropriate antiulcer therapy should be instituted and the patient further evaluated for the source of bleeding.

Case 5.21   Severe Deep Venous Thrombosis

A 60-year-old woman with advanced carcinoma of the cervix with extension into the left pelvic wall presents with an acute episode where her left leg became very edematous, cyanotic, and painful.

◆ **What diagnosis would you suspect?**

◆ This patient most likely has **phlegmasia cerulea dolens,** which is acute interruption of the venous outflow from obstruction secondary to her pelvic malignancy (phlegmasia means inflammation, cerulea means cyanotic, and dolens means painful). A contributing factor may be a relatively hypercoagulable state as a result of her carcinoma.

　　If not treated immediately, phlegmasia cerulea dolens may lead to sensory and motor loss and possibly **venous gangrene.**

　　This condition is an extreme form of iliocaval DVT, with obstruction so severe that it can impair arterial inflow to the leg.

◆ **How would you manage this patient?**

◆ **Treatment involves anticoagulation and leg elevation,** with careful observation of the viability of the tissues. Once treatment is initiated, evaluation with duplex ultrasound and CT scan of the pelvis to confirm the diagnosis can proceed. Occasionally, contrast venography is necessary. The majority of patients with early phlegmasia improve with leg elevation and systemic anticoagulation. In rare instances, venous thrombectomy may be indicated.

Chapter 6

Upper Gastrointestinal Tract Disorders

Bruce E. Jarrell, John L. Flowers, Molly Buzdon, Eric D. Strauch

Key Thoughts

1. When evaluating a patient for acute abdominal pain, it is imperative that the clinician first determines whether the patient has an acute or "surgical" abdomen on examination. An acute abdomen is generally described as having diffuse severe tenderness and pain, rebound tenderness, and abdominal guarding. Other surgical indicators include the presence of extraluminal or free air on radiographic study, signs of ischemic tissue with acidosis, elevated lactate, tachycardia, and hypotension. If present, immediate intervention is indicated to control the acute process, such as a leak, ischemic bowel, or infection.

2. When faced with gastrointestinal hemorrhage, it is important to localize the location of the bleeding and formulate a plan to control it before surgery. In part, this is because it is very difficult to identify the source of bleeding in the operating room by evaluating the external surface of the gastrointestinal tract.

3. Although restoration of circulation and correction of coagulation defects is crucial to the care of the patient with gastrointestinal hemorrhage, controlling the hemorrhage is the most important step for patient resuscitation. Transfusing blood and blood products beyond several units results in increased morbidity and mortality.

4. Gastroesophageal reflux disease (GERD) is a clinical diagnosis. Esophagogastroduodenoscopy (EGD) is not required except for patients who are older or have weight loss, who are not responding to medical management, or who have dysphagia or other obstructive symptoms. If antireflux surgery is planned, it is critical to document that normal esophageal peristalsis is present.

5. Paraesophageal hernias should be surgically repaired.

6. Gastric ulcers are associated with risk for cancer.

7. Prophylaxis with proton pump inhibitors (PPI) for stress ulcer and upper gastrointestinal (UGI) bleeding should be considered for patients with mechanical ventilation, coagulopathy, sepsis, multiorgan failure, prior UGI bleed, and neurologic trauma, among others.

8. A duodenal ulcer that has recently bled, and which has a visible artery in its base, has a high risk for rebleeding.

9. Renal failure is associated with platelet dysfunction and elevated bleeding time and is partially corrected with fresh frozen plasma (FFP) or arginine vasopressin (DDAVP) during an acute bleed.

10. Liver failure has an elevated international normalized ratio (INR) due to deficiency of factors II, VII, IX, and X which is corrected with FFP in an acute bleed and vitamin K. It also is associated with thrombocytopenia due to hypersplenism.

11. *Helicobacter* infections are associated with mucosa-associated lymphoid tissue gastric lymphoma.

Deep Thoughts

In each of the cases presented in the next three chapters, the authors have classified disorders based on the anatomic location of involved organs. In real life, patients may present with a variety of signs and symptoms which may, or may not, align with the anatomic location of the abnormality.

For the acute bleeding cases, the thinking is relatively straightforward and is described in the cases.

For the acute pain cases, narrowing the source of pain down to an organ system is extremely important but the early steps may be very difficult to do accurately and can involve such a wide variety of organs and systems that they are not easily described in the cases. Thus, an initial step is to focus on the entire patient and expeditiously assess other pertinent systems. The authors' thinking would be as follows.

In addition to the common abdominal disorders, there are a number of common nonabdominal or nongastrointestinal disorders that can present with acute abdominal findings and which are important to consider as part of the initial assessment. In general, a good way to think about processes that may be outside the abdomen but produce abdominal pain is as follows:

◆ What anatomic structures lie in close proximity to the peritoneal cavity and thus the peritoneum?
◆ What acute inflammatory, infectious, neoplastic, and ischemic events can occur in those structures?
◆ Which of these combinations are common in people, particularly relative to their age, gender, environment, and lifestyle?
◆ How urgent is the complaint and is the patient presenting in the office or emergency department?

Examples of this thinking which are common and which can present with abdominal pain and other abdominal symptoms include the following:

◆ Acute myocardial infarction (MI) occurring on the inferior aspect of the heart (ischemic event that can irritate the central area of the diaphragm)
◆ Pneumonias and pulmonary infarcts occurring at the base of a lung (infectious or ischemic event that can irritate the peripheral areas of the diaphragm)
◆ Leaking abdominal aortic aneurysm (a mass effect from the bleed in the retroperitoneal location which involves the peritoneum, local nerves, muscles, and other structures)
◆ Other examples: renal stones, genitourinary infections, retroperitoneal processes (such as hematomas, abscesses, neoplasms), muscular and neural disorders of abdominal area (such as occult trauma, vertebral compressions), and metabolic disorders (such as diabetes)

The best way to approach any clinical patient would include a differential diagnosis. This list of possible diagnoses is a good starting point for evaluation of the patient. The differential diagnosis should include likely diagnoses as well as those diagnoses with high morbidity and mortality. Evaluation should begin with the most dangerous diagnoses by performing tests and interventions that are high yield and simple and fast to obtain. Many of these conditions are potentially life-threatening and must certainly be evaluated before proceeding to less urgent abdominal conditions. An approach combines general assessment with specific abdominal assessment. For example, if the patient is in moderate abdominal distress and cardiac examination and studies show evidence for acute ischemia, there are several possible paths to follow:

◆ With a soft abdominal exam, the patient may have a primary cardiac explanation producing the perception of abdominal pain. This initial suspicion would lead you down the cardiac path of evaluation as the first priority. Is there an acute MI?
◆ Whereas with diffuse severe abdominal pain but limited abdominal tenderness on exam and also with new onset atrial fibrillation, the patient may have a primary cardiac problem that has resulted in an arterial embolus to the bowel. This initial suspicion would lead you to urgently investigate the two possibilities—is there an acute MI and is the bowel ischemic or necrotic?
◆ Whereas with signs of chest pain and diffuse acute peritoneal tenderness and guarding, the patient may have an intra-abdominal cause (such as a perforated hollow viscus due to a gastric or duodenal ulcer) that is irritating the diaphragm and causing the cardiac abnormalities. This initial suspicion would lead you to urgently investigate for evidence of bowel perforation. Is there free intraperitoneal air or radiologic imaging evidence for an abdominal process (see Case 6.7 and its variations)?

These examples demonstrate that there is no single correct approach to abdominal pain. However, variables which point to a more urgent problem include the following:

◆ Higher intensity of the patient's distress, pain, and anxiety
◆ Significant past history for coexisting disease (such as peripheral vascular disease) or medications with risk (such as steroids or nonsteroidal anti-inflammatory drugs [NSAIDs])
◆ More concerning abdominal physical, such as abdominal wall rigidity
◆ Cardiac arrhythmia, severe hypertension, hypotension, marked dehydration, lethargy, and fever

Thus, if these types of findings are present, then the situation is more urgent and thinking such as that described earlier should be prioritized. If they are not, then less urgent conditions may be present. The following chapters are generally aimed to help you think through these less urgent conditions associated with abdominal pain.

Case 6.1 Acute Epigastric Pain No. 1

A 34-year-old man presents with acute onset of sharp epigastric pain that has developed in 4 hours. He has been previously healthy. On physical examination, he appears in mild distress with moderate tenderness in the epigastrium. No masses are palpable.

Deep Thoughts

It is important to determine if on physical examination the patient has any signs of peritonitis. If so, then immediate surgical exploration should be considered for a perforated viscus, leaking AAA, or necrotic tissue.

◆ **What are the most likely diagnoses?**

◆ The differential diagnosis includes pancreatitis, peptic ulcer disease (PUD), gastric ulcer, gastroenteritis, GERD, and cholelithiasis.

◆ **What findings on history, physical examination, and initial laboratory studies support these diagnoses?**

◆ A history of gallstones or ethanol abuse suggests pancreatitis, which should be confirmed with a serum amylase and lipase. A history of use of NSAIDs or steroids suggests PUD.

◆ **What routine screening studies are appropriate?**

◆ A complete blood count (CBC), urinalysis, amylase, lipase, and liver function tests are necessary, as well as an obstructive series, which includes an upright chest x-ray (radiograph) (CXR).

The CBC, amylase and lipase, and bilirubin and alkaline phosphatase are normal. Chest and abdominal radiographs are unremarkable.

◆ **What is the next step?**

◆ The management of this patient is dependent on the location of care (i.e., office vs. emergency department) and the attending physician. Primary care physicians often begin diagnosis and treatment because this is the most cost-effective strategy. Most of these diagnoses are not surgical emergencies and can be electively evaluated after initiation of therapy to control the acute symptoms. Initial differential diagnoses include gallstones, GERD, gastritis, and peptic ulcer disease.

Many physicians obtain an **abdominal ultrasound to rule out gallstones. If the ultrasound is negative, then an empirical treatment course with an H₂ blocker or PPI to treat GERD, ulcer, or gastritis** is often appropriate.

Cases of suspected GERD warrant lifestyle modifications, including weight loss and avoiding meals before sleeping. It also means avoiding situations associated with GERD such as eating foods that decrease lower esophageal sphincter (LES) tone (e.g., chocolate, tea, coffee, alcohol) and sleeping flat in bed. This strategy results in improvement in 60%–70% of patients.

◆ **What would you do if the patient improves with this therapy?**

◆ Most physicians would simply follow such a patient and advise no further diagnostic procedures.

◆ **What would you do if the patient's symptoms persist?**

◆ If the medical management trial fails, then UGI endoscopy (EGD) is necessary to establish a diagnosis. This approach allows visualization of the esophagus, stomach, and duodenum, as well as biopsies to rule out any malignancies and to detect *Helicobacter pylori*.

> **QUICK CUT** Many physicians perform EGD after the first episode of significant epigastric pain, especially in older individuals or those with a higher risk of tumor or infection (e.g., immunosuppressed patients).

You perform EGD. No significant pathology is evident.

◆ **How would you manage this patient?**

◆ This patient, who most likely has nonulcer dyspepsia, should receive **symptomatic treatment with H₂ blockers or PPI, as well as treatment for *Helicobacter* infection, if documented.**

Case 6.2   Acute Epigastric Pain No. 2

You are following a 45-year-old man who has had an episode of epigastric pain presumed to be GERD that did not resolve on medical therapy. He is otherwise healthy and sees you regularly. You decide that EGD is necessary.

◆ **How would you manage the following findings on EGD?**

Case Variation 6.2.1. **GERD, which is symptomatic even with maximal therapy**

◆ This patient has failed medical therapy and is a candidate for antireflux surgery if you confirm the diagnosis. Guidelines for preoperative evaluation recommend that all patients considered for antireflux surgery should have EGD with biopsy and esophageal manometry. EGD is done to confirm that GERD is the underlying cause of the patient's symptoms, to determine if there are any pathologic changes to the esophageal mucosa, and to determine esophageal length. Manometry is critical to successful surgery (Fig. 6-1). It is necessary to **demonstrate intact esophageal peristalsis before surgery** to ensure that patients are able to swallow normally postoperatively.

  If the manometry shows normal LES tone or atypical symptoms such as cough or asthma, 24-hour pH probe testing is appropriate. If the patient has dysphagia or a suspected short esophagus, a cine-esophagogram to visualize the entire esophagus is also warranted. The standard operation is a **Nissen fundoplication** (Fig. 6-2). This operation restores the gastroesophageal junction and the LES (distal 5 cm of esophagus) to the normal intra-abdominal position and wraps a segment of stomach around the distal esophagus. This wrap augments LES tone while preserving LES relaxation during swallowing; therefore, it is functionally similar to a LES. If the esophagus does not have normal peristalsis, a Nissen fundoplication, which is 360 degrees, may impair esophageal emptying and a partial wrap would result in better symptom relief.

Case Variation 6.2.2. **Distal esophagitis**

◆ Esophagitis is a complication of GERD. It may be due to an incompetent LES, insufficient esophageal clearance of acid, or gastric dysfunction, causing increased intragastric pressure. Many patients with GERD have a hiatal hernia (the gastroesophageal junction is in the chest). However, most patients with a hiatal hernia do not necessarily have pathologic GERD. A 24-hour pH probe can be used to document the presence of acid reflux. Manometry is also performed to measure LES pressure and the length of the LES and to characterize the amplitude and coordination of esophageal contractions. **Medical therapy usually resolves GERD; a medical approach is warranted first.** This includes propping up the head of the patient's bed at night, eating frequent small meals, and not eating a late meal before bedtime. Mild to moderate esophagitis usually responds to 8–12 weeks of treatment with PPI. This causes complete remission in 85% of patients.

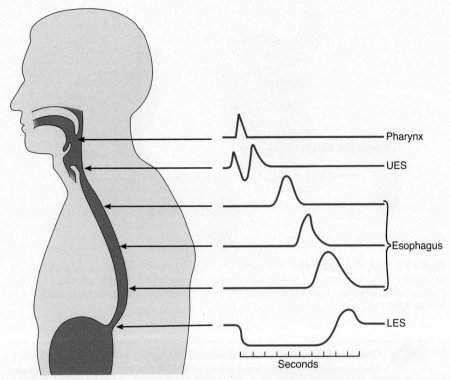

Figure 6-1: Intraluminal pressure of the esophagus using manometry. Swallowing is initiated as the upper and lower esophageal sphincters relax. A peristaltic contraction begins in the pharynx and travels progressively down through the esophagus. UES, upper esophageal sphincter; LES, lower esophageal sphincter. (From Castel DO, Richter JE, eds. *The Esophagus*, 3rd ed. Philadelphia: Lippincott Williams & Wilkins; 1999:102.)

 QUICK CUT Severe esophagitis, especially erosive esophagitis, that fails medical management warrants treatment with an antireflux procedure.

Case Variation 6.2.3. *Biopsy of the distal esophagus that shows Barrett esophagus*

◆ Barrett esophagus, which occurs in 10%–15% of patients with esophagitis, results from chronic gastroesophageal reflux. The condition involves the replacement of normal squamous epithelium of the distal esophagus by columnar epithelium, which is also termed metaplasia. It leads to an increased risk of esophageal adenocarcinoma.

A finding of Barrett esophagus warrants evaluation of biopsy for presence and **degree of dysplasia**. For minimal to mild dysplasia, the treatment is the same as for reflux esophagitis (e.g., acid reduction, bed elevation). Currently, only modest data support the concept that antireflux surgery induces regression of Barrett esophagus. Nissen fundoplication is indicated for the usual indications of reflux such as intractable symptoms, severe esophagitis, and esophageal stricture and may be recommended for the treatment of Barrett esophagus in the future.

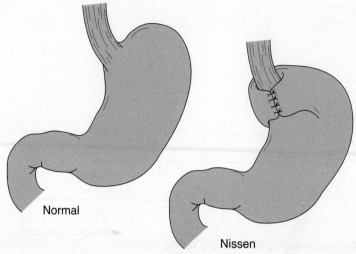

Figure 6-2: Nissen fundoplication. The upper stomach is wrapped around the esophagus to create a valve mechanism. (From McKenney MG, Mangonon PC, Moylan JA, eds. *Understanding Surgical Disease: The Miami Manual of Surgery.* Philadelphia: Lippincott-Raven; 1998:110.)

 QUICK CUT Surveillance endoscopy and biopsies are recommended every 18–24 months to determine if a Barrett esophagus progresses to dysplasia.

If a diagnosis of severe dysplasia is reached, a second pathologist experienced in this disorder should confirm the biopsy because of the implications of the diagnosis.

Case Variation 6.2.4. Biopsy of the distal esophagus that shows Barrett esophagus with severe dysplasia

◆ This finding is associated with a **high risk of occult adenocarcinoma in the distal esophagus. Esophageal resection should be considered.**

Case 6.3 Acute Epigastric Pain No. 3

You are following the patient in Case 6.2, a patient who has had an episode of epigastric pain that did not resolve on medical therapy. EGD is necessary, and a hiatal hernia is apparent.

◆ **How would you manage each of the following types of hiatal hernia (Fig. 6-3)?**

Case Variation 6.3.1. Type I hiatal hernia

◆ A type I hiatal hernia, or sliding hiatal hernia, which is discovered on routine evaluation, may affect patients with reflux symptoms. This common hernia usually causes no other symptoms. **These patients should receive treatment for GERD** without surgery.

Case Variation 6.3.2. Paraesophageal hiatal hernia

◆ A paraesophageal hiatal hernia has the gastroesophageal junction below the diaphragm and the stomach or other abdominal contents herniating through the esophageal hiatus into

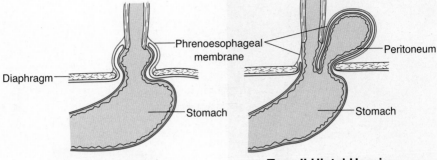

Type I Hiatal Hernia **Type II Hiatal Hernia**

Figure 6-3: A type I, or sliding, hiatal hernia compared to a type II, or paraesophageal hiatal hernia. In the type I hernia, the gastroesophageal junction is in the chest as part of the sliding segment of stomach that herniates into the mediastinum. In the paraesophageal hiatal hernia, the gastroesophageal junction is in a normal location, and a segment of stomach herniates up through the phrenoesophageal membrane into the chest. (From Castell DO, Richter JE, eds. *The Esophagus*, 3rd ed. Philadelphia: Lippincott Williams & Wilkins; 1999:385.)

the mediastinum. These hernias, unlike the sliding hiatal hernia, are at risk for volvulus or ischemia of the herniated organs particularly the stomach.

> **QUICK CUT** In a paraesophageal hernia, a portion of the stomach herniates into the chest, but the GE junction remains in the normal location. This hernia is extremely dangerous because the entire stomach can necrose if it becomes involved in the hernia sac and becomes strangulated (also called a gastric volvulus) (Fig. 6-4).

Case 6.4 Acute Epigastric Pain No. 4

You are following the patient in Case 6.2, who has had an episode of epigastric pain that did not resolve on medical therapy. EGD is necessary.

◆ **How would you manage the following findings on EGD?**

Case Variation 6.4.1. Pyloric channel ulcer (Fig. 6-5)

◆ Pyloric ulcers are associated with **increased acid production**. It is widely accepted that most peptic ulcers are associated with *H. pylori* **infection**. Elimination of *H. pylori* leads to ulcer healing and reduces the chance of ulcer recurrence.

A diagnosis of *H. pylori* involves the use of serum antibody testing or gastric biopsy for culture, bacterial staining (Warthin-Starry silver stain), or urease testing (*Campylobacter*-like organism test). The urea breath test, which does not require a gastric biopsy, is another diagnostic tool. **Treatment of *H. pylori* involves one of several regimens.** One recommended therapy includes a PPI such as omeprazole (20 mg twice a day [bid]) along with metronidazole (500 mg bid) and clarithromycin (250 mg bid). Amoxicillin may be substituted for clarithromycin. When taken for 2 weeks, these drugs have an eradication rate of 90%–96%. An alternative therapy involves bismuth, another agent that acts as an antimicrobial agent against *H. pylori*; it interferes with adhesion of the organism to the gastric epithelium and inhibits the organism's urease, phospholipase, and proteolytic activity. When taken for 2 weeks, bismuth

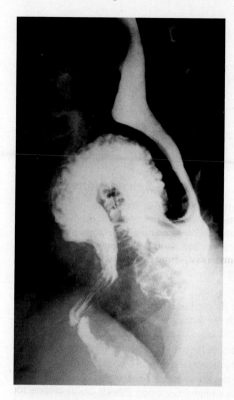

Figure 6-4: Contrast radiograph of a paraesophageal hernia and demonstration of gastric volvulus, which can result in necrosis of the stomach. This is a surgical emergency. (From Eubanks WS, Swanstrom LL, Soper NJ, eds. *Mastery of Endoscopic and Laparoscopic Surgery*. Philadelphia: Lippincott Williams & Wilkins; 2000:166.)

(262 mg four times a day [qid]) in combination with tetracycline (500 mg qid), metronidazole (500 mg three times a day), and omeprazole (20 mg bid) achieves a 98% eradication rate.

Case Variation 6.4.2. Duodenal ulcer

◆ Management is the same as with the pyloric channel ulcer (see Case Variation 6.4.1). You institute this therapy, and the test returns positive for *H. pylori*.

After you treat the patient for *H. pylori*, he remains symptomatic.

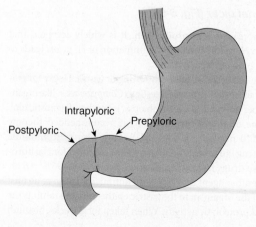

Intrapyloric
Postpyloric
Prepyloric

Figure 6-5: Location of pyloric channel ulcers in stomach and postpyloric ulcers in duodenum. (From Yamada T, Alpers DH, Laine L, et al, eds. *Textbook of Gastroenterology*, 3rd ed. Philadelphia: Lippincott Williams & Wilkins; 1999:1534.)

◆ **What is the appropriate treatment?**

◆ **Most physicians treat mild PUD for 4–6 weeks and extend the duration of treatment to 8–12 weeks for severe disease.** If the patient remains symptomatic after treatment for *H. pylori*, upper endoscopy is necessary, with re-evaluation of *H. pylori* infection.

QUICK CUT It is important to ask the patient about the use of ulcerogenic drugs such as NSAIDs or steroids; discontinuation of these agents, if possible, is warranted.

The patient completes treatment, but his symptoms persist. You repeat the EGD, and it reveals enlargement of the ulcer.

◆ **What is the next step?**

◆ Current medical therapies are highly effective in treating PUD. However, if the ulcer persists after adequate treatment for *H. pylori*, **medical therapy has failed**, and surgery is a reasonable choice. Highly selective vagotomy (HSV), truncal vagotomy and pyloroplasty (V&P), or vagotomy and antrectomy (V&A) are the commonly accepted procedures (Figs. 6-6 through 6-8). The best operation for PUD is a subject of debate. HSV has a low mortality rate, with the lowest rate of postoperative dumping symptoms, when compared to either V&P or V&A; however, HSV is associated with a higher rate of ulcer recurrence. In this case, most surgeons would not perform a V&A because of the high rate of complications (e.g., anastomotic leak, postoperative dumping syndrome) but would choose a **V&P or HSV**, whichever they are most comfortable with technically.

QUICK CUT All things being equal, HSV is the procedure of choice for uncomplicated PUD.

In this situation, it is also necessary to measure serum gastrin levels to rule out Zollinger-Ellison syndrome because high gastrin levels are associated with recurrent peptic ulceration.

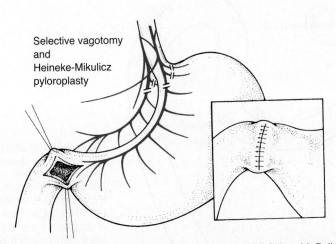

Selective vagotomy and Heineke-Mikulicz pyloroplasty

Figure 6-6: Truncal vagotomy and pyloroplasty. (From Lawrence PF, Bilbao M, Bell RM, et al, eds. *Essentials of General Surgery*. Baltimore: Lippincott Williams & Wilkins; 1988:180.)

Proximal
gastric vagotomy

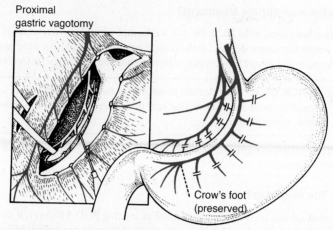

Crow's foot
(preserved)

Figure 6-7: Highly selective vagotomy. The gastric fundus and body are denervated, and the antrum and pylorus innervation is left intact, allowing gastric mixing and emptying to occur in a normal fashion. (From Lawrence PF, Bilbao M, Bell RM, et al, eds. *Essentials of General Surgery*. Baltimore: Lippincott Williams & Wilkins; 1988:182.)

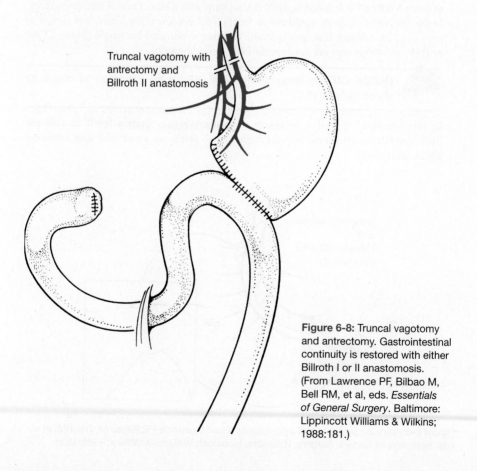

Truncal vagotomy with
antrectomy and
Billroth II anastomosis

Figure 6-8: Truncal vagotomy and antrectomy. Gastrointestinal continuity is restored with either Billroth I or II anastomosis. (From Lawrence PF, Bilbao M, Bell RM, et al, eds. *Essentials of General Surgery*. Baltimore: Lippincott Williams & Wilkins; 1988:181.)

Case 6.5   Acute Epigastric Pain No. 5

You are following the patient in Case 6.2, who has had an episode of epigastric pain that did not resolve on medical therapy. EGD is necessary, and a gastric ulcer is evident.

◆ **How does the location of the ulcer relate to gastric acid production?**

◆ There are four types of gastric ulcer (Fig. 6-9). Types I and IV are associated with relatively low acid output, and types II and III are associated with relatively high acid output.

◆ **How would you manage a gastric ulcer on the lesser curvature of the body of the stomach (type I)?**

◆ **Gastric ulcers, which are related to a breakdown in the gastric mucosal protective barrier, are associated with relatively low acid production.** It is necessary to ask the patient about the use of NSAIDs or steroids; if possible, avoidance of these medications is warranted. **Because gastric ulcers are associated with a significant risk of gastric cancer,** management must be designed with this in mind. At endoscopy, it is necessary to perform 8–12 biopsies from the edge of the ulcer. If the gastric ulcer is benign, **medical treatment** with antacids, H₂ blockers, and possibly with an *H. pylori* regimen is warranted. The optimal duration for treatment, which has not been adequately defined, ranges from 12 to 18 weeks.

You institute this therapy, and the patient's **symptoms resolve**. The gastric biopsy demonstrates a benign pathology.

◆ **What is the next management step?**

◆ This patient can be **followed** as long as he remains free of symptoms, and the ulcer has been shown to resolve.

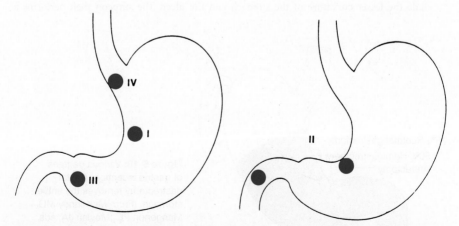

Figure 6-9: Types of gastric ulcer. A type I ulcer occurs at the incisura angularis on the lesser curvature, a type II ulcer is associated with a simultaneous duodenal ulcer, a type III ulcer is a prepyloric ulcer, and a type IV ulcer is a gastric cardia ulcer. (From Yamada T, Alpers DH, Laine L, et al, eds. *Textbook of Gastroenterology*, 3rd ed. Philadelphia: Lippincott Williams & Wilkins; 1999:1537.)

You institute this therapy, and the patient's **symptoms do not resolve**. The gastric biopsy demonstrates a benign pathology.

◆ **What is the next management step?**

◆ All patients with a history of gastric ulcers who have failed to become asymptomatic on medical management should have **repeat endoscopy**, with repeat biopsies for patients with nonhealed gastric ulcers.

 QUICK CUT Benign, nonhealed gastric ulcers may be further treated medically; however, if after approximately 18 weeks ulcers remain unhealed, many surgeons recommend that they be surgically resected.

The standard operation for benign, nonhealed gastric ulcers is **partial gastrectomy**, usually described as **antrectomy**; surgeons should be certain to remove the ulcer as part of the specimen. This recommendation is based on a concern for unrecognized cancer in the ulcer. In addition, many surgeons recommend earlier surgery on giant gastric ulcers (>5 cm) because of a higher risk of bleeding as well as a higher failure rate of healing (Fig. 6-10). **No vagotomy is performed.**

◆ **How would the proposed management change for a gastric ulcer at the gastroesophageal junction (type IV)?**

◆ Treatment of gastric ulcers at the gastroesophageal junction (type IV) should be similar to that just described. Again, it must be stressed that all gastric ulcers should be biopsied to rule out malignancy. If the ulcer has not healed after medical therapy, the patient should undergo repeat endoscopy at 8–16 weeks. If the ulcer is persistent but remains benign on biopsy, the clinician may continue medical therapy cautiously or refer the patient for surgery.

Surgical therapy of ulcers at the gastroesophageal junction is technically challenging. One option is a distal gastric resection with a vertical extension of the resection to include the lesser curvature of the stomach and the ulcer. The surgeon then performs a

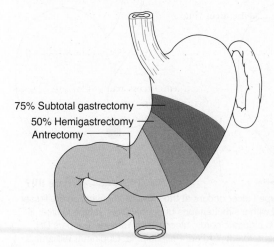

75% Subtotal gastrectomy
50% Hemigastrectomy
Antrectomy

Figure 6-10: Various degrees of gastric resection. A total gastrectomy removes the entire stomach. (From McKenney MG, Mangonon PC, Moylan JA, eds. *Understanding Surgical Disease: The Miami Manual of Surgery*. Philadelphia: Lippincott-Raven; 1998:123.)

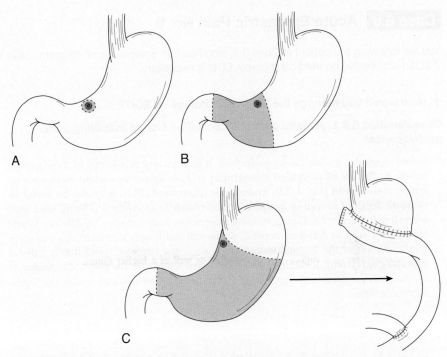

Figure 6-11: Three methods for resection of benign gastric ulcers. **A:** The ulcer is excised, and the gastric walls are closed. **B:** An antrectomy is performed, and the gastrointestinal tract is reconstructed with either a Billroth I or II reconstruction. **C:** Gastric ulcer that occurs high and near the gastroesophageal junction is resected. Note that no vagotomy is performed for gastric ulcers.

gastrojejunostomy. A more aggressive technique is a distal gastrectomy with removal of a portion of the esophageal wall and ulcer and a Roux-en-Y esophagogastrojejunostomy. **In either case, it is necessary to excise the ulcer** (Fig. 6-11).

◆ **How would you manage a patient with a type II ulcer of the stomach body associated with a duodenal ulcer?**

◆ Most surgeons consider this to be an ulcer associated with excess acid production. Thus, if surgery is necessary, an acid-reducing procedure is warranted. The most common procedure is **antrectomy with removal of the ulcer**. One notable difference between the surgery for types I and IV ulcers, compared to that for types II and III ulcers, is the **addition of a truncal vagotomy**; this greatly lowers acid production.

◆ **How would you manage a patient with a prepyloric gastric ulcer (type III)?**

◆ The **management of a type III ulcer**, which is associated with increased acid production, **is similar to a type II ulcer**. A commonly performed alternative procedure is a **V&P**. The surgeon must still be certain that the ulcer does not represent cancer.

Case 6.6   Acute Epigastric Pain No. 6

You are following the patient in Case 6.2, who has had an episode of epigastric pain that did not resolve on medical therapy. EGD is necessary.

♦ **How would you manage the following findings on EGD?**

Case Variation 6.6.1. A distal gastric ulcer, with a biopsy indicating early gastric cancer

♦ Before surgical resection can be performed, **it is necessary to attempt to stage gastric cancer by the use of computed tomography (CT) to assess for distant metastasis or lymph node spread (Fig. 6-12). Endoscopic ultrasound (EUS) may also be useful to evaluate depth of spread or lymphatic involvement.** Laparoscopy is being used with increasing frequency for staging. In some prospective studies, staging laparoscopy is better than CT scan in detecting hepatic, peritoneal, and lymphatic metastases. For early gastric cancers of the antrum or middle stomach, the treatment of choice is a **distal subtotal gastrectomy**, including 80% of the stomach, and regional lymphadenectomy. If the tumor is confined to the mucosa and does not involve the lymph nodes, the 5-year survival is 90%.

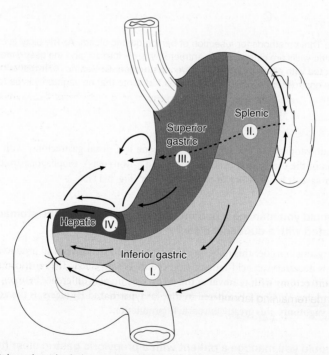

Figure 6-12: Lymph node drainage of the stomach as it relates to the location of the primary gastric cancer. The *arrows* indicate the direction of lymphatic flow from segments of the stomach to hepatic and coeliac lymph nodes. (From McKenney MG, Mangonon PC, Moylan JA, eds. *Understanding Surgical Disease: The Miami Manual of Surgery.* Philadelphia: Lippincott-Raven; 1998:119.)

Case Variation 6.6.2. A biopsy indicating infiltrating gastric carcinoma.

◆ Several factors relate to the prognosis of gastric cancer. Histologic classifications are difficult due to their heterogeneous morphology. In general, gastric carcinomas are described as either diffuse or intestinal. **Intestinal types** tend to form glands and have a **more favorable prognosis.** The **diffuse form** of gastric adenocarcinoma tends to extend widely in the submucosa and has a **worse prognosis.**

 QUICK CUT Penetration of gastric cancer through the submucosa and the presence of positive lymph nodes worsens prognosis.

In general, resection usually involves resection of the stomach, omentum, and perigastric lymph nodes. At least 15 lymph nodes are required for adequate nodal sampling and staging. The benefits of extended lymphadenectomy, involving nodes along the aorta and esophagus, have not been proven beneficial in the United States.

Case Variation 6.6.3. A biopsy indicating infiltrating gastric carcinoma and the wall of the stomach that appears fixed and rigid in its entirety.

◆ **Diffusely infiltrating gastric carcinoma is termed linitis plastica** and has a poor prognosis. It involves all layers of the stomach wall with a marked desmoplastic reaction. **Total gastrectomy with splenectomy** is sometimes advocated, but if the stomach is rigid and fixed throughout, **cure is rare.**

Case Variation 6.6.4. A biopsy indicating gastric carcinoma at the gastroesophageal junction.

◆ The incidence of gastric cancer at the gastroesophageal junction has increased over the past 15 years. Currently, about 40% of gastric adenocarcinomas involve the proximal stomach. The prognosis for these cancers is **less favorable** than those located in the antrum. The recommendation for **gastric resection** is at least 6 cm distally beyond the tumor to prevent tumor recurrence at the anastomosis. If the cancer extends into the gastroesophageal junction, it may be necessary to perform an **esophagogastrectomy** with anastomosis in the cervical or thoracic position using either colon or a free graft small bowel as an interposition graft (Fig. 6-13).

Case 6.7 Acute Epigastric Pain No. 7

A 40-year-old man presents to the emergency department with a 4-hour history of epigastric pain that has become very severe in the past hour. He has a low-grade fever and normal blood pressure (BP). Examination is normal, except for the abdomen, which reveals marked tenderness with involuntary guarding (**rigid abdomen**) and rebound tenderness. His white blood cell (WBC) count is 18,000/mm³ with a left shift, and the remaining laboratory studies are normal.

◆ **What study would you perform first?**

◆ An obstructive series with an upright CXR should be performed first to examine for **free air** under the diaphragm, indicating perforation of the gastrointestinal tract. A rigid abdomen is typical for chemical peritonitis (acid and bile) as usually seen in a perforated ulcer.

The patient's upright CXR demonstrates free air in the peritoneal cavity (Fig. 6-14).

Figure 6-13: Esophagogastrectomy for resection of a distal esophageal cancer occurring at the gastroesophageal junction. *Dotted line* indicates line of gastric transection. (From Wanebo HJ, ed. *Surgery for Gastrointestinal Cancer*. Philadelphia: Lippincott-Raven; 1997:235.)

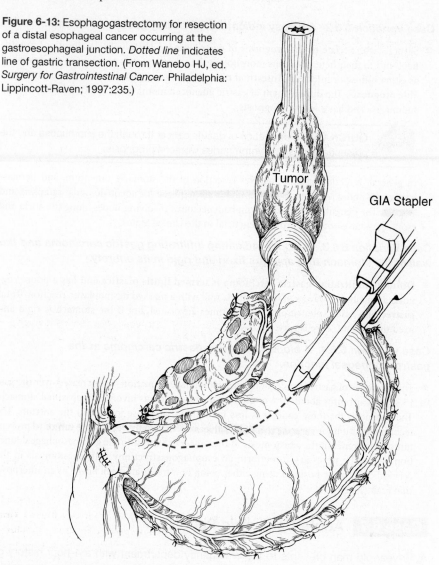

Tumor

GIA Stapler

QUICK CUT On an upright abdominal radiography or CXR, free air appears as air under the diaphragm. On a left lateral decubitus film, it is seen as air above (i.e., lateral to) the liver.

◆ **How would you use this information to make a management decision about this case?**

◆ Free air under the diaphragm is a sign of perforation; it is an indication to go to the operating room after resuscitation.

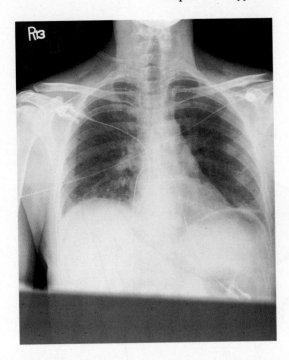

Figure 6-14: Upright and decubitus film of the abdomen showing free air.

You proceed to the operating room. You find a 1-cm perforation in the anterior portion of the duodenum.

◆ **How would you interpret the following additional finding, and what operation would you perform?**

Case Variation 6.7.1. ***There are fresh gastric contents in the peritoneal cavity, and the perforation appears several hours old.***

◆ If this patient has no prior history of ulcer disease, management of a perforation that is only several hours old involves **closure of the perforation**. This usually involves use of a **Graham patch**, which consists of a piece of omentum placed over the perforation and sutured in place. Postoperative treatment to heal the ulcer and prevent recurrence is then appropriate (Fig. 6-15). Most surgeons recommend omental patch closure only for perforated ulcers with postoperative treatment for *H. pylori* rather than a formal acid-reducing operation. This is always true when the patient has evidence of sepsis or hemodynamic instability. A formal acid-reducing operation such as a vagotomy and pyloroplasty incorporating the perforation can be done if there is significant evidence that the patient will not be compliant with postoperative therapy or has recurrent disease.

Case 6.8 Upper Gastrointestinal Bleeding No. 1

You are caring for a 30-year-old woman with pneumonia in the intensive care unit. She has had an ileus and has required nasogastric (NG) tube drainage. On morning rounds, you note that her NG drainage contains coffee-ground–type material and occasional blood streaks.

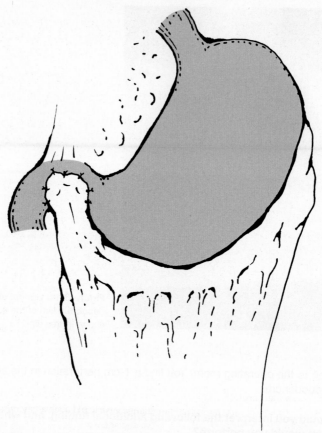

Figure 6-15: Repair of a perforated duodenal ulcer using an omental patch. In contrast, a gastric ulcer is not patched but resected. (From Yamada T, Alpers DH, Laine L, et al, eds. *Textbook of Gastroenterology*, 3rd ed. Philadelphia: Lippincott Williams & Wilkins; 1999:1541.)

◆ **How would you manage this patient?**

◆ Initiation of a PPI, H_2 blockade, sucralfate, or antacids with gastric pH monitoring is appropriate. If the patient is taking NSAIDs, misoprostol may also be necessary (Table 6-1). Misoprostol, a synthetic prostaglandin E_1 analog, has gastric mucosal protective properties and inhibits gastric acid secretion with coffee-ground bleeding. UGI endoscopy is not mandatory for this type of bleeding.

◆ **Are there patients in the hospital setting that you would manage with "ulcer prophylaxis"?**

◆ This patient, like many patients in an intensive care setting who are at increased risk for UGI bleeding due to ulceration and gastritis (stress gastritis or ulceration), definitely needs ulcer prophylaxis. The biggest risk factors for developing stress ulcerations are coagulopathy, mechanical ventilation for more than 2 days, and history of gastrointestinal ulceration or bleeding within the past year. The best prophylaxis is enteral feeds. PPIs are the most effective but the most costly, whereas H_2 blockers are slightly less effective but less costly.

Table 6-1: Drug Therapy for Peptic Ulcer Disease

Agent	Effect	Advantages and Disadvantages
Decrease Gastric Acidity		
Antacids	Neutralize gastric acid; also may increase mucosal resistance	Inexpensive; readily available
H_2 receptor antagonists (e.g., cimetidine)	Inhibit histamine receptor on parietal cell, which decreases acid output	Excellent results; mainstay therapy; once-daily evening dosing for maintenance therapy
Proton pump inhibitors (e.g., omeprazole)	Inhibit ATPase proton pump, which is final step in acid secretion from parietal cell	Quicker healing but more expensive than preceding agents
Increase Mucosal Defense		
Cytoprotective topical agent (e.g., sucralfate)	Binds to proteins in ulcer to form protective mucosal barrier	Not proven for gastric ulcers
Antibiotics (e.g., amoxicillin)	Eradicate *Helicobacter pylori*	Inexpensive; important in preventing recurrences in patients with *H. pylori*

ATPase, adenosine triphosphatase.
From Jarrell BE, Carabasi RA, Radomski JS. *NMS Surgery*, 4th ed. Philadelphia: Lippincott Williams & Wilkins; 2000:217.

There is concern that raising the gastric pH can increase the risk of nosocomial pneumonia, compared to prophylactic agents that do not change gastric pH such as sucralfate. However, PPI and H_2 blockers are more effective prophylactic agents.

1. Wait for bleeding to occur and then treat.
2. Treat every patient.
3. Attempt to **identify patients at higher risk for UGI bleeding and treat them prophylactically**, but do not treat the lower risk patients (more selective approach). Most surgeons would institute selective therapy. Several conditions place patients at higher risk (Table 6-2).

Table 6-2: Conditions that Put Individuals at High Risk for Upper Gastrointestinal Bleeding

Duodenal ulcer
Gastric ulcer
Diffuse erosive gastritis
Esophageal or gastric varices
Mallory-Weiss tear of the gastroesophageal junction
Gastric carcinoma
Arteriovenous malformations

From Jarrell BE, Carabasi RA, Radomski JS. *NMS Surgery*, 4th ed. Philadelphia: Lippincott Williams & Wilkins; 2000:198.

You institute therapy but do not perform any diagnostic procedures. Later in the day, bright-red blood appears in the patient's NG tube.

◆ What are the next steps in evaluation?

◆ The first steps in evaluation of UGI bleeding involve resuscitation. Placement of two large-bore intravenous (IV) lines is necessary, along with a blood draw for type and cross-match and hematocrit. Lavage of the NG tube until blood no longer returns is essential. IV fluids are essential, and close monitoring for signs of hypotension is appropriate. The administration of PPI or H_2 blockers and monitoring of gastric pH are also necessary. Once the patient has been stabilized, **upper endoscopy** to determine the precise source of bleeding is necessary.

◆ How would you manage the following findings?

Case Variation 6.8.1. A duodenal ulcer with a clean, white base and no active bleeding

◆ An ulcer with a white base has not bled recently. It can be observed without endoscopic treatment. The risk of rebleeding is low. Biopsy for *H. pylori* should be done at this time.

 QUICK CUT In all cases of duodenal ulcers, it is necessary to attempt to maintain a gastric pH above 5 to reduce the risk of rebleeding.

An H_2 blocker or a PPI effectively maintains the gastric pH at 5.

Case Variation 6.8.2. A duodenal ulcer with a fresh clot adherent to the ulcer

◆ This ulcer, which exhibits evidence of recent bleeding, has a 10%–15% chance of rebleeding. Endoscopic hemostatic therapy is warranted. The commonly accepted indications for endoscopic therapy include evidence of active or recent bleeding, large initial blood loss, and a high risk of rebleeding or death with the bleed. Endoscopic therapy includes a variety of methods, including injection of epinephrine and sclerosing agents, thermal contact methods (heater probe and argon plasma coagulation), laser therapy, and newer mechanical methods such as suturing. Biopsy for *H. pylori* should be done at this time.

Case Variation 6.8.3. A duodenal ulcer with fresh clot and a visible artery at its base

◆ This type of ulcer has the **highest risk of rebleeding (as high as 40%)**. A visible artery indicates that a vessel has been exposed by the ulcerative process and that rebleeding could be massive.

 QUICK CUT Most of the time, this type of ulcer is in the posterior duodenum and involves the gastroduodenal artery.

It would be appropriate to inject the area around the artery and attempt local control. Many surgeons would electively **operate** in the next 24–48 hours if a significant bleed had occurred before endoscopy because of the concern for the need for immediate surgical intervention if another bleed occurs (Fig. 6-16).

Case Variation 6.8.4. A duodenal ulcer with fresh bleeding in a patient with the onset of hypotension

◆ If the patient becomes **hypotensive** during the performance of endoscopy, immediate resuscitation with normal saline and packed red blood cells (RBCs) is necessary. The patient

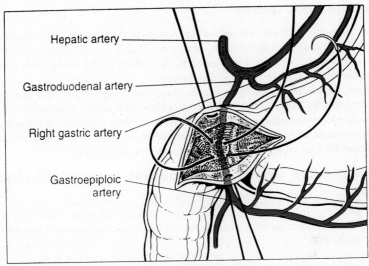

Figure 6-16: Suture ligature of a bleeding gastroduodenal ulcer in a posterior duodenal ulcer. Note that the stomach is opened and the artery ligated from within the lumen of the duodenum. (From Yamada T, Alpers DH, Laine L, et al, eds. *Textbook of Gastroenterology*, 3rd ed. Philadelphia: Lippincott Williams & Wilkins; 1999:1540.)

will most likely need to **go to the operating room.** Many surgeons recommend urgent oversewing of the vessel before exsanguinating hemorrhage occurs.

Case Variation 6.8.5. *A duodenal ulcer in a patient with acute renal failure and a creatinine of 6 mg/dL*

◆ This patient may have **platelet dysfunction caused by uremia**, which would make bleeding more likely. The platelet dysfunction can be lessened by dialysis and by desmopressin (ddAVP). Otherwise, the previously described treatment for UGI bleeding is appropriate.

Case Variation 6.8.6. *A duodenal ulcer in a patient with chronic alcoholic cirrhosis*

◆ This patient may have an **elevated prothrombin time** (PT) secondary to deficiency of factors II, VII, IX, and X, which can be temporarily corrected by FFP. In addition, the patient may have thrombocytopenia due to congestive splenomegaly, which can be partially corrected by platelet transfusion. Otherwise, the previously described treatment for UGI bleeding is appropriate.

Case Variation 6.8.7. *A gastric ulcer*

◆ **Management of bleeding gastric ulcers is similar to that of duodenal ulcers but with one difference.** All gastric ulcers warrant biopsy because gastric cancer may accompany ulcers. However, it is necessary to postpone biopsy for several days to weeks until the immediate bleeding has resolved and the patient has stabilized. Malignant gastric ulcers commonly appear as exophytic masses with heaped-up margins or necrotic ulcer craters, with bleeding from the edge of the craters. If the bleeding is controlled, you should plan to re-evaluate the patient within 2 weeks with repeat endoscopy.

 QUICK CUT If surgery is necessary for GU bleeding, excision of the ulcer rather than oversewing, as with duodenal ulcers, is warranted.

Case Variation 6.8.8. *Gastritis*

◆ Gastritis involves **multiple, nonulcerating erosions in the stomach**, often associated with ventilator dependence, major trauma, sepsis, severe burns, and renal failure. It is necessary to keep the gastric pH above 5 with antacids, H_2 blockers, or PPI. Studies have shown that sucralfate also decreases bleeding in this setting.

Most patients stop bleeding as a result of medical therapy, but on rare occasions, the bleeding does not cease. Endoscopic control of bleeding is usually unsuccessful because of the multiplicity of bleeding sites. In that case, it is necessary to perform a subtotal gastrectomy to control the bleeding. Lesser resections fail to control the bleeding in 50% of cases. The mortality of stress gastritis remains high regardless of treatment.

Case Variation 6.8.9. *Gastritis and gastric varices in a patient with a history of cirrhosis*

◆ Gastritis and gastric or esophageal varices may occur with alcoholic cirrhosis (Fig. 6-17). Often, the bleeding arises from gastritis and not the varices, and treatment should be instituted for gastritis.

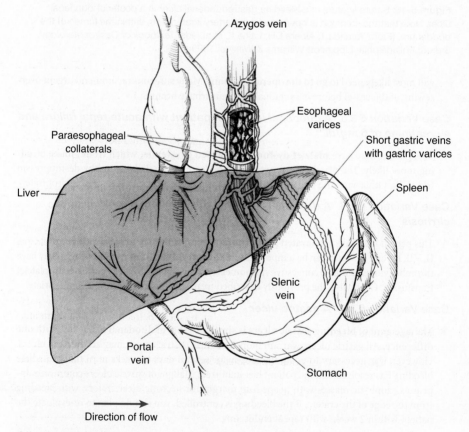

Figure 6-17: Vessels and blood flow involved in esophageal and gastric varices. (From Kaplowitz N. *Liver and Biliary Diseases*, 2nd ed. Baltimore: Lippincott Williams and Wilkins; 1996:551.)

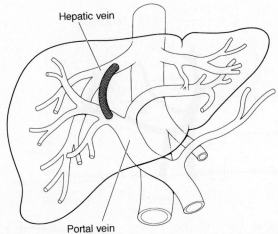

Hepatic vein

Portal vein

Figure 6-18: TIPS, in which an intrahepatic portion of a hepatic vein is cannulated percutaneously followed by the creation of an artificial tunnel between the hepatic vein and the portal vein. The tunnel is then dilated and held open with an expandable stent. (From Yamada T, Alpers DH, Laine L, et al, eds. *Textbook of Gastroenterology*, 3rd ed. Philadelphia: Lippincott Williams & Wilkins; 1999:723.)

QUICK CUT Gastric varices are more difficult to treat and do not respond to banding or sclerotherapy as often as esophageal varices.

Gastric varices may respond to injection with cyanoacrylate glue if available. If gastric variceal bleeding is severe and uncontrollable, management with **either portosystemic shunting (surgical or transjugular intrahepatic portosystemic shunt [TIPS]) or splenectomy** is necessary (Figs. 6-18 and 6-19).

Case Variation 6.8.10. **Gastritis and gastric varices with a history of chronic pancreatitis**

◆ In this situation, the gastric varices may be the result of splenic vein thrombosis, resulting in left-sided portal (sinistral) hypertension. A **splenectomy** is indicated if bleeding is persistent.

Case Variation 6.8.11. **Esophageal varices and a history of cirrhosis**

◆ Management of bleeding from esophageal varices entails treating the underlying coagulation abnormalities with FFP and vitamin K. Vasopressin or octreotide (somatostatin analog) may also be used to lower portal pressure.

QUICK CUT Endoscopic sclerotherapy or variceal banding controls the bleeding in 80%–95% of patients; however, patients rebleed in approximately 25% of cases. Endoscopy is usually repeated in 48 hours to sclerose or band (ligate) any remaining vessels.

Both sclerotherapy and band ligation have been effective in controlling bleeding and reducing the rate of rebleeding, but banding is preferred because it causes less injury to the esophagus (Fig. 6-20).

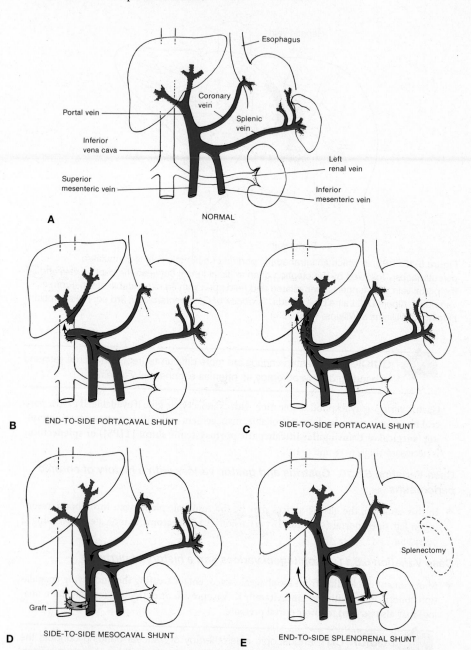

Figure 6-19: Surgical shunts are rarely performed today except for exception circumstances. Portosystemic shunts commonly used in the surgical treatment of portal hypertension. **A:** Normal arrangement. **B:** End-to-side portacaval shunt. **C:** Side-to-side portacaval shunt. **D:** Side-to-side mesocaval shunt. **E:** End-to-side splenorenal shunt. (*continued*)

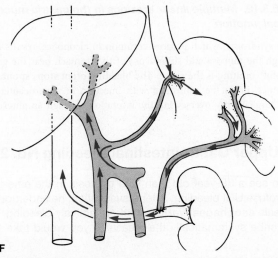

F

Figure 6-19: (*continued*) **F:** Distal splenorenal shunt. (From Yamada T, Alpers DH, Laine L, et al, eds. *Textbook of Gastroenterology*, 3rd ed. Philadelphia: Lippincott Williams & Wilkins; 1999:724–725.)

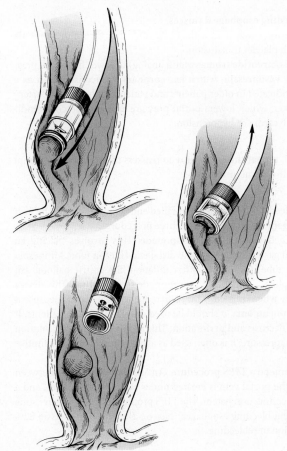

Figure 6-20: Endoscopic band ligation of an esophageal varix. This is the preferred treatment for a varix. (From Yamada T, Alpers DH, Laine L, et al, eds. *Textbook of Gastroenterology*, 3rd ed. Philadelphia: Lippincott Williams & Wilkins; 1999:722.)

*Case Variation 6.8.12. **Multiple linear erosions in the gastric mucosa at the gastroesophageal junction***

◆ **Mallory-Weiss** syndrome, which is more common in alcoholics, results from longitudinal tears through the mucosa and submucosa of the stomach near the gastroesophageal junction. Forceful vomiting is the cause. **The bleeding often stops spontaneously.** If the bleeding continues, it can be controlled with injection or electrocautery. Severe cases can be treated surgically by oversewing the laceration through an anterior longitudinal gastrostomy.

Case 6.9   Upper Gastrointestinal Bleeding No. 2

You are asked to see a 35-year-old man with cirrhosis in the emergency department who has profuse UGI bleeding. After resuscitation, he undergoes UGI endoscopy, which reveals **esophageal varices** that are actively bleeding. Your resident asks you to describe systematically the measures you would take to control the bleeding.

◆ **How would you answer?**

1. **Initial steps**
   - Attempt to **band the bleeding esophageal varices**.
   - **Correct the coagulopathy** (high PT with FFP) and the **thrombocytopenia** (<50,000 cells/mm^3) with platelet transfusion.
   - Treat the patient with **IV octreotide** (somatostatin analog) to lower his portal pressure. Alternatives are **IV vasopressin**, which has **coronary vasoconstriction as a side effect** and is contraindicated in older patients and patients with coronary artery disease, and a beta-blocker, which lowers portal pressure and may be contraindicated with profound bradycardia or hypotension.

2. **Intermediate step**
   If the patient continues to bleed, **repeat the endoscopy** to reassess the source and attempt control again with banding or other local procedures.

3. **Final steps**
   If the patient still continues to bleed, and the patient has failed endoscopic therapy. The next best step is controversial. Management involves one of three procedures.
   Some surgeons would proceed with **balloon tamponade**. This involves placing an NG tube with an esophageal and gastric balloon on the distal end (Linton tube, Minnesota tube, or Sengstaken-Blakemore tube) (Fig. 6-21). After inflation, the gastric balloon can be pulled against the gastroesophageal junction to **tamponade the bleeding**. This device usually provides hemostasis only when inflated, with recurrence when deflated. Because it carries a high risk of aspiration pneumonia, it should be used only in intubated patients. It also carries a risk of esophageal necrosis and perforation. This is only a temporary solution and does nothing to lower portal pressure; it is often used as a bridge until a more definitive procedure is done.
   Many surgeons would recommend a **TIPS procedure**. An artificial connection between a hepatic vein and a branch of the portal vein is created under radiologic guidance, and a stent is inserted to maintain the connection patent. The TIPS procedure is now the first-line therapy for refractory or recurrent bleeding esophageal varices. The procedure has an 82% 1-year patency rate and prevention of rebleeding.

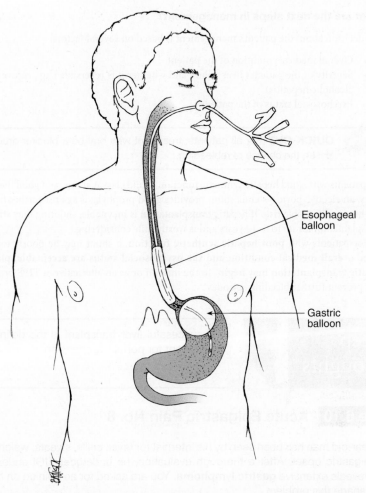

Esophageal
balloon

Gastric
balloon

Figure 6-21: A balloon tamponade tube, which is used in massive, uncontrollable bleeding for temporary tamponade. After insertion through the nose or mouth into the stomach, the gastric balloon is inflated to tamponade the varices. On occasion, it is necessary to inflate the esophageal balloon. (From Chen H, Sonnenday CJ, Lillemoe KD, eds. *Manual of Common Bedside Surgical Procedures*, 2nd ed. Philadelphia: Lippincott Williams & Wilkins; 2000:155.)

Rarely, some surgeons would emergently proceed to the operating room to perform a **portosystemic shunt**. However, this has a mortality of 50% or more and is not preferred by most surgeons, especially with a Child classification of class C. Portosystemic shunts are usually for patients with portal hypertension without cirrhosis or whose liver function is preserved and does not need a liver transplant.

As the result of one of these maneuvers, many patients stop bleeding. However, some patients exsanguinate despite the best medical and surgical efforts.

After the first treatment step, the patient stops bleeding and recovers. He is ready for discharge.

◆ **What are the next steps in management?**

◆ The decision about the patient's management is based on several factors:

- Overall medical condition of the patient
- Severity of the patient's liver failure and whether it is reversible (e.g., recovery from alcoholic hepatitis)
- Psychosocial status of the patient

 QUICK CUT For all patients, treatment with oral beta-blocker drugs may lessen the chance of rebleeding.

For patients with good hepatic synthetic function, Child class A status, and good life expectancy, an elective portosystemic shunt provides good prophylaxis against further bleeding and has an acceptable risk. If hepatic transplantation is inevitable, shunting may still delay transplantation for up to 5–10 years and is worthwhile considering.

For patients with **poor hepatic synthetic function**, a shunt may be poorly tolerated. **If the overall medical condition and the psychosocial status are acceptable, planning hepatic transplantation may begin.** In the interim or as an alternative, a TIPS procedure may prevent further bleeding episodes.

Deep Thoughts

A successful liver transplant is the definitive treatment for portal hypertension.

Case 6.10 **Acute Epigastric Pain No. 8**

A 48-year-old man has been seen by his internist for fever, chills, sweats, weight loss, and epigastric upset. After a thorough evaluation, he undergoes UGI endoscopy, which reveals extensive **gastric lymphoma**. You are asked for an opinion on how to best manage this problem.

◆ **How would you respond?**

◆ Although the stomach is the most common site of extranodal lymphoma, lymphomas are rare cancers of the stomach, comprising only 2% of all gastric cancers. The lymphoma has **usually reached a large size** before symptoms are apparent. Preoperatively, one must determine the degree of spread. Typically, a chest and abdominal CT, biopsy of enlarged peripheral nodes, and bone marrow biopsy are necessary. A careful examination of the oropharynx to detect abnormalities (additional lymphoma) in the Waldeyer ring is also appropriate. Survival is dependent on stage of disease, extent of penetration of the gastric wall, and histologic grade of the tumor.

◆ **What treatment would you recommend?**

◆ Therapy for gastric lymphomas is controversial and based on stage. Patients with mucosa-associated lymphoid tissue lymphoma usually respond to *Helicobacter* eradication and require surgery only if they fail to respond. The role of gastrectomy for staging and treatment of gastric lymphomas has significantly diminished and most patients are successfully treated with chemotherapy with or without radiation.

Chapter 7

Pancreatic and Hepatic Disorders

Bruce E. Jarrell, Eric D. Strauch

Key Thoughts

1. The natural history of asymptomatic gallstones is benign, and cholecystectomy is not recommended.

2. Acute cholecystitis should be treated with antibiotics followed by cholecystectomy within several days in most cases.

3. Painful jaundice is typically secondary to biliary obstruction due to common bile duct stones.

4. Painless jaundice is associated with distal biliary obstruction from tumors.

5. Biliary obstruction due to stones should be treated with removal of the stones by endoscopic retrograde cholangiopancreatography (ERCP) in most cases followed by cholecystectomy or operative common duct exploration at the time of cholecystectomy.

6. Gallstone pancreatitis usually resolves with hydration and observation. Treatment includes evaluating the common bile duct for the presence of stones, usually without the need for ERCP, and removing the gallbladder after the pancreatitis improves to prevent recurrence.

7. Acute cholangitis is suggested by right upper quadrant (RUQ) pain, fever, and jaundice. The patient should receive antibiotics and fluid resuscitation, followed by ERCP and relief of the obstruction. Cholecystectomy is performed after recovery from the sepsis and acute illness.

8. Resected ampullary cancer has the best long-term survival of the pancreatobiliary cancers obstructing the distal common bile duct.

9. Most pancreatic pseudocysts resolve spontaneously.

10. Cystic liver lesions are usually simple cysts, are not usually symptomatic, and do not require surgery. In the presence of fever and sepsis and internal echoes in the cyst on ultrasound, it may represent an abscess, which is usually drained percutaneously.

11. The most common solid liver masses are hemangioma, which do not require surgery.

12. The most common malignant tumor of the liver is metastatic carcinoma. The primary should be sought. Resection of metastatic colonic carcinoma to the liver, with no metastasis outside the liver, can result in long-term survival.

13. Hepatocellular carcinoma is the most common primary liver cancer, is associated with cirrhosis, and has an elevated serum alpha fetoprotein.

COMMON PANCREATICOBILIARY DISORDERS

Case 7.1 Asymptomatic Gallstones

A 24-year-old woman with a family history of polycystic kidney disease is being screened by ultrasound to determine if she has the disease. She does not have the disease, but ultrasound examination shows several small gallstones (Fig. 7-1). Further history and review of symptoms find no evidence of symptomatic gallstone disease.

◆ **How would you manage this patient?**

 QUICK CUT Studies have found that the natural history of asymptomatic gallstones is benign.

◆ Generally, less than 10% of patients with asymptomatic gallstones develop symptoms requiring surgery over a 5-year period. For this reason, **cholecystectomy is not generally recommended** in asymptomatic patients except in certain individuals. Exceptions may include immunocompromised patients because they are prone to more serious complications of gallstone disease; patients with a porcelain gallbladder (calcified gallbladder); and patients with gallstones larger than 3 cm, which are associated with the development of gallbladder carcinoma. Experts once believed that it was necessary to remove gallstones in asymptomatic diabetic persons because of high complication rates; however, this practice is no longer performed.

Case 7.2 Right Upper Quadrant Pain No. 1

A 24-year-old woman presents to the emergency department with a 12-hour history of pain in her upper right abdomen, nausea, vomiting, and anorexia. Physical examination shows guarding and tenderness in the RUQ.

◆ **What are the most likely diagnoses?**

◆ The most likely diagnosis is one of three conditions: symptomatic **cholelithiasis, biliary colic, or acute cholecystitis**. Without fever, acute cholecystitis is unlikely. In a young

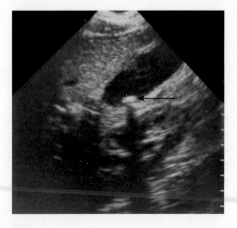

Figure 7-1: Ultrasound study shows a sonolucent density (*arrow*) in the gallbladder.

woman, the differential diagnosis of RUQ pain includes gastroenteritis, peptic ulcer disease (PUD), acute hepatitis, renal colic, pleural-based pneumonia, and pyelonephritis.

◆ **What specific items in the history or physical examination would you look for to support these diagnoses?**

◆ The factors that predispose to gallstone formation include increasing age, family history of gall-stones, female sex, obesity, history of recent pregnancy, and previous diagnosis of gallstones.

Symptoms of gallstone disease include fever, pain or guarding in the RUQ, and biliary colic. Examination of the abdomen may elicit **Murphy sign**, which is inspiratory arrest during deep palpation of the RUQ due to pain (Fig. 7-2).

◆ **What would make you suspicious that another diagnosis is more likely?**

◆ A history of indigestion, long-term NSAID use, antacid use, tarry stools, or ethanol abuse prompt consideration of **PUD or gastritis**.

The patient has no suspicious history or physical examination findings that suggest a diagnosis other than gallstone disease.

◆ **How would you establish the diagnosis?**

◆ The most efficient method of diagnosis is an **ultrasound** of the RUQ. Findings on ultra-sound suggestive of gallbladder disease include thickening of the gallbladder wall, pericho-lecystic fluid, and presence of gallstones (Fig. 7-3).

◆ **What blood chemistries would you expect to be abnormal with a diagnosis of cholelithiasis?**

◆ Blood tests should include a complete blood count (CBC) with differential, amylase, lipase, and liver function tests. **Mild leukocytosis** is present in some patients, a white blood count (WBC) of 12,000–15,000/mm³, who have uncomplicated cholelithiasis. **Mild jaundice** with a bilirubin as high as 2–3 mg/dL may be present in 20% of patients; it is secondary to

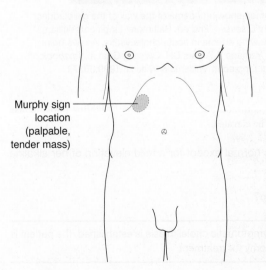

Murphy sign
location
(palpable,
tender mass)

Figure 7-2: Location of the Murphy sign. While the patient is taking a breath, there is an arrest of inspiration due to pain on palpation of the right upper abdomen.

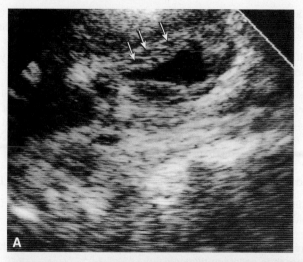

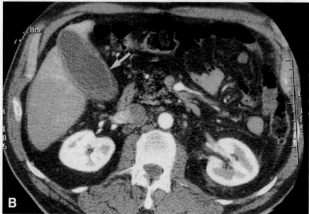

Figure 7-3: A: Ultrasound of the abdomen showing edema of the wall of the gallbladder. (From Kaplowitz N, ed. *Liver and Biliary Diseases*, 2nd ed. Baltimore: Lippincott Williams and Wilkins; 1996:257.) **B:** CT scan showing edema in acute cholecystitis. *Arrows* point to edematous gallbladder wall.. (From Yamada T, Alpers DH, Owyang C, et al. *Textbook of Gastroenterology*, 3rd ed. Philadelphia: Lippincott Williams & Wilkins; 1999:3037.)

inflammation and cholestasis, not common bile duct obstruction. **Alkaline phosphatase and transaminase** levels may also be elevated.

The patient's blood studies return normal except for a mild elevation of her alkaline phosphatase.

◆ **What would be your next step?**

QUICK CUT Once symptomatic cholelithiasis is established, the patient is offered a cholecystectomy for treatment.

Deep
Thoughts

Patients have the right to participate in their own treatment plans and can decide if the symptoms and risks of the disease outweigh the risks of the intervention.

◆ **Should the patient receive antibiotics?**

◆ Most patients with uncomplicated, symptomatic cholelithiasis **do not need antibiotics** at presentation. A cholecystectomy is considered to be a clean-contaminated situation, and a single, preoperative dose of a first-generation cephalosporin is recommended. Antibiotics may be appropriate for longer term use in patients who have a high risk of developing septic complications following cholecystectomy. This typically includes patients older than 70 years of age, patients with acute cholecystitis, and patients with a history of obstructive jaundice, common duct stones, or jaundice. Patients who have undergone preoperative ERCP also warrant treatment with preoperative antibiotics.

The patient decides to proceed with a cholecystectomy.

◆ **What type of cholecystectomy would you recommend?**

◆ The commonly accepted standard procedure is **laparoscopic cholecystectomy**. Open cholecystectomy is usually done when laparoscopic cholecystectomy cannot for technical or medical reasons.

◆ **What are the basic steps in a cholecystectomy?**

◆ Entry to the abdomen occurs through an incision or through trocars for the laparoscopic procedure. After exploration of the abdomen, the surgeon removes the gallbladder from the fundus to the junction of the cystic and common duct (retrograde cholecystectomy) or vice versa. The important parts of the procedure include removing the fundus from the bed of the liver, identifying and ligating the cystic duct without injury to the common duct, and ligating the cystic artery. Many surgeons believe that an operative cholangiogram to visualize the biliary tree and rule out other disease such as common duct stones is also important if there is any doubt about the anatomy (Fig. 7-4).

◆ **What are the major complications of a cholecystectomy?**

◆ **Injury to the common duct** is a serious complication that may result in chronic biliary strictures, infection, and even cirrhosis and is more common during laparoscopic cholecystectomy compared to open cholecystectomy. Injury to the hepatic artery is also a serious concern that may lead to hepatic ischemic injury or bile duct ischemia and stricture.

You perform a laparoscopic cholecystectomy.

◆ **What is your postoperative management plan?**

◆ Observe the patient for recovery from general anesthesia. Within 7–24 hours, most patients are ready for discharge, and they can be seen in the office in 7–10 days.

Case 7.3 Right Upper Quadrant Pain No. 2

You see a 30-year-old woman in the emergency department with RUQ pain, nausea, vomiting, and a temperature of 102°F. An ultrasound study reveals gallstones

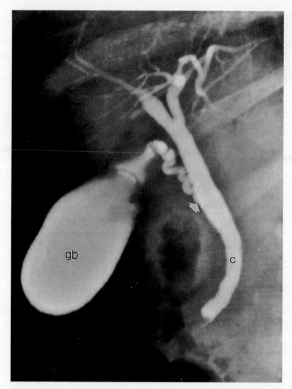

Figure 7-4: Intraoperative cholangiogram showing a normal common duct and filling of the duodenum. *gb*, gallbladder; *c*, common bile duct; *arrow*, junction of cystic duct with common bile duct. (From Yamada T, Alpers DH, Owyang C, et al. *Textbook of Gastroenterology*, 3rd ed. Philadelphia: Lippincott Williams & Wilkins, 1999:2721.)

and a thickened, edematous gallbladder wall. Blood work indicates a WBC count of 19,000/mm^3 and an elevated alkaline phosphatase; the remaining studies are normal.

◆ **What is the most likely diagnosis?**

◈ The patient most likely has **acute cholecystitis with cholelithiasis** (acute calculus cholecystitis).

◆ **What is the next step?**

◈ It is necessary to start **antibiotics** after obtaining blood cultures. Generally, antibiotics that cover **gram-negative rods and anaerobes** are warranted preoperatively and for 24 hours postoperatively in patients undergoing cholecystectomy. The most frequent organism cultured from patients is *Escherichia coli*, followed by *Enterobacter*, *Klebsiella*, and *Enterococcus*. A second-generation cephalosporin is adequate for most high-risk cases. Most patients need intravenous (IV) resuscitation and are placed on nothing-by-mouth (NPO) feeding. A nasogastric (NG) tube is necessary if they have persistent nausea or vomiting.

◆ **What course do you expect the patient to follow over the next 1–2 days?**

◈ With antibiotics and fluids, the patient's temperature will most likely return to normal. Her condition will improve.

◆ **What is your management plan?**

◆ The patient should have a **laparoscopic cholecystectomy within 72 hours of symptom onset**.

Case 7.4 | Right Upper Quadrant Pain No. 3

You admit a woman with symptomatic cholelithiasis. In addition to an elevated alkaline phosphatase and gallstones on ultrasound, her bilirubin is elevated at 4 mg/dL.

◆ **How does this finding change the proposed management plan?**

◆ You should suspect common bile duct obstruction when a patient presents with jaundice or has elevated liver enzymes. It is also necessary to determine whether the ultrasound shows dilated bile ducts, which is evidence for obstruction of the common bile duct.

> **QUICK CUT** It is essential to clear the common duct of stones if they are present, either using ERCP preoperatively or intraoperatively by common bile duct exploration and stone extraction.

Management may involve several approaches. In the past, an open cholecystectomy with exploration of the common bile duct was more common. Currently, either of the following treatment plans is recommended: **ERCP followed by laparoscopic cholecystectomy or laparoscopic cholecystectomy, with intraoperative cholangiogram, and common duct exploration or laparoscopic cholecystectomy and postoperative ERCP (Fig. 7-5)**.

Case 7.5 | Right Upper Quadrant Pain No. 4

A woman who is 6 months pregnant is admitted with symptomatic cholelithiasis.

◆ **What is the appropriate management plan?**

◆ Gallstones are present in 3%–11% of pregnant women and in most cases are asymptomatic.

> **QUICK CUT** Symptomatic cholelithiasis as well as gallstone pancreatitis can be managed nonoperatively in the majority of pregnant patients with hydration and pain management.

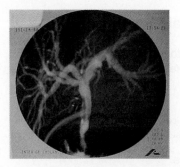

Figure 7-5: A T-tube cholangiogram, following a common duct exploration, showing free flow of dye into the duodenum.

If the patient has recurrent episodes of pain or an episode of biliary colic, acute cholecystitis, obstructive jaundice, or peritonitis, surgery or ERCP is justifiable. If possible, cholecystectomy is safest during the second trimester. In selected cases, ERCP and sphincterotomy are usually safe. After delivery, the gallbladder is removed.

Deep
Thoughts

The health of the mother is the most important factor in a fetus's care. That is if the mother is sick, the fetus is significantly affected.

Case 7.6 ♦ Right Upper Quadrant Pain No. 5

A 35-year-old woman is admitted with symptomatic cholelithiasis and gallstones visible on ultrasound. Blood studies show that she has an elevated amylase.

◆ **How does this laboratory finding influence management?**

◆ Most patients with an elevated amylase have mild pancreatitis, which is probably irrelevant unless significant signs and symptoms of the condition are present. The pancreatitis may result from either edema and inflammation of the distal bile duct and pancreas due to the gallbladder inflammation or a common duct stone. Usually, the amylase returns to normal quickly, and the patient improves by the next day. **Cholecystectomy and operative cholangiography may then be performed (Fig. 7-6).**

QUICK CUT A high quality cholangiogram is mandatory with biliary pancreatitis. Noninvasive imaging such as MRCP may be preferred because ERCP is associated with inducing pancreatitis in a small percentage of patients.

◆ **How would the proposed management change if the patient appears ill secondary to acute pancreatitis?**

◆ If the patient has significant complications from the pancreatitis, such as high fluid requirements, hypocalcemia, oliguria, hypotension, or pulmonary complications, **it is necessary to delay the cholecystectomy**. If she also has a dilated common bile duct or a stone in her distal duct, then consideration of ERCP is appropriate because of the probability of distal bile duct obstruction. Relieving the obstruction is important for rapid recovery.

Case 7.7 ♦ Right Upper Quadrant Pain No. 6

A 60-year-old man has marked RUQ pain and gallstones on ultrasound examination. He has a temperature of 104°F and a blood pressure (BP) of 100/60 mm Hg.

◆ **What is the most likely diagnosis?**

◆ The high fever may indicate **acute cholecystitis or a complication** of gallbladder disease such as cholangitis, empyema of the gallbladder, or a pericholecystic abscess.

You begin resuscitation with IV fluids and antibiotics.

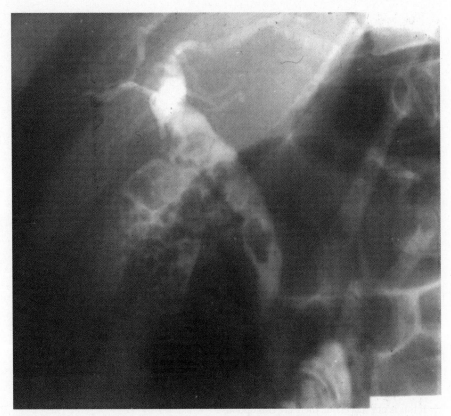

Figure 7-6: Intraoperative cholangiogram showing distal obstruction due to a retained stone.

◆ **What studies would you perform to establish a diagnosis?**

◆ An **ultrasound examination** would still be the first study.

You perform an ultrasound and find that the gallbladder is distended with fluid that has internal echoes and gallstones.

◆ **What is the next step?**

◆ This is most likely an empyema of the gallbladder. This condition generally requires IV antibiotics and **emergent exploration** with cholecystectomy, depending on the prior health of the patient. When the patient's general health is poor, percutaneous cholecystostomy to drain the gallbladder is an option with a lower operative risk (Fig. 7-7).

◆ **How would the proposed management change if the ultrasound study showed previous removal of the gallbladder, a dilated common bile duct, and air in the biliary system?**

◆ This suggests a serious complication such as **suppurative cholangitis**, which results when bacterial infection occurs with bile duct obstruction. In this case, the bacteria are gas-forming organisms. Patients commonly demonstrate jaundice and require urgent decompression of the bile duct. Quick stabilization with IV fluids and antibiotics is essential.

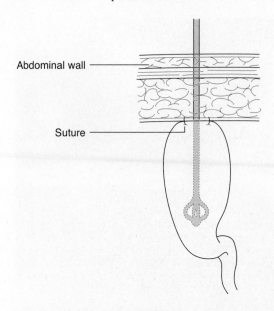

Abdominal wall ───

Suture ───

Figure 7-7: Percutaneous cholecystostomy for temporary drainage of an infected gallbladder.

QUICK CUT In cases of suppurative cholangitis, the best treatment is resuscitation, antibiotics and emergent ERCP with sphincterotomy, decompression of the biliary tree, and stone removal if feasible (Fig. 7-8).

If this is not successful, there are two options.

1. A transhepatic cholangiogram and stone extraction, which may be performed by an interventional radiologist *OR*
2. If this procedure is not successful, cholecystectomy and common bile duct drainage

Many surgeons do not perform cholangiography in this situation because it may worsen the patient's sepsis and potentially cause injury to the common duct due to poor visualization of the common duct due to inflammation.

Case 7.8 Right Upper Quadrant Pain No. 7

A 78-year-old man who presented to the emergency department with a 12-hour history of RUQ pain and tenderness has been admitted. He appears quite ill.

◆ **How would you evaluate and manage the following situations?**

Case Variation 7.8.1. A temperature of 104°F, a BP of 90/60 mm Hg, and a WBC count of 20,000/mm³

◆ This patient may have acute biliary sepsis and needs emergent evaluation, antibiotics, and resuscitation. Possible diagnoses include empyema of the gallbladder, CBD obstruction with cholangitis, liver abscess, among others. It is necessary to establish a diagnosis and institute definitive therapy. If the cause is biliary in nature, urgent drainage or surgery is essential in most cases.

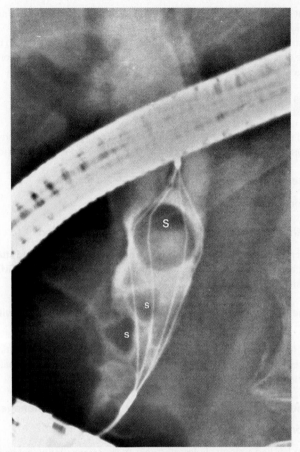

Figure 7-8: ERCP showing a distal common bile duct obstruction due to a stone (*S*) and extraction of stone. (From Yamada T, Alpers DH, Owyang C, et al. *Textbook of Gastroenterology*, 3rd ed. Philadelphia: Lippincott Williams & Wilkins; 1999:2723.)

Case Variation 7.8.2. A temperature of 96°F and a WBC count of 3,900/mm³

◆ The patient should be treated in a similar manner as previously described (see Case Variation 7.8.1).

 QUICK CUT Elderly patients may manifest signs of sepsis with hypothermia and leukopenia.

Case Variation 7.8.3. A tender 3-cm–diameter palpable mass in the RUQ, a temperature of 103°F, and mental obtundation

◆ This mass is most likely an **inflamed gallbladder** with omentum attached to the gallbladder that "walls it off." When the gallbladder is palpable, typically in sick elderly patients, many surgeons term the condition a "palpable gallbladder." The implication is that an emergent cholecystectomy is necessary as soon as resuscitation occurs because there is a high risk of gallbladder rupture, which carries a high mortality. The mental obtundation is a sign of sepsis.

If the patient is too sick to undergo surgery, then the gallbladder can be drained via percutaneous radiologic guidance or with a small cut down under local anesthesia.

Some similar older patients have air in the wall of the gallbladder, which indicates that a gas-forming organism has invaded the tissues. This is obviously a serious complication and requires urgent surgery. It is termed an **emphysematous gallbladder**.

Case 7.9 Right Upper Quadrant Pain No. 8

You are asked to see a 51-year-old man who presented to the emergency department with recent onset of jaundice (bilirubin, 9 mg/dL), fever, and RUQ pain and tenderness.

◆ **What is the most likely diagnosis?**

◆ The condition most likely is **acute cholangitis**.

◆ **What are the basic steps in the patient's initial evaluation?**

◆ The basic steps are **resuscitation, antibiotics, and an urgent ultrasound study of the biliary tree**. If obstruction or dilation of the common bile duct is seen, then **ERCP and biliary decompression** are warranted.

◆ **What is the likelihood that this patient has pancreatic cancer with distal bile duct obstruction?**

◆ This cancer is very unlikely. Biliary sepsis does not usually develop in patients with pancreatic cancer, even after instrumentation. Patients present with abdominal or back pain, weight loss, and jaundice.

◆ **How do the following situations influence the proposed management?**

Case Variation 7.9.1. **Previous cholecystectomy**

◆ If the patient has had a recent cholecystectomy, there is a possibility that he has a **retained stone in the common bile duct**.

> **QUICK CUT** A common duct stone occurring within 2 years after a cholecystectomy is termed a retained stone, whereas a stone appearing after 2 years is termed a primary common bile duct stone.

An RUQ ultrasound is appropriate, and if it is positive, attempted ERCP or percutaneous transhepatic cholangiography with stone extraction is necessary. If this procedure is not successful, the patient should return to the operating room, where bile duct exploration can be performed.

The patient may also have a diagnosis of a **biliary stricture** resulting from an injury that occurred during cholecystectomy. The evaluation is the same, but the treatment is surgical exploration and bypass of the stricture, usually with a choledochojejunostomy (Figs. 7-9 and 7-10). Endoscopic dilatation is another option for treatment, although studies have found that it is less beneficial.

Case Variation 7.9.2. **No previous cholecystectomy**

◆ The most likely diagnosis is a **common duct stone with biliary obstruction**. An RUQ ultrasound evaluation to examine the gallbladder and the common bile duct is appropriate.

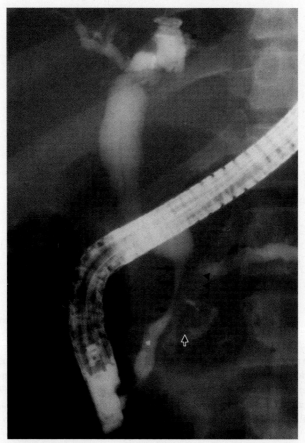

Figure 7-9: Cholangiogram of a distal bile duct stricture. The *arrows* indicate the area of stricture. This stricture could be a benign scar or a malignant tumor.

An ultrasound is good for detecting gallstones and bile duct dilation but not as good at visualizing distal bile duct stones. If the patient is found to have gallstones, IV antibiotics are warranted, followed by ERCP with stone extraction. A cholecystectomy is necessary afterward.

Case 7.10 Complications of Laparoscopic Cholecystectomy

You perform a laparoscopic cholecystectomy for cholelithiasis in a 40-year-old man.

◆ **What is the appropriate management in each of the following postoperative situations?**

Case Variation 7.10.1. Postoperative fever and abdominal pain

◆ Most patients have an uneventful recovery after laparoscopic cholecystectomy, although they may have significant **fever or pain, which may indicate an infection or biliary leak**.

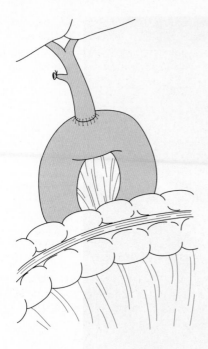

Figure 7-10: Choledochojejunostomy.

The two most useful tests are an **abdominal ultrasound study and hepatobiliary imino-diacetic acid** (HIDA scan). This scan involves the IV injection of hepatoiminodiacetic acid. The dye is excreted into the biliary tract as long as the serum bilirubin is below 8–10 mg/dL. A HIDA scan is a particularly good test for detecting biliary leaks, as well as acute cholecystitis (the gallbladder fails to visualize in acute cholecystitis) (Fig. 7-11). If no biliary leak or

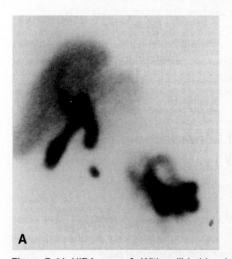
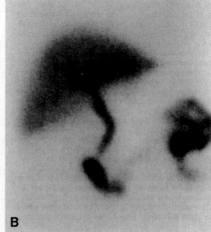

Figure 7-11: HIDA scans **A:** With gallbladder visualization. **B:** Without gallbladder filling but good filling of the duodenum. The HIDA scan is useful for detecting biliary leaks, obstructed cystic ducts, and common bile duct obstructions. (From Lawrence PF, Bilbao M, Bell RM, et al, eds. *Essentials of General Surgery*. Baltimore: Lippincott Williams & Wilkins; 1988:236.)

collection is evident on ultrasound, and the scan reveals normal hepatic excretion, then it is appropriate to follow the patient. If a collection is found and it is of significant size, it should be drained completely. If a biliary leak or obstruction is seen, the patient should undergo an ERCP to define the biliary anatomy. Some surgeons also obtain a computed tomography (CT) scan to rule out a hepatic abscess proximal to hepatic duct obstruction.

Case Variation 7.10.2. Jaundice

◆ The workup is similar to that previously described (see Case Variation 7.10.1).

Case Variation 7.10.3. A leak on HIDA scan and a cystic duct stump leak on ERCP (Fig. 7-12)

◆ Management usually involves **biliary drainage with a temporary stent** placed during ERCP (see Fig. 7-21 later in this chapter). Exploration is necessary in the patient who fails to improve rapidly.

◆ **How would the proposed management change if both the HIDA scan and the ERCP demonstrate complete obstruction of the bile duct?**

◆ Re-exploration and some sort of **biliary drainage procedure** are necessary. Occasionally, primary repair of the ductal injury is possible, but more often, a new anastomosis with the gastrointestinal (GI) tract is essential. The typical operation is a choledochojejunostomy.

Case 7.11   Painless Jaundice

You are asked to evaluate and manage a 55-year-old man with jaundice of recent onset. He denies pain but has marked pruritus. Blood studies reveal a direct bilirubin

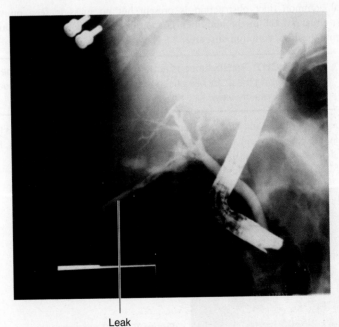

Leak

Figure 7-12: ERCP and cholangiogram showing extravasation of dye near the cystic duct remnant and along the undersurface of the liver.

of 6 mg/dL, normal aspartate aminotransferase (AST [serum glutamic-oxaloacetic transaminase]) and alanine aminotransferase (ALT [serum glutamate pyruvate transaminase]), and an alkaline phosphatase of six times normal.

◆ **What are the most common diagnoses?**

◆ The pattern indicates an **obstructive process to the biliary tree**. The differential diagnosis is **cancer of the head of the pancreas; periampullary carcinoma; cholangiocarcinoma (Klatskin tumor); stricture of the common bile duct; and, occasionally, a common bile duct stone impacted in the ampulla**. Pancreatic adenocarcinoma and cholangiocarcinoma, which may be associated with tobacco use, are usually accompanied by weight loss. In addition, these cancers may be accompanied by vague abdominal or back pain. Strictures of the common bile duct typically occur in chronic alcoholics who have chronic pancreatitis or patients who have had prior biliary surgery. **Common bile duct stones that are impacted in the ampulla typically result in intermittent symptoms of abdominal pain, jaundice, fever, and chills; thus, they do not fit this picture.** However, on occasion, presenting features may be similar to those of patients with carcinoma.

◆ **How would you further define the problem?**

◆ An **abdominal ultrasound study** is a good initial step to visualize the common bile duct as well as stones in the gallbladder or duct.

An ultrasound study indicates a dilated common bile duct and no gallstones or pancreatic masses.

◆ **What is the next management step?**

◆ If distal common duct obstruction is present but no mass is seen on ultrasound, contrast-enhanced **CT of the abdomen** is appropriate. CT is better than ultrasound at visualizing the distal common duct area.

 QUICK CUT Transcutaneous abdominal ultrasound is not the best method for visualizing the distal bile duct and pancreatic head area because intestinal gas obscures the view.

It may be possible to visualize the mass further with finer CT cuts of the pancreas (Fig. 7-13), but often, the pathology can still not be elucidated. If a mass can be visualized, ERCP may further define the lesion and allow the gathering of brushings for cytology.

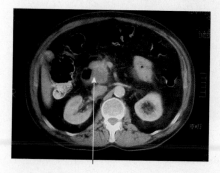

Figure 7-13: CT scan showing a mass (*arrow*) in the head of the pancreas.

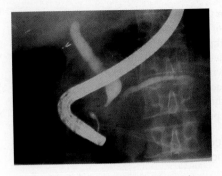

Figure 7-14: ERCP showing a narrowing of the distal common bile duct and a "double duct" sign, which is a dilated common bile duct and pancreatic duct.

You perform a CT scan of the abdomen and see no mass in the pancreas.

◆ **What is the next management step?**

◆ In this setting, upper GI endoscopy and **endoscopic ultrasound (EUS)** performed through the duodenal wall commonly allow an excellent assessment of the pancreatic head. It is possible to combine ERCP with EUS if further information is necessary. CT and EUS also both allow **assessment of the tumor to discover whether local metastasis, positive lymph nodes, portal vein involvement, or liver metastases are present (Fig. 7-14).**

An EUS allows you to visualize a 2-cm mass in the head of the pancreas (Fig. 7-15).

◆ **Is biopsy of the mass appropriate?**

◆ **Most experienced pancreatic surgeons are comfortable proceeding with pancreatic exploration without a preoperative pathologic diagnosis.** The advisability of a percutaneous, preoperative biopsy is a matter of debate because of concern about cancer spread and conceivable prevention of a curable resection. Regardless, some surgeons prefer to biopsy

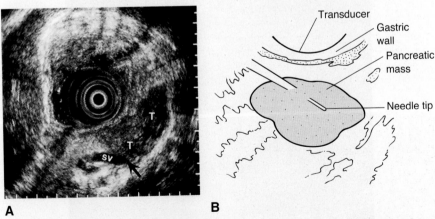

A   **B**

Figure 7-15: A: EUS showing a mass in the pancreas. *Arrow* is pointing to obstruction of the splenic vein by the tumor. **B:** Needle biopsy under EUS guidance. T indicates tumor, SV indicates Splenic Vein. (From Yamada T, Alpers DH, Owyang C, et al. *Textbook of Gastroenterology*, 3rd ed. Philadelphia: Lippincott Williams & Wilkins; 1999:3012, 3016.)

the lesion and have a definitive diagnosis prior to surgery. It is important to try and have or establish a tissue diagnosis at surgery but prior to pancreatic resection because the operation is extensive and the risk of significant complications is high.

Establishing a tissue diagnosis is particularly difficult in patients with **chronic pancreatitis**, where a thickened, scarred pancreatic head can feel like cancer. In contrast, pancreatic cancer can be associated with adjacent pancreatic areas with chronic scarring due to a local inflammatory process, making the biopsy look similar to chronic pancreatitis and misleading the surgeon into thinking the process is benign.

Final evaluation using an endoscopic transduodenal biopsy reveals a definitive diagnosis of pancreatic adenocarcinoma involving the head of the pancreas.

◆ **What preoperative findings would make the patient inoperable?**

◆ To tolerate this procedure, the patient must have an **acceptable general medical condition, with no evidence of distant metastasis** and a normal chest x-ray (CXR) and no neurologic symptoms or bone pain. Further evaluation is necessary if any of these conditions is present. The CT scan and EUS require careful evaluation to check for evidence of **local invasion** of the portal vein, nearby structures, or local lymph nodes (Fig. 7-16). The **liver must be free of metastatic lesions (Fig. 7-17).** The use of laparoscopy assists in staging the patient. This allows direct visualization of some of these structures and confirms any metastases by biopsy. Confirmed metastases are a sign of incurable disease. In essence, the best chance for resectability is a small lesion that is limited to the pancreas.

There are no obvious metastases on CT scan or EUS, and you determine that the patient is operable.

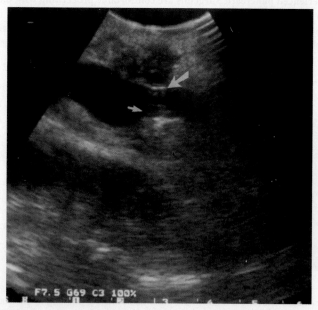

Figure 7-16: Ultrasound showing superior mesenteric vein involvement with pancreatic cancer. *Arrows* point to tumor. *Dark space* is vein. (From Wanebo HJ, ed. *Surgery for Gastrointestinal Cancer.* Philadelphia: Lippincott-Raven; 1997:179.)

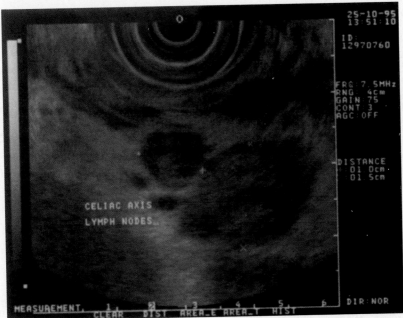

Figure 7-17: Endoscopic ultrasound showing metastatic lymph nodes in the celiac axis region. (From Wanebo HJ, ed. *Surgery for Gastrointestinal Cancer*. Philadelphia: Lippincott-Raven; 1997:213.)

◆ **What operative decisions are necessary?**

◆ It is often difficult to determine the resectability of pancreatic cancer preoperatively. Local invasion of visceral vessels may not always be apparent on CT or EUS. A CT scan may miss liver lesions smaller than 2 cm and peritoneal and omental metastases. Therefore, the **first phase of surgery involves assessing for distant metastasis** by examining the liver and peritoneal surfaces, with biopsy of suspicious lesions for frozen section diagnosis. Lymph node metastases in the periaortic or celiac region indicate the tumor is beyond the limits of resection and should be confirmed with biopsy.

Other determinations of unresectability include tumor involvement of the inferior vena cava, aorta, and superior mesenteric artery. **If these findings indicate no metastasis and no local invasion, pancreaticoduodenectomy may proceed.**

◆ **What are the basic steps in pancreaticoduodenectomy?**

◆ After evaluation for metastasis and resectability, the head of the pancreas is mobilized from the retroperitoneum and superior mesenteric vein and portal vein. The common bile duct and the first portion of the duodenum are transected in order to preserve the pylorus. The pancreatic neck is transected, followed by detachment of the head and uncinate process from the posterior structures. The jejunum at the ligament of Treitz is transected, the specimen removed, and the GI tract reconstructed (Fig. 7-18).

Tumor resection is successful. The pathology returns with complete removal of the primary adenocarcinoma of the pancreas with negative margins and no local or metastatic disease. The patient asks about his prognosis.

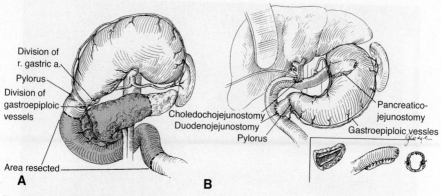

Figure 7-18: A: Pancreaticoduodenectomy, with organs resected using a pylorus-preserving method. **B:** Reconstruction of the gastrointestinal tract connecting the pancreas, bile duct, and proximal duodenum to the bowel. (From Wanebo HJ, ed. *Surgery for Gastrointestinal Cancer*. Philadelphia: Lippincott-Raven; 1997:395.)

◆ **How would you respond?**

◆ Most surgeons believe that the **cure rate at 5 years is very low**, in the range of 5%–10%. However, in some studies, the reported 5-year survival rate for resected pancreatic ade-nocarcinomas in the head of the pancreas has been as high as 35%–48% in patients with negative nodes. Several factors favor long-term survival, such as tumor diameter less than 3 cm, negative nodal status, diploid tumor DNA content, tumor S-phase fraction less than 19%, negative resection margins, and the use of postoperative adjuvant chemotherapy and radiotherapy.

◆ **How would your response change if you had performed a palliative biliary and gastric bypass after finding unresectable pancreatic adenocarcinoma with local spread (Fig. 7-19)?**

◆ Surgical palliation with biliary and gastric bypass may prevent gastric outlet or duodenal obstruction and bile duct obstruction. Abdominal and back pain can be decreased by celiac axis injection with alcohol to ablate the nerves. **The mean survival in patients undergoing surgical palliation is less than 8 months. Surgical palliation can often be avoided with biliary and duodenal stents.**

Case 7.12   Painless Jaundice due to Obstruction at the Common Bile Duct Bifurcation

You are asked to evaluate a 60-year-old man with painless jaundice. An abdominal ultrasound shows dilated intrahepatic ducts but no dilation of the common bile duct.

◆ **What is the next step?**

◆ If intrahepatic biliary obstruction but no extrahepatic biliary obstruction is present, this may represent a cholangiocarcinoma or Klatskin tumor. Klatskin tumors are tumors of the biliary tree at the bifurcation of the hepatic ducts. Because they are not always seen as a mass on CT, the next best step is either **ERCP or percutaneous transhepatic cholangiography**

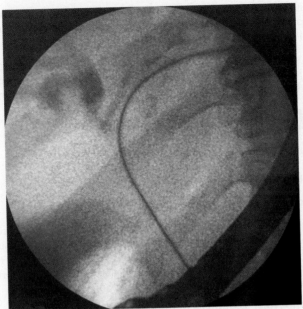

Figure 7-19: Biliary stent in a patient with a distal bile duct obstruction due to unresectable cancer. (From Kaplowitz N, ed. *Liver and Biliary Diseases*, 2nd ed. Baltimore: Lippincott Williams & Wilkins; 1996:721.)

to demonstrate the level of obstruction. For lesions higher in the bile duct, percutaneous transhepatic cholangiography is preferable because it visualizes the proximal hepatic ducts better than ERCP. **Biopsies and cytology** may also be performed during these procedures to make the diagnosis of cancer.

On percutaneous transhepatic cholangiography, you find a constricting lesion typical of a Klatskin tumor. The biopsy returns cholangiocarcinoma.

◆ What is the next step?

◆ Klatskin tumors are associated with a poor prognosis because of the high rate of vascular invasion, unresectability, and metastatic disease. If **no evidence for unresectability or metastasis** is evident on CT, **exploration with resection** of the bile ducts and gallbladder is appropriate. Tumors may extend into the left or right hepatic duct, in which case a hepatic lobectomy or trisegmentectomy may be necessary. **However, most tumors are unresectable.**

On exploration, no local metastatic disease is present. You perform a complete resection of the primary cholangiocarcinoma at the hepatic duct bifurcation. The patient recovers and asks about his prognosis.

◆ What is your response?

◆ The survival rate for patients with Klatskin tumors is poor; most tumors are unresectable at the time of diagnosis. Although recent improvements have been made in the treatment of these tumors, **the 5-year survival rate is still 15%** for patients undergoing curative resection.

◆ How would your response change if you performed only palliative stenting of the hepatic duct strictures after finding unresectable cholangiocarcinoma with local spread?

◆ The 5-year survival rate in patients undergoing palliative stenting for cholangiocarcinoma is **less than 5%.** The most common cause of death is locally invasive disease. Neither radiation nor chemotherapy has any proven long-term benefit in the treatment of cholangiocarcinoma.

Case 7.13 Other Biliary Tract Cancers

You are evaluating a 50-year-old woman for jaundice.

◆ How would you manage the following situations?

Case Variation 7.13.1. Diagnosis of ampullary adenocarcinoma

◆ The patient should have a complete evaluation similar to the preceding patient (see Case 7.12). If no metastases are present, exploration is necessary. Most ampullary cancers require a pancreatoduodenectomy (Whipple procedure) to remove the lesion. In contrast to pancreatic cancer, ampullary cancer has a higher cure rate, with reported survival at 5 years as high as 65% (much higher than that for any other biliary cancer).

Case Variation 7.13.2. Diagnosis of duodenal adenocarcinoma

◆ The management of duodenal tumors depends on the size and location of the lesion. If the tumor involves the ampulla, it is necessary to perform a pancreatoduodenectomy. Removal of a lesion in the first or fourth part of the duodenum may be possible with segmental resection. Patients with duodenal cancers have a worse prognosis because their carcinomas usually involve nearby structures.

Case Variation 7.13.3. A mass in the gallbladder fossa visible on ultrasound

◆ A mass in the gallbladder fossa is usually a malignant gallbladder adenocarcinoma. These tumors may cause symptoms similar to gallstones. CT is appropriate to evaluate the mass further and look for evidence of metastasis (Fig. 7-20).

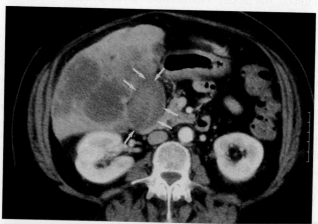

Figure 7-20: CT scan of a gallbladder cancer (*arrows*). (From Yamada T, Alpers DH, Owyang C, et al. *Textbook of Gastroenterology*, 3rd ed. Philadelphia: Lippincott Williams & Wilkins; 1999:3037.)

If CT reveals an infiltrating mass in the gallbladder with no evidence of metastatic disease, it is advisable, if possible, to perform **an open cholecystectomy, a wide resection of the surrounding liver, and a hilar lymph node resection**. Most surgeons advocate a wedge resection of the liver with a 2–3-cm margin around the gallbladder. Laparoscopic cholecystectomy is probably not appropriate because of the inability to remove hepatic tissue.

Recurrent cancer may occur at the trocar sites. The most common means of spread in carcinoma of the gallbladder is by direct extension into the liver. Unfortunately, **the discovery of most of these cancers occurs late in their course, when they involve a large portion of the liver, making them unresectable**.

Case Variation 7.13.4. *A 3-cm polyp in the gallbladder*

◆ Observation of small polyps is usually appropriate. Cholecystectomy is warranted for removal of larger polyps (>2 cm) because of the 7%–10% risk of developing adenocarcinoma of the gallbladder.

Case Variation 7.13.5. *A calcified gallbladder*

◆ A calcified gallbladder, also called a porcelain gallbladder, has a 50% association with adenocarcinoma and should be removed.

Case 7.14 Acute Epigastric Pain No. 10

You are following a 29-year-old man who had an episode of epigastric pain. His serum amylase and lipase are three times normal, and no gallstones are visible on ultrasound examination of the abdomen.

◆ **What management is appropriate?**

◆ This patient most likely has pancreatitis based on initial assessment. To be certain that you are not missing other possible diagnoses, an obstructive abdominal series is necessary to rule out other common disorders such as a perforated ulcer with free air. Findings in pancreatitis include a generalized ileus (usual), as well as a localized ileus of the second and third portions of duodenum secondary to a localized inflammatory process. CT of the abdomen is not mandatory for patients with uncomplicated pancreatitis.

 QUICK CUT The usual treatment for pancreatitis involves NPO feeding, IV hydration, pain control, and observation.

Deep Thoughts	It is important to diagnose the cause of the acute pancreatitis to guide therapy and prevent future recurrence.

Many patients recover quickly as a consequence of this therapy. If a particular patient does not improve rapidly, it may be necessary to administer total parenteral nutrition (TPN) to maintain good nutrition.

◆ **How would the presence of gallstones influence the proposed management?**

◆ Gallstone pancreatitis is generally managed in a similar way. The serum amylase level is monitored over the next 24–48 hours. When the amylase decreases and the patient improves, **laparoscopic cholecystectomy** is warranted.

Case 7.15   Acute Epigastric Pain No. 11

A 34-year-old man has severe abdominal pain that has been progressively increasing over the past several hours. His amylase value is elevated. You admit him and begin therapy. Over the next hour, you note that he appears severely ill; hypotension, hypoxemia, and multiorgan failure develop rapidly.

◆ **What is the most likely diagnosis?**

◆ The patient most likely has **severe necrotizing pancreatitis** with massive third-space fluid loss due to local pancreatic inflammation. In addition, he has systemic inflammatory response syndrome, resulting in multiorgan system failure. It is hypothesized that this syndrome is mediated by cytokine release, resulting in acute respiratory distress syndrome (ARDS), multiorgan system failure, and hemodynamic instability.

◆ **What steps are necessary next?**

◆ Major **fluid resuscitation in a critical care unit** is essential. CT of the abdomen is useful to assess the extent of local inflammation and to search for additional causes of decompensation, including bowel necrosis and perforation, abscess formation, and biliary obstruction with infection (Fig. 7-21).

After receiving 6 L of normal saline over 12 hours, the patient remains hypotensive with a very low urine output—10 mL/hr in the past **4** hours.

The patient may need more IV fluids for adequate resuscitation. Pressor support could increase organ perfusion and prevent further organ injury. Septic shock is associated with vasodilation and hypovolemia. Adequate fluid resuscitation is necessary to restore organ perfusion. Vasoconstriction with pressors such as norepinephrine coupled with appropriate fluid resuscitation can be critical to restore organ perfusion.

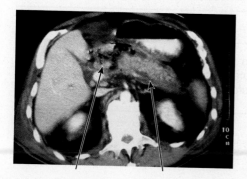

Figure 7-21: CT scan of the abdomen showing the head and body of the pancreas (*arrows*) severely edematous and inflamed.

◆ **What is your plan for fluid resuscitation?**

◆ The adequacy of resuscitation should still be a concern. The patient may need a **pulmonary artery catheter** if his hemodynamic status cannot be resolved using the central venous pressure (CVP) as a guide to determine how much fluid and what pressor support is best to optimize organ perfusion.

The patient has labored breathing and a pulse oximeter reading of 90%.

◆ **What is the best way to assess the patient's pulmonary status and manage his ventilation?**

◆ This patient warrants immediate physical examination with chest auscultation, an arterial blood gas (ABG), and a CXR. Supplemental oxygen and continuous pulse oximeter monitoring are necessary during this examination. This patient's problems may be due to **pulmonary edema from overhydration, ARDS from a systemic response to the pancreatitis, atelectasis, or pneumonia**, which are often difficult to distinguish by CXR. An ABG provides important information on oxygenation (Po_2) as well as adequacy of ventilation (Pco_2), which helps decide the need for mechanical ventilation. Experienced clinicians usually intubate before the patient's condition becomes serious. The decision to intubate is usually made based on a combination of ABGs and clinical status.

Your resident student wants to know the correlation between serum amylase and severity of the pancreatitis.

◆ **What would you say?**

◆ **Amylase levels do not correlate with the severity of pancreatitis** or the prognosis. Ranson (Table 7-1) prognostic signs can be used to ascertain the severity of the pancreatitis.

Table 7-1: Ranson Prognostic Signs Associated with Acute Pancreatitis

On admission
Age older than 55 years
White blood cell (WBC) count >16,000 cells/mm^3
Glucose >200 mg/dL
Lactate dehydrogenase (LDH) >350 IU/L
Aspartate aminotransferase (AST) >250 IU/L
After 48 hours
Hematocrit decrease = 10%
Blood urea nitrogen (BUN) increase = 5 mg/dL
Ca^{2+} level <8 mg/dL
Pao_2 <60 mm Hg
Base deficit >4 mEq/L
Fluid sequestration >6 L

You decide that the pulmonary failure in this patient requires intubation and ventilation. Over the next 2 days, **signs and symptoms of sepsis** develop, with fever, leukocytosis, and septic shock.

◆ **What is the next step?**

◆ You should be most concerned about the extent of pancreatic necrosis or **pancreatic abscess**, although other sources of sepsis such as pneumonia, IV access infection, and urinary tract infection (UTI) warrant investigation. To evaluate for pancreatic abscess, a dynamic CT scan is the most reliable examination (Fig. 7-22). This CT scan includes the use of radiographic contrast material timed to determine the vascularity of the pancreas.

A CT scan shows a peripancreatic collection.

◆ **What is the next step?**

 QUICK CUT For a peripancreatic collection with internal loculation or debris, sampling by a percutaneous route under CT scan or ultrasound guidance is necessary, if possible. For a large number of WBCs or bacteria, the diagnosis of an abscess is appropriate, and abscess drainage is essential. Drainage may occur either surgically or percutaneously with a catheter.

◆ An experienced clinician should decide which type of drainage to use because some collections contain a large amount of debris and cannot be drained with a catheter. Appropriate antibiotics, usually for gram-negative and anaerobic coverage, are necessary. If adequate percutaneous drainage is not possible, open surgical drainage is required.

The patient is recovering from percutaneous pancreatic abscess drainage when he suddenly becomes hypotensive and the drainage becomes bloody.

◆ **What condition do you suspect, and how do you manage it?**

◆ The most likely diagnosis is **erosion of the catheter or abscess into a major artery** such as the splenic, gastroduodenal, or superior mesenteric arteries or a pancreatic vessel. Diagnosis involves **angiography; control consists of embolization** in most cases.

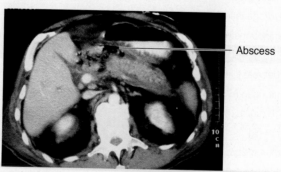
— Abscess

Figure 7-22: CT scan of a pancreatic abscess with air in the cavity.

Suppose a severe case of pancreatitis occurred in a 70-year-old patient.

◆ **Would you change your approach?**

◆ In older patients with abdominal pain and increased amylase levels, it is necessary to consider diagnoses other than pancreatitis. Abdominal catastrophes such as **mesenteric ischemia and volvulus** could manifest similarly. The pain pattern of mesenteric ischemia may be less localized to the epigastric region, but in obtunded patients, this could be difficult to determine. A serum amylase elevation by itself is not a reliable enough marker of pancreatitis in severely ill patients. CT is very useful in assessing the intra-abdominal process.

In practice, any patient who is severely ill with suspected pancreatitis warrants close examination to rule out some other cause. CT is one good way to reassure oneself of the presence of pancreatitis because it shows edema of the pancreas and surrounding tissue. If that is not present, then one should be suspicious of the diagnosis. If after the CT the diagnosis remains uncertain, exploratory laparotomy may be appropriate.

◆ **What is the expected course of a patient with severe pancreatitis?**

◆ The sicker the patient, the more likely the development of serious complications involving other organs and tissues. The mortality of severe pancreatitis remains high.

Case 7.16 Acute Epigastric Pain No. 12

A 34-year-old alcoholic man who has developed acute pancreatitis initially improves, but his symptoms fail to resolve completely. Instead, he **continues to have moderate abdominal pain, anorexia, persistent elevation of serum amylase, and inability to eat due to early satiety.**

◆ **What is the suspected diagnosis?**

◆ The presumptive diagnosis is a **pancreatic pseudocyst**, which is a collection of fluid near the pancreas presumably due to leakage of pancreatic fluid and edema. It can cause pain due to a local compressive effect, especially on the posterior wall of the stomach, which causes the early satiety.

◆ **How would you confirm this diagnosis?**

◆ This is best visualized by **CT of the abdomen**, although an abdominal ultrasound study can also be useful (Fig. 7-23). Small pseudocysts are common with pancreatitis and do not usually cause this picture.

The CT shows a pseudocyst in the lesser sac that is 8 cm in diameter.

◆ **What is the next step?**

◆ The common practice would be **NPO feeding, TPN, and observation**, as long as no signs of infection are present.

You institute this therapy, and the patient improves over the next 10 days. The pain resolves, the amylase returns to normal, and the pseudocyst shrinks to 2 cm.

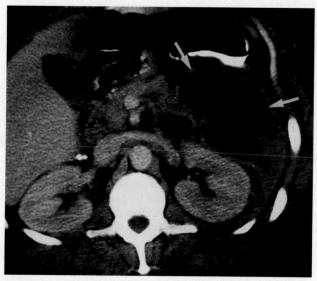

Figure 7-23: CT scan of the abdomen showing a pancreatic pseudocyst (*arrows*).

◆ **What is the next step?**

◆ Treatment involves beginning feeding and following the patient's symptoms and serum amylase. If these are stable, the **pseudocyst is resolving**, and the patient feels better and can be discharged.

◆ **How would you manage the patient if the pain and other symptoms continued or recurred and the serum amylase remained elevated?**

 QUICK CUT If a pseudocyst is present on CT and the patient fails to improve by 6 weeks, intervention is appropriate.

◆ The 6-week waiting period is observed for two reasons: Many pseudocysts resolve in 6 weeks, and the cyst wall must contain enough fibrous tissue to allow surgical suturing to occur. There are many ways to treat pancreatic pseudocysts. The best way has not been scientifically determined and each approach has its own advantages and disadvantages. These include percutaneous drainage by radiologic guidance, which is technically easy to do but has a high recurrence rate, may lead to infection of the pseudocyst and the development of a pancreaticocutaneous fistula. Stenting the pancreatic duct with ERCP past the ductal injury can be done. Many feel the procedure of choice involves internal drainage of the fluid collection into the GI tract. Internal drainage of a pancreatic pseudocyst can be performed endoscopically or surgically. Endoscopic drainage is performed through and endoscope using EUS guidance. A stent or stents are placed from the duodenal or gastric lumen through the enteric wall and pseudocyst wall into the pseudocyst itself allowing pseudocyst contents to drain into the stomach. This approach is less invasive than a surgical approach but is less likely to be successful if the pseudocyst has a large amount of debris and complex fluid. Surgically, the most common procedure is a **cystogastrostomy** (Fig. 7-24). The surgeon opens the stomach anteriorly

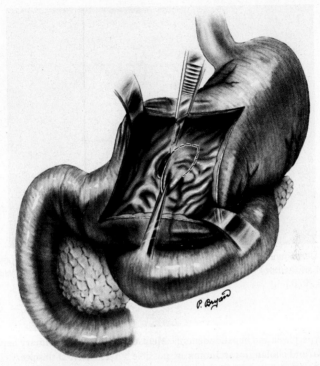

Figure 7-24: Cystogastrostomy for pancreatic pseudocyst. (From Howard JM, Idezuki Y, Ihse I, et al, eds. *Surgical Diseases of the Pancreas*, 3rd ed. Baltimore: Lippincott Williams & Wilkins; 1998:428. After Bradley EL III, Zeppa R. The pancreas. In: Sabiston DC, ed. *Davis-Christopher Textbook of Surgery*, 13th ed. Philadelphia: WB Saunders; 1986.)

and locates the cyst with a needle and syringe through the posterior stomach. Because the cyst is contiguous with the posterior stomach wall in most cases, it is necessary to make a communication with the cyst through the posterior wall. This procedure is very effective in resolving the pseudocyst. A **biopsy** is always taken to ensure that the cyst is inflammatory in origin rather than **cystadenoma or cystadenocarcinoma of the pancreas.**

COMMON HEPATIC DISORDERS

Case 7.17 Hepatic Mass

A 37-year-old woman is seen for vague RUQ pain. Laboratory studies are normal. An RUQ ultrasound study reveals no gallstones but does show a 3- × 4-cm mass in the right lobe of the liver.

◆ What are the common diagnoses?

◆ **Most likely, this lesion is benign.** If **cystic** on ultrasound, it is probably a **simple cyst.** If **solid,** the most common diagnosis is a **hemangioma.** Other likely tumors include focal

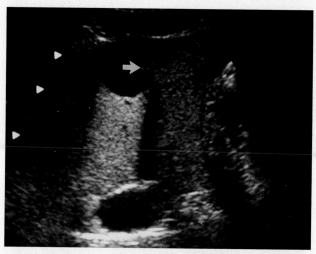

Figure 7-25: Ultrasound of the liver showing a hepatic cyst. (From Yamada T, Alpers DH, Owyang C, et al. *Textbook of Gastroenterology*, 3rd ed. Philadelphia: Lippincott Williams & Wilkins; 1999:2978.)

nodular hyperplasia and hepatic adenoma. **Metastatic carcinoma, primary hepatocellular carcinoma, and cholangiocarcinoma** are possible but less likely at this age.

◆ **What special history features or physical findings are appropriate?**

◆ Inquiries regarding history of use of oral birth control pills, exposure to environmental toxins, hepatitis B and C, previous injury to the liver, and known primary tumors are necessary. On physical examination, signs of chronic liver disease, including cirrhosis, polycystic kidney disease, and primary kidney tumors, should be sought.

◆ **How would you evaluate and manage the following types of lesions?**

Case Variation 7.17.1. Cystic lesion with no internal echoes suggestive of a simple cyst (Fig. 7-25)

◆ Although a simple cyst can cause symptoms of RUQ discomfort, it is **asymptomatic** in most cases. Rarely, a hepatic cyst may develop hemorrhage, secondary bacterial infection, or obstructive jaundice. Generally, a simple cyst needs **no further management**. If symptoms persist, treatment of the cyst with aspiration followed by a sclerosant or by simple excision is warranted. If multiple cysts are present in the liver in a patient who also has polycystic kidney disease, the patient has polycystic liver disease. Treatment is similar to that for simple cysts of the liver.

Case Variation 7.17.2. Multilocular cyst with calcifications in the wall and internal echoes (Fig. 7-26)

◆ A suspected **echinococcal cyst,** which results from *Echinococcus granulosus,* a GI parasite, may be present. The serologic test for *Echinococcus* is usually positive. Treatment is aimed at **operative sterilization** of the cyst by injecting the cyst under controlled operative conditions using hypertonic saline (a scolocidal agent), followed by **excision of the cyst.** It is

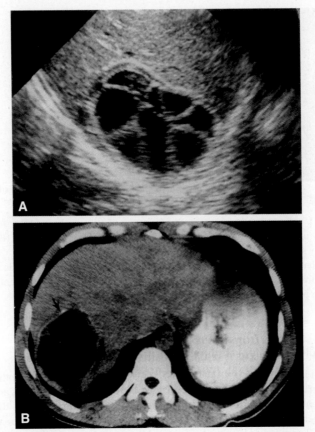

Figure 7-26: CT scan of the liver showing *Echinococcus* cyst. **A:** Ultrasound study of echinococcal cyst showing a multiseptated cystic structure. **B:** CT scan without contrast shows a cystic structure (*arrows*) with internal walls and calcification of the fibrotic wall. (From Kaplowitz N, ed. *Liver and Biliary Diseases*, 2nd ed. Baltimore: Lippincott Williams & Wilkins; 1996:241.)

necessary to take care not to spill the cyst contents into the peritoneum, which could allow them to infect the peritoneal cavity or produce an anaphylactic reaction.

Case Variation 7.17.3. *Cystic lesion suggestive of an abscess*

◆ A hepatic abscess usually presents with fever, elevated WBC count, and abdominal tenderness. Treatment of a pyogenic (ie, bacterial) abscess should consist of **IV antibiotics and CT-guided drainage.** In most cases, resection can be avoided. An **amebic abscess** may be treated with **metronidazole alone** and no surgery.

Case Variation 7.17.4. *Solid-appearing lesion (Fig. 7-27)*

◆ The differential diagnosis for a solid liver lesion includes **hemangioma, focal nodular hyperplasia, hepatic adenoma, metastatic cancer, and hepatocellular carcinoma.** The history is important. Pertinent findings include oral contraceptive use, which is present in a high percentage (as high as 90%) of patients with hepatic adenoma and occurs less

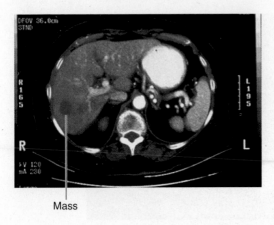

Mass

Figure 7-27: CT scan of solid liver lesion.

frequently in patients with focal nodular hyperplasia. A history of hepatitis (B or C) or cirrhosis may suggest hepatocellular carcinoma.

Note that serum-based liver studies may be unremarkable in individuals with any one of these three conditions. Alpha-fetoprotein, as well as hepatitis B surface antigen, may be positive in patients with hepatocellular carcinoma.

The lesion is solid. You suspect a hemangioma.

◆ How would you establish the diagnosis?

◆ This lesion is a collection of ectatic vascular cavernous spaces lined by endothelium. Magnetic resonance imaging (MRI) with IV gadolinium is the best test to diagnose a hepatic hemangioma, which has a characteristic appearance of a vascular lesion that fills from the periphery to the center (Fig. 7-28). A labeled red blood cell scan or a bolus-enhanced dynamic CT scan is also highly reliable in making the diagnosis of a hemangioma.

The discovery of most hemangiomas is incidental; it occurs during an ultrasound examination to check for gallstones. Hemangiomas are usually asymptomatic and almost never present with spontaneous hemorrhage. Thus, removal is not warranted. Most surgeons use the following as a general **guideline for surgical removal of benign hepatic masses**.

 QUICK CUT Significant symptomatic lesions, lesions with a risk of spontaneous rupture, and lesions with uncertainty as to the diagnosis warrant removal.

Biopsy of a hepatic lesion should only be performed after it is certain that the lesion is not a hemangioma because of a high risk of bleeding. Hepatic adenoma also has a high bleeding risk with biopsy. Thus, biopsy is only performed selectively to confirm a diagnosis.

You obtain an MRI. It is negative for hemangioma.

◆ What is the next step?

◆ CT is an appropriate test to differentiate between the other possible diagnoses. Patients with **focal nodular hyperplasia** occasionally demonstrate **a central stellate scar on CT scan** but require a liver biopsy to establish a diagnosis (Fig. 7-29). **No treatment** for **focal nodular hyperplasia** is indicated.

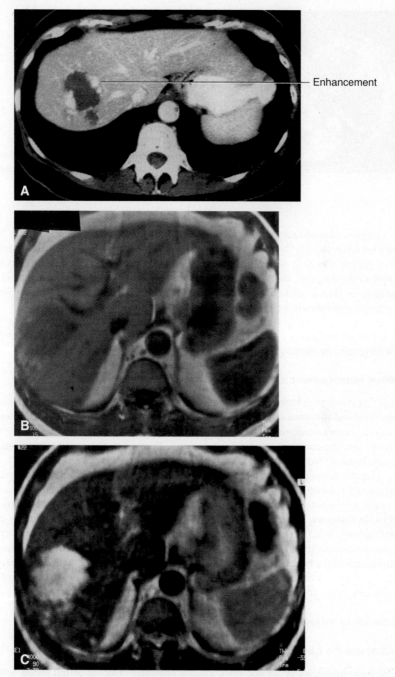

Enhancement

Figure 7-28: A: CT scan showing peripheral enhancing hepatic lesion. (From Yamada T, Alpers DH, Owyang C, et al. *Textbook of Gastroenterology*, 3rd ed. Philadelphia: Lippincott Williams & Wilkins; 1999:3031.) **B:** MRI on T1 weighted image shows minimal signal from the lesion. **C:** MRI on T2 weighted image shows an intense signal typical of hemangioma. (Parts **B** and **C** from Kaplowitz N, ed. *Liver and Biliary Diseases*, 2nd ed. Baltimore: Lippincott Williams & Wilkins; 1996:245.)

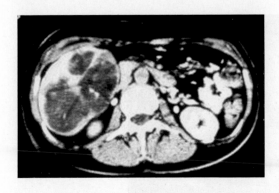

Figure 7-29: CT scan of the liver showing focal nodular hyperplasia.

Hepatic adenoma may be difficult to distinguish from hepatocellular carcinoma, but its risk for malignancy is low. **Hepatic adenomas are associated with** oral contraceptives **and may regress after their discontinuation. Persistent or large lesions** should be resected to confirm the diagnosis and to prevent spontaneous rupture, which is a significant risk with pregnancy. Hepatic adenomas are thought to have an especially high risk of rupture during pregnancy and therefore should be treated prior to pregnancy.

The CT scan suggests hepatocellular carcinoma. You perform a biopsy, and the pathology returns hepatocellular carcinoma.

◆ **What management is appropriate?**

◆ The first step is to **determine whether metastatic disease exists**, usually with a **CT scan of the chest and abdomen** to examine for lung metastasis and other abnormalities. Abdominal metastases are typically in the hepatic hilar lymph nodes and celiac nodes, and they extend locally into the diaphragm and other structures. **If no metastases exist, then a surgical assessment** of the hepatic lesions is appropriate.

Hepatic resection is most commonly performed for primary hepatocellular carcinoma and colorectal cancer metastatic to the liver. For both tumors, the prognosis is favorable for patients with lesions that are **resectable with a 1-cm margin, solitary, less than 5 cm in diameter, in noncirrhotic livers, without vascular invasion, and of low-grade malignancy.** When **resection** is appropriate, surgeons should perform it aggressively because it offers the patient the **highest rate of cure; similar factors are shown for colorectal metastasis to the liver (Table 7-2).** If these criteria are not met, resection is not warranted. In that case, it is treated medically except for special cases where hepatic transplantation protocols can be considered.

You decide to remove the mass.

◆ **What are the basic principles of hepatic resection?**

◆ The basic principles of hepatic resection are **complete removal of the lesion without patient death** (Fig. 7-30). The hepatic inflow and outflow are isolated and occluded to the resected segment. Liver tissue is then transected in a location where a 1-cm margin is obtained, maintaining hemostasis while crossing the liver. In the hands of experienced surgeons, otherwise healthy patients tolerate the procedure well.

Table 7-2: Prognostic Factors in Resectable Colorectal Metastasis to the Liver

Factors that Influence Resectability of Liver Tumors		
	Positively	**Negatively**
Number of lobes	Single lobe	Bilobar
Extrahepatic metastasis	No	Yes
Medical condition	Good	Poor
Cirrhosis	No	Yes
Factors that Influence the Prognosis of Resected Liver Lesions		
	Positively	**Negatively**
Number	Solitary	Multiple
Size of lesions	Small (≤5 cm)	Large (>5 cm)
Chronicity	Metachronous with primary tumor	Synchronous with primary tumor
Surgical margin	>1 cm	<1 cm
Stage (primary tumor)	I or II	III
Location of primary tumor	Colon primary	Rectal primary

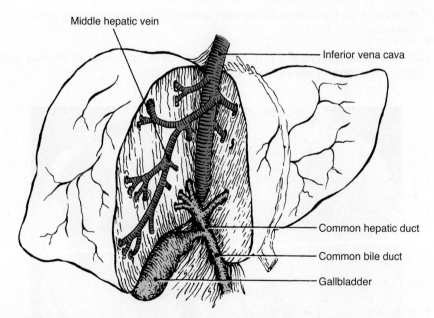

Figure 7-30: Planes of resection of the liver. (From Jarrell BE, Carabasi RA III, Radomski JS. *NMS Surgery*, 4th ed. Philadelphia: Lippincott Williams & Wilkins; 2000:261.)

Case 7.18 Fever and Pain in the Right Upper Quadrant

A 37-year-old man with a history of IV drug abuse is hospitalized for an extensive upper extremity abscess. He receives treatment incision and drainage and IV antibiotics. Despite 3 days of IV antibiotics, he remains febrile (temperature to 103°F).

◆ **What are the possible causes of this patient's fever?**

◆ It is necessary to drain the wound adequately and treat it properly. Other processes that may cause fever in IV drug abusers are endocarditis, intra-abdominal abscess, pancreatitis, pneumonia, UTI, or infected indwelling catheters. HIV–related infections are also a possibility in IV drug users who share needles. You should examine the patient for these possibilities and send blood cultures.

On examination, the patient's abdomen is tender in the RUQ. Laboratory studies reveal that his WBC count is 24,000/mm³ and his alkaline phosphatase is elevated.

◆ **How would you work up this patient?**

◆ Findings of RUQ tenderness and fever with leukocytosis point to a hepatobiliary condition. This could include **complications of gallstones or infectious processes** such as cholangitis or liver abscess. Appropriate tests include ultrasound or spiral CT. An ultrasound demonstrates many hepatobiliary processes, including liver abscesses and biliary obstruction or stones, whereas CT may be better at identifying hepatic abscesses near the dome of the liver and visualizing other lesions such as intra-abdominal abscesses or diverticulitis (Fig. 7-31).

A CT scan reveals multiple low-density lesions within both lobes of the liver with peripheral rim enhancement indicative of liver abscesses.

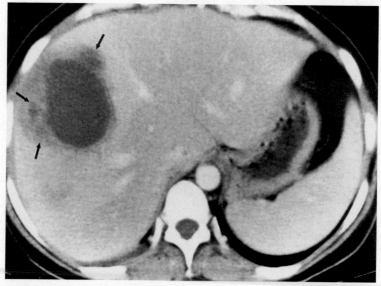

Figure 7-31: CT scan of a solitary hepatic abscess.

◆ **What treatment is appropriate?**

◆ Liver abscesses may be either **pyogenic (caused by bacterial spread) or amebic (caused by** *Entamoeba histolytica*). Typically, liver abscesses result from a partial or complete obstruction of the biliary system with spread of bacteria up the biliary tree. Bacterial translocation from a perforated abdominal viscus into the portal vein or arterial embolization of bacteria via the hepatic artery due to IV drug abuse is also likely in this case. Abscesses can be small and multiple or large and singular.

> **QUICK CUT** The preferred treatment of multiple, small pyogenic abscesses is broad-spectrum IV antibiotics for 4–6 weeks. Generally, initial therapy of large, single pyogenic liver abscesses is percutaneous drainage via radiologic guidance.

For proper treatment with antibiotics, it is necessary to obtain a sample culture. Larger abscesses are treated by percutaneous drainage. It is appropriate to leave the catheter in place for 2–3 weeks and give IV antibiotics simultaneously. **If coexisting biliary pathology exists, the drained abscess fails to improve, or surgery is necessary for any other reason, open drainage is warranted.**

◆ **If the patient has a large, single liver abscess and serologies positive for** *E. histolytica*, **how does this alter the proposed treatment plan?**

◆ The treatment for **amebic abscesses is metronidazole** alone; bacterial superinfection may occur with aspiration of uncomplicated amebic abscesses.

Chapter 8

Lower Gastrointestinal Disorders

Bruce E. Jarrell, Molly Buzdon, Daniel Bochicchio, Eric D. Strauch

Key Thoughts

1. Many small bowel obstructions are due to adhesions and will resolve with bowel rest, correction of the fluid and electrolytes, and time. Surgery is usually indicated if it fails to resolve or if certain clinical findings are present: localized abdominal tenderness, a hernia, fever, markedly elevated white blood cell (WBC), acidosis, large fluid requirements, or a closed loop obstruction on radiograph or hernia. Tumors of the small bowel such as carcinoid tumor can present with obstruction.

2. Acutely ischemic bowel is a difficult diagnosis and should be suspected when atrial fibrillation, acute myocardial infarction (MI), hypercoagulable state, low-flow states, or an abdominal bruit is present with severe abdominal pain.

3. The common complications of inflammatory bowel disease that may lead to surgical intervention include obstruction, bleeding, fistula formation, perforation, toxic megacolon (typically ulcerative colitis), and failure of medical therapy.

4. Ulcerative colitis has an increasing risk for dysplasia and colonic malignancy for active disease over 10 years. Cancer develops in flat areas in contrast to the polyp–cancer progression in the usual colon cancers.

5. A retrocecal appendix may not exhibit the usual clinical course of right lower quadrant (RLQ) pain.

6. Adjuvant chemotherapy (postoperatively) improves survival in stage III colon cancer.

7. Rectal cancer has a high risk of local recurrence at the site of resection.

8. Rectal cancers respond to radiation therapy, whereas colonic cancers do not.

9. Anal cancers respond to combination chemo and radiation therapy, which is primary therapy for anal cancer.

10. Anal cancer and lower rectal cancers (may) metastasize to inguinal nodes.

11. Patients with clinical diverticulitis must have colon cancer ruled out (after the acute event is subsides).

12. Massive lower gastrointestinal (GI) bleed is usually secondary to diverticulosis or arteriovenous malformations of the cecum.

13. The site of lower GI bleeding must be confirmed before surgery.

SMALL INTESTINAL DISORDERS

Case 8.1 Crampy Abdominal Pain No. 1

A 45-year-old woman has a 3-day history of **nausea and crampy abdominal pain** followed by vomiting and **abdominal distention**. She has had **no bowel movements** in the past 3 days. She has no other significant history except for a previous appendectomy.

On physical examination, mild tachycardia and mild orthostatic hypotension are present. The patient is otherwise normal, **except for the abdomen, which is distended, tympanitic, and mildly tender throughout but without rebound or localized tenderness**. The bowel sounds have a crescendo–decrescendo quality with periods of hyperactivity and periods of silence. There is no stool in the rectum. WBC count is 14,000/mm^3, and hematocrit is 44%.

◆ **What is the most likely diagnosis?**

◆ A small bowel obstruction is the most likely possibility, although a number of other problems such as ileus could have a similar clinical picture.

The next step is to obtain an abdominal radiograph.

◆ **What abdominal radiograph is warranted?**

◆ An obstructive series, which usually includes an **upright posterior-anterior and lateral chest radiograph (CXR) and a flat and upright abdominal radiograph**, is necessary.

◆ **How should you interpret this series (Figs. 8-1 and 8-2)?**

◆ This radiograph, which is most typical of small bowel obstruction, shows multiple air-fluid levels in the small bowel and no evidence of air in the colon or rectum. There is no evidence of a complication such as perforation or necrosis of the bowel (see Figs. 8-1 and 8-2).

◆ **What is the patient's predicted fluid and electrolyte status?**

◆ Dehydration due to vomiting and poor oral intake is expected. In addition, the usual metabolic picture involves a contraction alkalosis with hypokalemia, which develops as a result of a multistep process. When H$^+$ is secreted into the stomach, HCO$_3^-$ is secreted into the plasma. To maintain neutrality, Cl$^-$ is also secreted into the stomach. With vomiting, there is loss of H$^+$, Na$^+$, Cl$^-$, and water, which leads to alkalosis and volume contraction. In response to this state, the kidney preferentially retains Na$^+$ at the expense of H$^+$ and K$^+$, which is lost in the urine.

◆ **How would you correct this metabolic problem?**

◆ Correction of this deficit requires rehydration with sodium and potassium-containing intravenous (IV) fluids. The alkalosis usually corrects itself after rehydration if renal function is normal.

◆ **What is the overall management plan?**

◆ Rehydration and assessment of the patient's overall condition are necessary. It is **usually safe to manage small bowel obstructions with nasogastric (NG) drainage and IV fluids if there is no clinical sign of ischemic intestine or peritonitis.** This management strategy may last for several days **in the absence of marked leukocytosis, fever, acidosis, or localized tenderness** and no radiographic findings suggestive of ischemia, closed loop obstruction, or perforation. **Serial physical examination, laboratory studies, and abdominal radiography** are important parts of the observation plan.

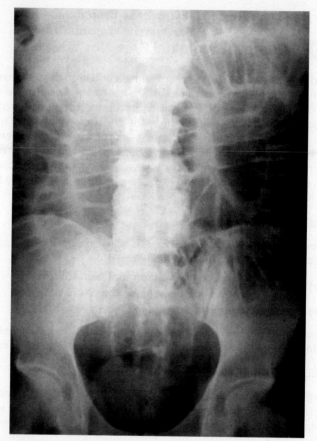

Figure 8-1: Plain radiograph of the flat abdomen showing bowel obstruction. Note the large amounts of air in the supine position. (From McKenney MG, Mangonon PC, Moylan JA, eds. *Understanding Surgical Disease: The Miami Manual of Surgery*. Philadelphia: Lippincott-Raven; 1998:139.)

The patient improves over the next several days. Her pain and distention resolve, and her appetite returns.

◆ **What would be the management plan at this point?**

◆ Removal of the NG tube and feeding should begin. If the patient tolerates the food, then discharge is appropriate. No further radiographs or other evaluation is necessary.

 QUICK CUT Many small bowel obstructions, particularly adhesive small bowel obstructions or incomplete obstructions, resolve with nonoperative management.

The final diagnosis is adhesions secondary to the prior appendectomy; this diagnosis is presumptive in that there is no way to prove this specific diagnosis except at laparotomy. The patient should return if symptoms recur.

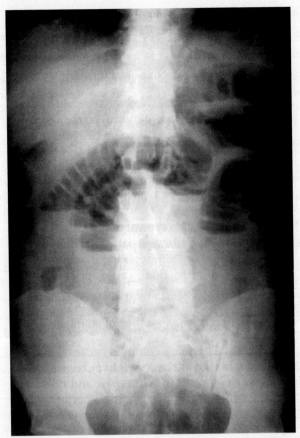

Figure 8-2: Upright abdominal radiograph showing bowel obstruction. Note the air-fluid levels. Together, Figures 8-1 and 8-2 make up an "obstructive series." (From McKenney MG, Mangonon PC, Moylan JA, eds. *Understanding Surgical Disease: The Miami Manual of Surgery*. Philadelphia: Lippincott-Raven; 1998:139.)

◆ **Does the initial assessment and management change in any way as a result of the following findings?**

Case Variation 8.1.1. *1-day duration of present illness*

◆ You would be more suspicious of a more proximal obstruction in the GI tract. Proximal obstructions tend to have less abdominal distention on physical examination. The management remains unchanged.

Case Variation 8.1.2. *No previous abdominal surgery*

◆ Adhesions may develop with no prior surgery, but other causes such as a **hernia, small or large bowel tumors, tumors metastatic to the bowel, or inflammatory processes** should also be suspected.

Case Variation 8.1.3. Heme-positive stool in rectum

◆ Increased suspicion of an **obstructing tumor or ischemic bowel is** warranted.

Case Variation 8.1.4. No bowel movements but still passage of flatus

◆ If the patient has no bowel movements but continues to have flatus, this is termed a **partial small bowel obstruction**. The radiographic picture may show the usual findings but also may show air in the colon or rectum. Partial small bowel obstruction is more likely to resolve without surgery and is less likely to have a complication such as ischemia or perforation.

Case Variation 8.1.5. Small amount of diarrhea

◆ This finding is also typical of a **partial obstruction**. You should also suspect a fecal impaction and severe constipation as a cause of the diarrhea. Gastroenteritis is another possible explanation, although the overall picture is not typical of this diagnosis. Examination for fecal impaction is appropriate. You should otherwise manage the patient for a partial small bowel obstruction.

Case Variation 8.1.6. Presence of an inguinal hernia

◆ An inguinal hernia, a common cause of obstruction, may go unrecognized preoperatively in patients who are overweight or have altered consciousness (Fig. 8-3). If present, this condition requires **urgent repair and relief of the bowel obstruction** because of the risk of strangulation.

Case Variation 8.1.7. A Clark level 4 melanoma that was excised 2 years ago

 QUICK CUT Melanoma is the most common tumor that metastasizes to the intestine.

◆ Melanoma frequently manifests as a bowel obstruction and can present many years or even decades later. Tumor-related obstructions often **do not resolve with nonoperative management**, and surgery is indicated. Even so, the tumor is often extensive, and surgical resection is not possible. The patient should be explored to establish a diagnosis and to relieve the obstruction.

Even a patient with known tumor may have an obstruction due to another cause such as adhesions. However, if it is an unresectable tumor, the prognosis is poor.

Case Variation 8.1.8. Ovarian cancer that had been previously excised

◆ Ovarian cancer can **recur locally or as peritoneal studding**, resulting in obstruction. Treatment is similar to melanoma (see Case Variation 8.1.7). **Debulking incurable ovarian tumors may improve survival** and warrants consideration.

Case Variation 8.1.9. Metastatic breast cancer treated with chemotherapy 1 year ago

◆ Metastatic breast cancer can also manifest as bowel obstruction. Treatment is similar to that used in Case Variation 8.1.7.

Case Variation 8.1.10. Localized abdominal tenderness with rebound

◆ **Localized tenderness** with other signs and symptoms of bowel obstruction should alert the clinician that a **potential serious complication** such as a closed loop obstruction, perforation, ischemia, or an abscess is present. Localized tenderness is an **indication that surgical exploration** rather than observation is necessary.

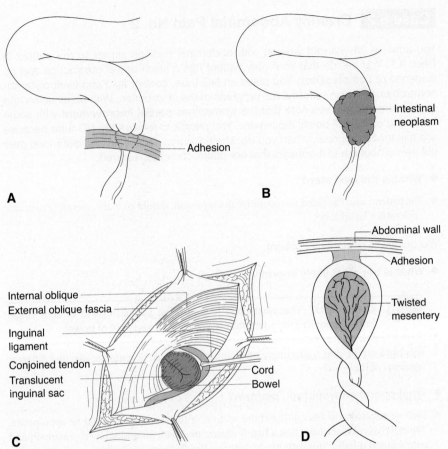

Figure 8-3: Common causes of bowel obstruction. **A.** Adhesion, **B.** neoplasm **C.** groin hernia. **D.** Closed loop obstruction. (From Greenfield LJ, Mulholland MW, Oldham KT, et al, eds. *Surgery: Scientific Principles and Practice*, 2nd ed. Philadelphia: Lippincott Williams & Wilkins; 1997:818, 820.)

Case Variation 8.1.11. *WBC count of 24,000/mm^3*

◆ Marked leukocytosis is another indicator of a serious complication and warrants exploration.

Case Variation 8.1.12. *Moderate metabolic acidosis*

◆ Metabolic acidosis with no other obvious cause warrants suspicion of **ischemic or necrotic bowel**. Depending on the patient's overall status and the radiographic findings, there are two options: (1) urgent exploration or (2) mesenteric arteriography to check for an arterial occlusive lesion before exploration can be done; if clinically, the intestine does not appear necrotic or perforated.

Case Variation 8.1.13. *Temperature of 103°F*

◆ This degree of temperature, which indicates a bowel perforation or ischemic process with sepsis, warrants exploration.

Case 8.2 Crampy Abdominal Pain No. 2

You admit a 38-year-old woman with abdominal findings similar to the patient in Case 8.1. You decide that your new patient has a small bowel obstruction and no evidence of complications. You place an NG tube, correct fluid and electrolyte abnormalities, and plan to follow the progress of the obstruction. With observation and serial examinations, you note that the woman has **partial improvement** with some flatus and one small bowel movement. You decide to remove the NG tube because she has made progress. When you do, she becomes nauseated and distended over the next 6 hours, and it appears that her obstruction has recurred.

♦ **What is the next step?**

♦ The patient, who has failed nonoperative management, should go to the operating room for exploratory laparotomy.

You decide to explore this patient.

♦ **What is the most likely operative finding?**

> QUICK CUT The most likely finding is an adhesive band of scar tissue from the earlier procedure that is occluding a segment of bowel.

♦ This band can be single, affecting a small amount of bowel, or multiple, affecting different segments of the bowel.

♦ **What operation would you perform?**

♦ Lysis of adhesions to free up the entire section of involved bowel would be appropriate. Typically, you find one band that is highly obstructing, with distended bowel proximally and empty bowel distally. This definitively confirms the diagnosis of small bowel obstruction.

♦ **What is your postoperative plan?**

♦ The patient remains nothing by mouth (NPO) with an NG tube for several days until bowel function returns. After she resumes eating, you may discharge her. Most patients who have undergone a lysis of adhesions are cured of obstruction in the short term. Follow-up primarily consists of wound observation to check for any signs of infection. No currently known therapy prevents recurrence of the adhesions or obstruction over the long term.

Case 8.3 Crampy Abdominal Pain No. 3

You are asked to see a 46-year-old woman in the emergency department who has the signs and symptoms of a small bowel obstruction.

♦ **How would each of the following radiographs influence your decision making?**

Case Variation 8.3.1. *Closed loop obstruction (see Fig. 8-3)*

♦ Typically, an adhesive band occludes the inlet and outlet of a loop of bowel, allowing secretions and air to accumulate in the loop and distend it. The loop can become ischemic due to blood flow obstruction from either twisting the blood supply or the adhesive band obstructing the blood supply. The loop can also perforate. The patient should be urgently explored after resuscitation.

On exploring the patient in Case Variation 8.3.1, you find a single loop of bowel that has twisted around an adhesion, causing an obstruction of the loop. You untwist the loop and cut the adhesion. On reinspection of the previously twisted segment of bowel, you note that it appears viable but edematous and obviously injured.

◆ **What options would you consider in the management of this patient?**

> **QUICK CUT** The primary issue is whether the bowel is viable. If observation does not provide a definitive indication, either resection and reanastomosis or a "second-look" operation is necessary. A "second-look" operation is a planned re-exploration 24 hours later to inspect the questionable bowel. Resection of any ischemic or necrotic bowel followed by anastomosis reestablishes bowel continuity.

◆ Many surgeons prefer this "second-look" operation, a proven, safe method of patient management. The major pitfall in management is delaying the second operation. Clinicians may convince themselves that patients are doing well after the first operation and do not need the second surgery. If in fact, ischemic bowel is present, it may not make patients sick for several days, and by the time it is evident, they are much sicker. Thus, the delay significantly jeopardizes patients.

Case Variation 8.3.2. *Crampy abdominal pain and free air in the peritoneal cavity*

◆ Exploration is necessary to resolve this problem. If the free air occurred during observation for a small bowel obstruction, it is most likely due to either an ischemic perforation or perforation due to overexpansion of the bowel. Thus, part of the process of observation includes monitoring the degree of intestinal distention on the radiographs.

◆ **How might the operative findings differ in the same patient, with free air on abdominal radiograph?**

◆ The operative findings in this patient might be similar to the previous patient with the additional finding of a perforation in the distended loop of bowel. This would most likely require resection.

Case Variation 8.3.3. *Crampy abdominal pain and an inguinal hernia*

◆ **This patient has evidence of a small bowel obstruction and bowel within a hernia sac. Urgent exploration is necessary after resuscitation.**

You decide to explore a patient with an incarcerated inguinal hernia and a small bowel obstruction.

◆ **What are the options for operative management?**

◆ Management may differ depending on how sick the patient appears.

- In a relatively stable patient with no signs of systemic illness, exploration through a hernia incision in the groin is appropriate. The surgeon can explore the hernia, inspect the bowel and return it to the peritoneal cavity if viable, and repair the hernia.

- In a patient who appears ill, exploration through a midline abdominal incision is preferred. This allows a more thorough inspection of the entire bowel. If the bowel is questionable or necrotic, either observation until it is viable or resection and re-anastomosis are possible. The surgeon may repair the hernia entirely or partially (to prevent immediate recurrence followed by formal repair at a later date when the patient has recovered).

Case 8.4　Injury to the Bowel during Lysis of Adhesions

You are exploring a 60-year-old man with a small bowel obstruction that involves particularly dense adhesions. In the process of lysing one, you enter the bowel lumen.

◆ **What are the management options?**

◆ An unplanned enterotomy is an undesirable event when it occurs during lysis of adhesions. If holes are small, primary repair is appropriate. If holes are large, multiple, or involve densely adherent bowel, the segment of affected bowel may require resection.

◆ **What problems might you anticipate in the postoperative period?**

◆ The greatest risk of an enterotomy is a postoperative leak and development of a **small bowel fistula**.

Case 8.5　Crampy Abdominal Pain No. 4

You are asked to see a 49-year-old man on the medical service who is recovering from pneumonia. Abdominal distention, nausea, and crampy abdominal pain have recently developed.

◆ **What might be causing the distention?**

◆ Patients with multiple other diseases such as heart failure, sepsis, or chronic obstructive pulmonary disease (COPD) may look as if they have a bowel obstruction. This man could have a small bowel obstruction; if this is present, treatment as described in the previous cases is warranted. However, distention has many additional causes, including **paralytic ileus, air swallowing, and constipation**. An ileus is a paralytic state in which the bowel fails to maintain peristalsis. Nausea, vomiting, and abdominal distention develop, and, from a functional standpoint, nothing can pass through the bowel.

◆ **If you are uncertain of the diagnosis of bowel obstruction in a complex situation such as this, is there any way you can confirm the diagnosis of a small bowel obstruction without an operation?**

◆ If you are uncertain of the diagnosis or if NG drainage leads to only partial improvement, **an upper GI series with small bowel follow-through or a computed tomography (CT) scan with oral contrast prior to the decision to explore the patient** is warranted. If the bowel is obstructed, the contrast stops at the obstruction, and this establishes the diagnosis.

　Severe constipation should also be evident with this study, although a colon full of stool is usually visible on a plain radiograph of the abdomen. If the contrast finds its way to the colon and eventually to the rectum, there is no mechanical bowel obstruction, and surgery will not help. Treatment of constipation involves enemas and disimpaction, not surgery. Paralytic ileus from many causes may also produce obstructive symptoms. It may lead to poor peristalsis and a slow transit time as seen on the small bowel follow-through.

Case 8.6 Abdominal Pain No. 5

A 70-year-old woman presents to the emergency department with a 1-day history of nausea, vomiting, and increasingly severe abdominal pain. She has a low-grade fever as well as mild distention of the abdomen, which is nontympanitic and mildly tender. Her pain seems much more severe than her abdominal findings. Her abdominal radiograph shows a nonspecific ileus.

On initial evaluation, the patient is stable, with a blood pressure (BP) of 140/85 mm Hg (her baseline). She has a WBC count of 15,000/mm^3 and no acidosis.

◆ **What is the next step?**

◆ Based on the initial findings, a suspicion of **ischemic bowel** is appropriate. Two approaches are possible.

    1. Proceed to the operating room if you think the patient has necrotic bowel.
    2. Perform further evaluation prior to a management decision.

In this case, because the patient appears stable and has no strong evidence for necrosis, further evaluation is most likely safe. After **hydration, it is necessary to ensure that the patient is well oxygenated and perfused**. When a patient presents with pain out of proportion to physical examination findings, then mesenteric ischemia should be suspected. A CT angiogram or formal angiogram should be performed if mesenteric ischemia is suspected.

The patient undergoes an angiogram which shows non occlusive ischemia (Fig. 8-4). Clinically, she improves after antibiotics and hydration.

◆ **What is the next step?**

◆ She has most likely had an ischemic event that has resolved for the time being but is **likely to recur**. The next episode could be worse, resulting in colon necrosis. You have established an anatomic abnormality on angiogram. Repair of this defect would most likely prevent a recurrence of ischemia. She should undergo an urgent **revascularization** of her mesenteric circulation.

The patient undergoes revascularization successfully (see Fig. 5.23).

◆ **What long-term management plan is appropriate?**

◆ Most surgeons would place the patient on antiplatelet therapy with **aspirin**. In addition, evaluation for the presence of cardiac and peripheral vascular disease is warranted because it is probably present and will affect her survival (see Case 5.13).

Case 8.7 Abdominal Pain No. 6

A 75-year-old woman similar to the patient in Case 8.6 presents to the emergency department. Based on the history and physical examination, mesenteric ischemia is a possibility.

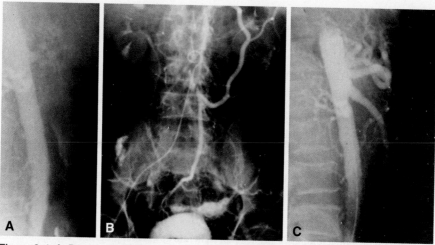

Figure 8-4: A: Preoperative lateral aortogram demonstrates total occlusion of the celiac and superior mesenteric arteries. **B:** Anteroposterior view with selective injection demonstrates large inferior to superior mesenteric artery collateral flow. **C:** Postoperative angiography demonstrates widely patent celiac and superior mesenteric arteries after transaortic endarterectomy. (Reprinted with permission from Mulholland MW, Lillemoe KD, Doherty G, et al. *Greenfield's Surgery*, 5th ed. Philadelphia: Lippincott Williams & Wilkins; 2010.)

◆ **How would the following findings influence your evaluation?**

Case Variation 8.7.1. *Significantly worsening pain over the next hour*

◆ Concern that the patient has necrotic bowel should prompt you to proceed to the operating room. A vascular surgeon should be consulted and ideally the patient placed on an operating room table where angiography and stenting can be done. Thus, evaluation of the mesenteric vessels and revascularization can be performed if indicated.

Case Variation 8.7.2. *WBC count of 24,000/mm³*

◆ Ischemia, necrosis, or perforation with infection should be suspected. Most surgeons would view this as an indication to proceed to the operating room.

Case Variation 8.7.3. *WBC count of 2,500/mm³*

◆ Your concerns should be similar to those in Case Variation 8.7.2. Elderly individuals, in particular, sometimes respond to overwhelming sepsis with leukopenia, often with a marked left shift.

Case Variation 8.7.4. *Moderate to severe metabolic acidosis*

◆ Your concerns should be similar to those of a patient who has a WBC count of 24,000/mm³ (see Case Variation 8.7.2).

Case Variation 8.7.5. *Atrial fibrillation*

◆ **Embolization** to the bowel from a thrombus in the left atrium associated with atrial fibrillation should be suspected. Depending on the patient's overall status, an angiogram of the mesenteric circulation before exploration is a possibility; exploration is most likely necessary. The embolus can be removed and arterial flow re-established if indicated.

Case Variation 8.7.6. *History of abdominal bruit*

◆ A bruit is an audible vascular sound associated with turbulent blood flow heard on auscultation. A bruit may suggest **stenosis of the celiac and mesenteric vessels among other diagnosis such as an aortic aneurysm**. An evaluation including an ultrasound or CT angiogram should be performed. Most patients with bowel ischemia do not have bruits.

Case Variation 8.7.7. *A hematocrit of 55%*

◆ Polycythemia is most likely to be **secondary to severe dehydration**, which could be corrected by rehydration. Treatment involves rehydration. Although polycythemia vera is less common in older patients, it may also occur. It is a **hypercoagulable state** and, like other hypercoagulable conditions, can cause stasis, low flow, and thrombosis in the mesenteric vascular beds. Treatment of primary polycythemia consists of phlebotomy and hydration. Angiography should still be performed for operative planning. Polycythemia as a secondary event may also be associated with COPD, and depending on the state of the patient, a pulmonary evaluation would be appropriate.

Case Variation 8.7.8. *History of congestive heart failure*

◆ Congestive heart failure can be associated with low-flow states in the mesenteric circulation. An angiogram can confirm a **low-flow nonocclusive state** in a suspected combination of congestive heart failure and mesenteric ischemia. Treatment of this condition involves direct mesenteric infusion of a vasodilator such as papaverine and efforts to improve cardiac output.

Case Variation 8.7.9. *History of thoracic aortic dissection*

◆ Aortic dissection can occlude any vessel orifice in the aorta. The combination of dissection and mesenteric ischemia suggests an occlusion related to the dissection. Angiography allows for diagnosis and the planning of surgical correction.

Case Variation 8.7.10. *BP of 90/60 mm Hg (in the emergency department)*

◆ The combination of suspected mesenteric ischemia and hypotension may indicate ischemia, causing sepsis and hypotension, or hypotension, causing nonocclusive ischemia due to low flow. Overall patient assessment, measurement of hemodynamics, angiography, or surgery may be necessary to diagnose the problem correctly.

Case Variation 8.7.11. *Bloody diarrhea*

◆ This suggests an **ischemic segment of colon with necrosis of at least the mucosa** and subsequent sloughing. The next step in evaluation is **sigmoidoscopy** to assess the colon. If full-thickness necrosis is present, **exploration** and resection are necessary. If only **mucosal ischemia** is present, it is possible to avoid resection by **optimizing hemodynamics, antibiotic administration, and close observation**.

Laboratory studies reveal that the patient is acidotic, with a blood pH of 7.14 and a WBC count of 25,000/mm^3. You decide that she may have necrotic bowel and that abdominal exploration is warranted.

◆ **How should you manage the following operative situations?**

Case Variation 8.7.12. *Necrosis of the left colon*

◆ Resection of the colon back to well-perfused edges is necessary. If the patient is stable and conditions are favorable, reanastomosis of the colon is appropriate. If not, a colostomy and Hartmann pouch operation (stapling the distal colon closed and placing back into the abdomen) are warranted (Fig. 8-5).

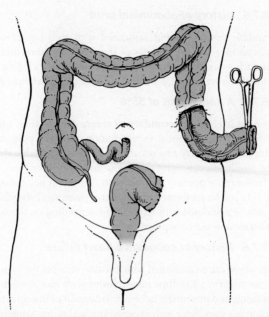

Figure 8-5: Hartmann procedure. The proximal bowel is brought out as a colostomy, and the distal bowel is stapled closed and left in the abdomen. (From Lawrence PF, Bilbao M, Bell RM, et al, eds. *Essentials of General Surgery*. Baltimore: Lippincott Williams & Wilkins; 1988:214.)

Case Variation 8.7.13. Necrosis of the intestines from the ligament of Treitz to the transverse colon

◆ In the majority of cases, this is a hopeless situation. Management should probably not involve resection with closure of the abdomen, thus allowing patients to succumb to the illness. Surgical resection and reanastomosis may be appropriate in younger individuals with no other illnesses. Resection of the majority of bowel is appropriate, leaving patients with a short bowel syndrome and the need for chronic total parenteral nutrition (TPN) or small bowel transplantation.

Case Variation 8.7.14. Necrosis of 2 ft of jejunum and ischemia of adjacent bowel

◆ Resection of the necrotic bowel back to healthy edge is necessary, with reanastomosis performed under favorable conditions. If there is doubt as to the viability of the remaining bowel, a "second-look" procedure should be performed the next day. In seriously ill patients, another alternative is an ileostomy, which allows direct observation of the viability of the bowel. Because there is no intestinal anastomosis, there is no risk of anastomotic breakdown. Patients may also benefit from postoperative mesenteric angiography to allow assessment of the vasculature.

Case Variation 8.7.15. Ischemia but no necrosis of the intestines and acute occlusion of the origin of the superior mesenteric artery

◆ In this situation, it is desirable to revascularize the bowel. The superior mesenteric artery should be exposed and the occlusion either removed or bypassed. The bowel can then be inspected for viability and managed accordingly. In addition, these patients are ideal subjects for preoperative mesenteric angiography.

Case Variation 8.7.16. Ischemia of the intestines with multiple small punctate areas of necrosis throughout the jejunum and ileum in a patient with a pulse in the superior mesenteric artery and mild chronic congestive heart failure

◆ This suggests either multiple small emboli or a low-flow state. Obviously, necrotic areas warrant resection. Postoperative optimization of hemodynamics and a "second-look" operation are a reasonable management scheme, although the outlook is poor. Angiography may demonstrate a low mesenteric flow rate.

Case Variation 8.7.17. Viable but ischemic intestines in a patient with a pulse in the superior mesenteric artery but evidence of a low-flow rate

◆ The hemodynamic status of this patient should be optimized. Preoperative angiography and recognition of the low-flow state would be better treated by optimizing vascular perfusion than with surgery. This would avoid an unnecessary operation.

INFLAMMATORY BOWEL DISEASE

Case 8.8   Abdominal Pain No. 7

You are asked to see a 24-year-old woman in the emergency department with crampy abdominal pain, nausea, and vomiting. Past history is significant for a 2-year history of Crohn disease of the terminal ileum. She initially received treatment with steroids and has been in remission on no steroids for 6 months.

The patient's abdomen is distended, and her obstructive series is compatible with a **small bowel obstruction**. She has no fever or localized pain and no signs of complications, including no acidosis and only a mild leukocytosis (WBC count = 13,000/mm^3).

◆ **What is the most likely diagnosis?**

◆ The suspected diagnosis is **a small bowel obstruction secondary to a stricture of the bowel involved with Crohn disease**. Crohn disease shares some similarities with ulcerative colitis (Table 8-1).

◆ **How could you confirm the diagnosis?**

◆ **CT of the abdomen** would be useful because it might demonstrate the area of stenotic bowel in the terminal ileum. It could also help determine the existence of any complications such as perforation or formation of an abscess or fistula. In addition, it might suggest another diagnosis (e.g., tumor).

A CT scan of the abdomen reveals a stenotic segment of bowel in the terminal ileum region and no other suggestions of complications.

◆ **What is the management plan?**

◆ If the stenosis is a fixed stricture, then resection is necessary because medical treatment will not improve the obstruction. If the obstruction is due to inflammation, then continued medical therapy may relieve the obstruction.

Table 8-1: **Inflammatory Disease of the Colon: Ulcerative Colitis and Crohn Disease**

Characteristics	Crohn Disease	Ulcerative Colitis
Usual location	Any segment of colon; ileocolic disease is most common.	Rectum, left colon, or entire colon
Anatomic and clinical features	Segmental distribution, skip areas Inflammation with deep fissures Thickened bowel wall, fibrous strictures Abscesses, fistulas Common, continuous rectal bleeding Noncaseating granulomas Mesenteric lymphadenopathy Focal aphthous ulcers Deep ulceration with cobblestone appearance Strictures Perianal disease	Continuous disease: ~50% involves rectum only, half is pancolitis, 10%–20% involve terminal ileum. Mucosal disease: epithelial ulceration and crypt abscesses Rectal bleeding Bowel stricture rate; should raise suspicion of cancer No perianal disease
Radiologic features	Upper gastrointestinal series with small bowel follow-through Enteroclysis study shows "string sign"—narrowing of terminal ileum from edema.	Mucosal ulcerations with islands of intact mucosa (pseudopolyps)
Medical management	Steroids for acute flare-ups Immunosuppressive drugs Metronidazole for perianal disease	Steroids for acute disease 5-Aminosalicylic acid for prevention of relapse
Natural history	Rarely goes into complete remission Tends toward obstruction, local infection, and fistulas Poor nutrition Increased incidence of carcinoma but less than with ulcerative colitis	Increased incidence of carcinoma that progressively increases with duration

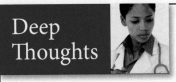

Deep
Thoughts

The goal of surgery for Crohn's disease is to relieve the obstruction while preserving as much normal bowel as possible. This would include the use of stricturoplasty, which opens a strictured area by cutting the stricture longitudinally and repairing it transversely to expand the lumen.

◆ **What problems should you anticipate in future years?**

◆ Reoperation may be necessary; in some series, the rate of reoperation is as high as 50% for additional problems related to Crohn disease. Resection of the terminal ileum may also lead to problems because it is responsible for the reabsorption of bile acids and vitamin B_{12}. Impaired bile acid absorption can **cause diarrhea, depletion of the bile salt pool, and malabsorption as well as oxalate stones.** Gallstones are more common, and vitamin B_{12} deficiency may occur.

◆ **How would the management change if the CT scan demonstrated an internal fistula between two segments of small bowel?**

◆ The management would remain unchanged. **Management is based on patient symptoms and active problems, not radiologic findings.**

Case 8.9 Perianal Disease in a Patient with Crohn Disease

You are asked to care for a 20-year-old woman with Crohn disease and perianal disease. On examination, you note a tender perineum and inflammation.

◆ **What management is appropriate?**

◆ This patient's condition poses a difficult problem, and surgery is generally indicated only to drain perirectal abscesses, if present. Management of superficial fistulas involves opening the tract. Setons are plastic tubes or sutures placed through the fistula that slowly allow the fistula to close. They are used for deeper fistula to allow healing to occur without injury to the sphincter. **Metronidazole** is useful in the management of the majority of patients with perianal problems.

Case 8.10 Management of Crohn Colitis

You are caring for a 19-year-old woman with Crohn disease that involves the colon.

◆ **How does Crohn disease in the colon differ from Crohn disease in the small bowel?**

◆ Crohn disease of the rectum is an unfavorable, unrelenting problem that often leads to fecal diversion. When the disease is limited to the colon, 5-acetylsalicylic acid compounds have some effect in addition to steroids. When the disease is limited to the small bowel, 5-acetylsalicylic acid compounds have little effect. If surgical complications are present, a subtotal colectomy is often needed and ileostomy if the rectum is involved. If not, then the ileum can be anastomosed to the sigmoid colon or rectum and continence retained.

Case 8.11 Complications of Long-Standing Ulcerative Colitis

A 36-year-old woman with a long-standing diagnosis of ulcerative colitis that has been managed medically consults you for advice on long-term prognosis and management.

◆ **What recommendations would you make?**

> **QUICK CUT** Individuals with ulcerative colitis are at an increased risk of developing colorectal cancer, which is related to the duration of their illness and the extent of disease.

◆ The risk for developing cancer is generally low for the first 10 years of the ulcerative colitis (2%–3%) but then increases by 1%–2% a year. Thus, the risk of colon cancer may be as high as 20% in a patient who has had ulcerative colitis for 20 years. The American Gastroenterological Association recommends that patients with pancolitis undergo colonoscopy every 1–2 years beginning after 8 years of the disease. For patients with colitis involving only the left colon, screening colonoscopy performed every 1–2 years beginning after 10 years of the disease is usually sufficient. Suspicious lesions such as strictures, polypoid lesions, and mucosal plaques warrant biopsy. Random biopsies are also necessary because the colon cancer of ulcerative colitis does not always follow the sequence of polyp to cancer; it may also develop on a flat mucosal surface. If **severe dysplasia** is identified on biopsy, **removal of the colon and rectum is indicated**.

Severe dysplasia is evident on several biopsies taken during a recent colonoscopy.

◆ **What surgical principles are important in dealing with the risk of cancer?**

> **QUICK CUT** Ulcerative colitis is a mucosal disease limited to the mucosa and submucosa, whereas Crohn disease involves the whole intestinal wall.

◆ Procedures that **remove the entire colonic and rectal mucosa are curative**, eliminating the risk of cancer. It is also important to **restore anal continence** and **establish a reservoir function** to allow defecation to occur at convenient times for the patient. In addition, it is necessary to use a procedure that accomplishes these goals in a highly **reliable fashion with low operative risk**.

◆ **What are the newer procedures?**

◆ Treatment of ulcerative colitis has involved several procedures. In the past, total proctocolectomy and ileostomy was the approach of choice. Regardless of whether the patient had a continent ileostomy, no ileostomy was desirable, and normal defecation was preferable. Subtotal colectomy, mucosectomy (removal of the rectal mucosa), and ileorectal anastomosis, which is still sometimes indicated for older patients, then became the procedure of choice. Its failure rate is as high as 20%–50% after 5–10 years.

Newer procedures, which preserve anal continence but remove the entire colon and rectum, are now in use. Currently, the **most acceptable procedure is total proctocolectomy, which removes the mucosa and thus the risk of cancer, with the creation of an ileal pouch (reservoir) and anastomosis of the pouch to the anus (restores continence)** (Fig. 8-6). Late complications are common for this difficult disease requiring a complex operation for long-term continence (Table 8-2).

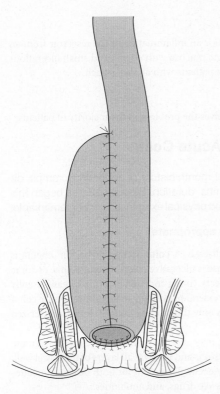

Figure 8-6: After total proctocolectomy for ulcerative colitis, gastrointestinal reconstruction is accomplished by creation of an ileal pouch and anastomosis of the pouch to the anus.

◆ **After the patient recovers from surgery, what long-term follow-up is appropriate?**

◆ If all of the patient's colon and rectum are removed, cancer is very rare but can occur because it is difficult to remove all mucosal cells and cancer can occur in the pouch. If residual rectal mucosa is present, proctoscopy at 6-month to 1-year interval is necessary as surveillance for colon carcinoma. (Any of the usual problems that may occur after complicated surgery could also develop, and she should receive education about these problems.)

She recovers from her total proctocolectomy and ileal pouch–anal anastomosis. She returns 6 months later with fever, blood-tinged diarrhea, and pain on defecation.

Table 8-2: Late Complications after Ileal Pouch–Anal Anastomosis

Pouchitis (30%–50%)
Small bowel obstruction (11%–26%)
Cuffitis (5%–14%)
Pouch failure (5%–10%)
Fistula (3%–12%)
Sexual dysfunction—male and female (5%–20%)
Cancer—cuff or pouch (rare)

From Greenfield LJ, Mulholland MW, Lillemoe KD, et al, eds. *Greenfield's Surgery*, 5th ed. Philadelphia: Lippincott Williams & Wilkins; 2010.

◆ **What is the most likely diagnosis?**

◆ The suspected diagnosis is **"pouchitis,"** which is an inflammation of the reservoir from an unknown cause. On endoscopy, a hemorrhagic mucosa with edema and small ulcerations is seen. This problem develops in up to half of patients with an ileal pouch.

◆ **What treatment is appropriate?**

◆ Treatment is with **metronidazole**, which resolves the problem in the majority of patients.

Case 8.12　Complications of Acute Colitis

A 29-year-old woman presents with a several-month history of abdominal cramps, diarrhea, and a 5-lb weight loss of several months' duration. Bloody diarrhea began this morning. Except for the diarrhea, the history and physical examination are unremarkable.

◆ **What evaluation and management are appropriate?**

◆ The patient may have inflammatory bowel disease. A **colonoscopy** or barium enema is necessary to determine if the pathologic disease is ulcerative colitis, Crohn colitis, or some other process. Ulcerative colitis typically affects young individuals. This disease usually begins in the distal colon and rectum and can extend proximally to involve the entire colon in about 50% of patients. Typically, it involves only the mucosa initially. It is characterized by crypt abscesses and raised ulcerations.

Crohn's disease an inflammatory disorder, may affect any part of the GI tract from the mouth to the anus. It typically occurs as skip lesions and involves all layers of the bowel wall. Severe perineal disease, including fistula, may occur. Treatment for both diseases includes corticosteroids, sulfasalazine, immunosuppressive drugs, and antibiotics.

After institution of therapy, the patient stabilizes and is placed on chronic therapy and followed clinically with a diagnosis of ulcerative colitis. Two months later, she returns to the emergency department acutely ill, with recurrence of bloody diarrhea, abdominal pain, and distention. Her temperature is 101°F, her BP is stable and normal, and her heart rate is 120 beats per minute. Her abdomen is distended and acutely tender.

◆ **What is the suspected diagnosis?**

◆ You would be concerned about **toxic megacolon** in a patient with ulcerative colitis and abdominal pain, distention, fever, and bloody diarrhea.

◆ **What is the initial evaluation?**

◆ Routine blood studies and an abdominal obstructive series to rule out bowel perforation are necessary. Many physicians would also perform CT of the abdomen to be certain that there is not an abdominal process such as an abscess or perforation. **A typical appearance on abdominal radiography usually establishes the diagnosis (Fig. 8-7).** Sigmoidoscopy may also be helpful but should be performed cautiously.

Her radiographs show a very dilated colon with mucosal edema and no signs of abscess or perforation.

◆ **How would you initially manage this patient?**

◆ **Provided that the patient is stable, a trial of medical therapy is indicated.** Treatment consists of placement of an NG tube, NPO feeding, TPN, and IV fluids and broad-spectrum antibiotics. Most physicians would also use high-dose **IV steroids**. The acute problem resolves in 50% or more patients with this therapy. **Close observation for worsening signs and symptoms,**

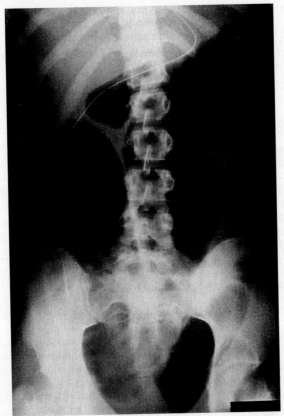

Figure 8-7: Plain film of the abdomen showing acute toxic megacolon. (From Greenfield LJ, Mulholland MW, Oldham KT, et al, eds. *Surgery: Scientific Principles and Practice*, 2nd ed. Philadelphia: Lippincott Williams & Wilkins; 1997:1097.)

with frequent abdominal examinations and radiographs, is necessary because the mortality of patients who have a bowel perforation from toxic megacolon ranges from 27% to 44%.

◆ **How would you manage the following findings?**

Case Variation 8.12.1. Free air on upright CXR

◆ The patient should be taken immediately **to the operating room**; this is evidence of perforation. The mortality rate is extremely high when perforation has occurred. The procedure of choice is **ileostomy with** formation of a **Hartmann pouch of the rectum and total abdominal colectomy** (see Fig. 8-5). This procedure, which leaves the rectum intact, may not cure the patient or remove the risk of cancer. Therefore, further discussion of management and subsequent definitive surgery is necessary once the patient recovers.

Case Variation 8.12.2. Air in the wall of the colon

◆ This also is a sign of impending perforation, and the patient may require operative intervention. The Hartmann procedure is used (see Case Variation 8.13.1).

Case Variation 8.12.3. Significant improvement over the next several days

◆ With improvement in the patient's condition, emergent surgery can be avoided.

Case Variation 8.12.4. **No changes over the next several days**

◆ If the patient fails to improve over 3–6 days, surgery is appropriate.

Case Variation 8.12.5. **A persistent, stormy course with worsening fever, leukocytosis, and pain**

◆ The patient is not responding to medical management, and surgery is necessary.

DISORDERS OF THE COLON

Case 8.13 **Right Lower Quadrant Pain No. 1**

You see a 25-year-old woman in the emergency department for abdominal pain, which has been present for 12 hours. The pain began in the middle abdomen, and it has now migrated to the lower abdomen on the right side. She has anorexia. On physical examination, the only finding is mild pain without guarding or rebound tenderness in the RLQ. Laboratory studies and abdominal radiographs are normal, and a pregnancy test is negative.

◆ **What evaluation is appropriate?**

◆ You should be suspicious for appendicitis as well as a gynecologic problem. Part of the physical examination should include rectal and pelvic examinations. **A rectal examination can detect pain in the right pelvis due to retrocecal appendicitis (Fig. 8-8).** The pelvic examination can detect ovarian pathology and pelvic inflammatory disease. If these parts of the examination are normal, management as for early appendicitis is appropriate, with hydration, NPO feeding, and observation with serial examinations, including a repeat complete blood count (CBC). Exploration with these mild symptoms is not appropriate. To avoid masking the progression of symptoms, pain medication should be avoided.

Most surgeons would also obtain an abdominal ultrasound to allow visualization of the fallopian tubes and ovaries to rule out gynecologic pathology. Some physicians would perform a CT scan of the abdomen to diagnose appendicitis, such as dilated appendix, thickened wall, intimation and fat stranding, appendolith, and abscess.

You decide to observe the patient, and she develops more pain, with localized rebound and guarding in the RLQ (Fig. 8-9).

◆ **How does this alter management?**

◆ With further localization and persistence of the worsening pain, this patient fits a picture of appendicitis. Management should involve weighing the risk of appendicitis and perforation

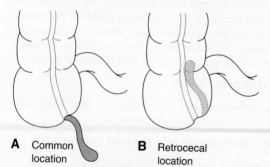

A Common location   **B** Retrocecal location

Figure 8-8: Position of normally located and retrocecal appendix. **A:** Common location. **B:** Retrocecal location.

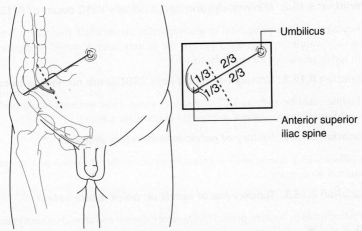

Figure 8-9: Location of pain in acute appendicitis. The *inset* shows the incision that is used for an appendectomy. (From McKenney MG, Mangonon PC, Moylan JA, eds. *Understanding Surgical Disease: The Miami Manual of Surgery*. Philadelphia: Lippincott-Raven; 1998:318.)

with the risk of an operation. Most surgeons would err on the side of a few unnecessary appendectomies rather than a few perforated appendices. The general guideline states that it is safe to perform 10%–15% of unnecessary appendectomies, with the hope that an appendix that ruptures while being observed will be rare.

There are two surgical options.

- Laparoscopy and visualization of the appendix, which is well tolerated and also allows removal of the appendix
- Exploration, which is performed through a McBurney incision and the appendix visualized and removed (see Fig. 8-9)

You decide to explore the patient. You find acute appendicitis and perform an appendectomy.

◆ **What is the postoperative plan?**

◆ As soon as the patient will tolerate feeding, it should begin. Discharge is usually appropriate at that time, and follow-up may continue in the office until the patient has made a complete recovery.

Case 8.14 Right Lower Quadrant Pain No. 2

You are asked to see a woman with a history and physical examination similar to that described in Case 8.14.

◆ **How might the following admission findings change the evaluation and management?**

Case Variation 8.15.1. *Dysuria and a urinary WBC count of 10,000/hpf*

◆ These findings are suggestive of a urinary tract infection (UTI) and could cause RLQ pain similar to appendicitis, but they could also be secondary to an appendiceal abscess in continuity with the bladder. It would be appropriate to continue to follow the patient for further signs of appendicitis, although these are less likely.

Case Variation 8.15.2. Minimal dysuria and a urinary WBC count of 8–10/hpf

◆ This finding would not be unusual in acute appendicitis, in which the local inflammatory process is in continuity with some part of the urinary tract. It would be appropriate to remain highly suspicious for appendicitis.

Case Variation 8.15.3. Urinary red blood cells (RBCs) too numerous to count

◆ This finding could be a severe UTI or a kidney stone. Most surgeons would perform an ultrasound or a CT scan without contrast (to examine for a stone).

Case Variation 8.15.4. History of pelvic inflammatory disease

◆ Pelvic inflammatory disease tends to recur. Appendicitis may still develop. A careful pelvic examination is necessary.

Case Variation 8.15.5. Tenderness of cervix on pelvic examination

◆ This finding tends to confirm pelvic inflammatory disease and should prompt gynecologic consultation.

Case Variation 8.15.6. Tenderness of adnexa on the right side

◆ This finding tends to confirm pelvic inflammatory disease, possibly with a tubo-ovarian abscess and should also prompt gynecologic consultation.

Case Variation 8.15.7. Cervical discharge

◆ This findings tends to confirm pelvic inflammatory disease. It is necessary to stain for gonococcus and obtain gynecologic consultation.

Case Variation 8.15.8. Other family members at home with gastroenteritis

◆ It is probable that this woman has been in contact with family members who have gastroenteritis. Although she could still have appendicitis, gastroenteritis is much more likely, and she should receive treatment for this latter condition.

Case Variation 8.15.9. Voiding symptoms in a 65-year-old man

◆ This patient may have bladder outlet obstruction and a large, distended bladder. With careful physical examination, percussion of the distended bladder may be possible. Treatment involves insertion of a Foley catheter, if possible, and re-examination.

Case Variation 8.15.10. Family history of inflammatory bowel disease (IBD)

◆ The presentation of IBD, which is sometimes familial, may be similar to appendicitis. With suspected IBD, further studies may be appropriate before exploration takes place. CT may show a thickened loop of bowel or enlarged nodes in the terminal ileum. **With certain IBD, exploration is not necessary.** It is appropriate to establish the diagnosis with colonoscopy or barium enema (Fig. 8-10). Initial treatment involves steroids, and maintenance therapy involves a 5-acetylsalicylic acid–containing medicine. It is prudent to remember that appendicitis may develop even in patients with established IBD. The addition of steroids to a missed appendicitis will surely create complications and delay or obscure the correct diagnosis of appendicitis.

Exploration of a patient with suspected appendicitis may reveal a normal appendix and establish the diagnosis of IBD (terminal ileitis). Gross findings such as an inflamed ileum, fat wrapping of the intestine, a thickened wall, and enlarged nodes are the basis of diagnosis of IBD. Because of the risk of anastomotic breakdown and GI fistula, most surgeons would not biopsy the bowel. It is possible to biopsy a local node, and if granulomas are present,

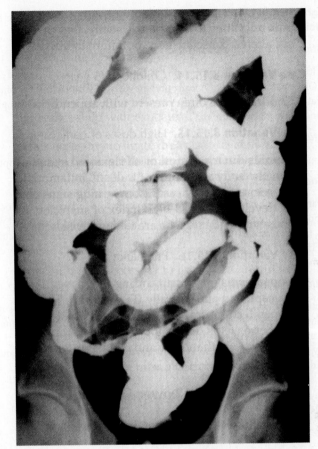

Figure 8-10: Barium enema showing the "string sign" typical of a distal ileal stricture due to Crohn disease. (From McKenney MG, Mangonon PC, Moylan JA, eds. *Understanding Surgical Disease: The Miami Manual of Surgery*. Philadelphia: Lippincott-Raven; 1998:135.)

make the diagnosis, but this is not necessary. Most surgeons remove the appendix if it is not involved with the inflammatory process; removal eliminates the possibility of a future diagnosis of appendicitis.

Case Variation 8.15.11. *2-month history of crampy pain and diarrhea*

◆ It is necessary to consider a cause other than appendicitis to account for this problem. IBD, constipation, and carcinoma are all possible diagnoses. A more complete workup with imaging and colonoscopy should be considered.

Case Variation 8.15.12. *Marked tenderness in the right pelvis on rectal examination*

◆ When an appendix is retrocecal or deeper in the pelvis, it may not cause localized pain in the anterior abdominal wall because it is not in contact with the parietal peritoneum. Tenderness on rectal examination may be the best clue to localize this problem. If this is present, the suspected diagnosis is appendicitis, and the patient should go to the operating room.

✦ **How might the following situations change the presentation of appendicitis?**

Case Variation 8.15.13. Advanced age (75 years)

✦ Appendicitis has a bimodal distribution, with peaks in incidence around 25 years and 65 years. Older patients do not typically present with the classical history of periumbilical pain migrating to RLQ pain. Usually, they present with vague abdominal complaints, sepsis, altered consciousness, or failure to thrive.

Case Variation 8.15.14. Childhood (5 years)

✦ Children more often present with appendicitis in which the appendix has ruptured.

Case Variation 8.15.15. High doses of corticosteroids

✦ Steroids can mask most or all signs and symptoms of any inflammatory process. In addition, the body's attempt to "wall off" inflammation and abscesses is blunted with steroids. Therefore, in many cases, the warning signs are absent until perforation occurs and sepsis develops. Thus, a high index of suspicion is necessary. It is essential to be very cautious with patients who are taking steroids.

Case Variation 8.15.16. Pregnancy

✦ Appendicitis may occur during pregnancy. As the uterus enlarges, it pushes the appendix cephalad and laterally (Fig. 8-11). Thus, the pain is in the upper lateral abdomen. Appendectomy can be safely performed during pregnancy with minimal risk to the mother or fetus. Early operation is appropriate. A perforated appendix carries a significant risk to both mother and child; peritonitis, not appendectomy, poses the risk.

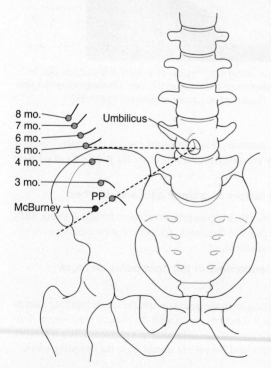

Figure 8-11: Location of pain of appendicitis in pregnancy. (From Yamada T, Alpers DH, LaMe L, et al, eds. *Textbook of Gastroenterology*, 3rd ed. Philadelphia: Lippincott Williams & Wilkins; 1999:1068.)

Case 8.16 Right Lower Quadrant Pain No. 3

You see a 28-year-old woman in the emergency department who has a typical history of appendicitis. The pain, which began in the periumbilical region and migrated to the RLQ, is now very localized. There is marked tenderness over the McBurney point. Because her condition has worsened, you decide that exploration is appropriate.

◆ **How would you manage the following operative findings?**

*Case Variation 8.16.1. **A red, inflamed appendiceal tip with exudate***

◆ This represents acute appendicitis, and it is necessary to ligate the appendix at its base and amputate the appendix, leaving a small stump beyond the ligature or stable line.

*Case Variation 8.16.2. **Acute gangrenous appendicitis with necrosis extending up to the base of the cecum***

◆ When the base of the appendix is necrotic, it is still necessary to ligate and amputate the organ using sutures. Most surgeons then bury the base of the appendix into the cecum with a suture to lessen the chance of a "blowout" of the stump. If the cecum also appears involved, it is safe to invert a larger segment of the base of the cecum in most cases. If the cecum is involved in an inflammatory process or mass that seems to originate from the appendix, then a right colectomy is appropriate. This procedure is essential both to remove the necrotic appendix and cecum safely and to not miss a perforated colon cancer.

*Case Variation 8.16.3. **Perforated appendicitis with localized abscess***

◆ The abscess can be treated with percutaneous drainage and antibiotics with or without interval (delayed 6–9 weeks) appendectomy or the patient can be treated operatively with drainage of the abscess and appendectomy either open or laparoscopically (Fig. 8-12).

*Case Variation 8.16.4. **Acute appendicitis with a 1-cm round, moveable mass***

◆ This may be a fecalith, which is associated with appendicitis. A seed or similar-sized object was ingested. Fecaliths also are apparent on abdominal radiographs in some patients; this establishes the diagnosis of appendicitis and simplifies the decision to operate.

*Case Variation 8.16.5. **Normal appendix***

◆ It is necessary to **examine for other** causes of the pain. These include mesenteric adenitis, inflammation of a Meckel diverticulum, terminal enteritis, ovarian and fallopian tube disorders, and diverticulitis. Except under unusual circumstances, removal of the appendix is appropriate to eliminate the diagnosis of appendicitis in the future.

Case 8.17 Right Lower Quadrant Pain No. 4

A 34-year-old man has suspected appendicitis. On exploration, you find a mass at the tip of the appendix.

◆ **What management is appropriate for the following findings?**

*Case Variation 8.17.1. **A 1-cm diameter, yellow firm mass at the tip of the appendix***

◆ This is most likely a **small carcinoid tumor** (Fig. 8-13). Biopsy is not necessary. If the tumor is at the tip of the appendix, less than 2 cm in diameter, and there is no evidence of spread to the cecum or nearby nodes, a routine appendectomy may be performed.

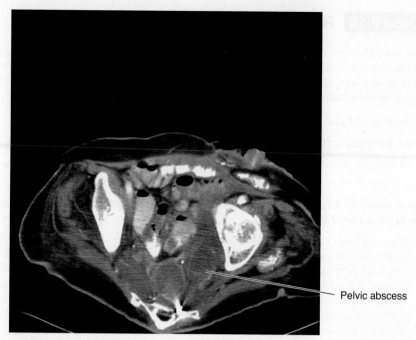

Pelvic abscess

Figure 8-12: CT scan showing a pelvic abscess.

Case Variation 8.17.2. A 2.2-cm diameter, yellow firm mass at the base of the appendix

◆ This is most likely a larger carcinoid tumor that involves the base of the cecum. Excision, not biopsy, is appropriate.

 QUICK CUT A carcinoid tumor with a size of 2 cm or more or involvement of the base of the appendix or cecum suggests malignant behavior and is an indication to perform a right colectomy.

An adenocarcinoma may appear similar, although the color is different. Colectomy may require an extension of the incision cephalad for adequate exposure. Reanastomosis of the ileum and colon can usually be performed safely.

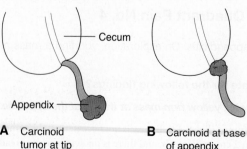

Cecum

Appendix

A Carcinoid tumor at tip

B Carcinoid at base of appendix

Figure 8-13: Location of carcinoid tumors of the appendix.

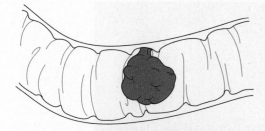

Figure 8-14: A pedunculated small bowel carcinoid tumor causing a small bowel obstruction.

Case Variation 8.17.3. A 3-cm round pedunculated mass in the terminal ileum that appears to be obstructing the lumen (Fig. 8-14)

◆ **Carcinoid tumors and adenocarcinomas** of the small intestine may manifest as **pedunculated masses** that cause intermittent small bowel obstruction that may mimic appendicitis. It is necessary to remove the involved ileum and regional lymph nodes. Examination of the remaining bowel for other lesions is also appropriate because of a **significant incidence of multiple carcinoid tumors in the bowel.**

The pathology for the appendiceal mass returns as carcinoid tumor.

◆ **What management plan is appropriate?**

◆ For each of the previously discussed carcinoid tumors (Case Variations 8.17.1 and 8.17.2), it is necessary to obtain a baseline urinary 5-hydroxyindoleacetic acid (5-HIAA) and serum serotonin level. The **principal determinants of malignancy involve the biologic behavior of the tumor** rather than its histologic appearance, location, and size. Thus, long-term follow-up of patients with such tumors is appropriate. If there is a question of recurrence, a **CT scan of the abdomen** and an octreotide scan, which localizes to neuroendocrine tumors, is warranted.

Case 8.18 Right Lower Quadrant Pain No. 5

A 60-year-old man with a ruptured appendix recovers from surgery and is discharged. One week later, he presents with fever, chills, anorexia, and malaise.

◆ **What evaluation is appropriate?**

◆ This could be a **pelvic abscess or a wound infection** if the wound has closed. If a wound infection is present, drainage is necessary. If not, then most surgeons would obtain a CT or ultrasound study of the pelvis to examine for an abscess. On palpation, a pelvic abscess feels like a tender mass on rectal examination.

You establish a diagnosis of a pelvic abscess (see Fig. 8-12).

◆ **What management plan is appropriate?**

◆ Management of a pelvic abscess varies. Many surgeons would **drain the abscess** with a percutaneously placed catheter if accessible, and others would use open surgical drainage. Occasionally, transrectal or transvaginal drainage is appropriate if the abscess is intimate with either of those structures (Fig. 8-15). Once drained, an abscess resolves in most cases, and an associated cecal fistula would be unusual.

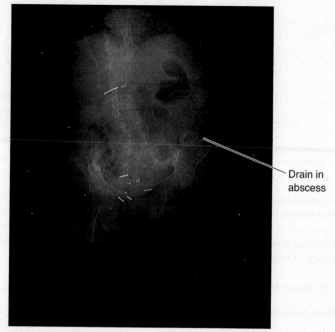

Figure 8-15: CT scan with guided drainage of a pelvic abscess.

MALIGNANT DISORDERS OF THE COLON, RECTUM, AND ANUS

Case 8.19   Screening for Colorectal Cancer

A 40-year-old man is concerned about colorectal cancer. He wants to know your recommendations for screening for colorectal cancer.

◆ **What do you tell him?**

◆ Screening is aimed at **detecting cancers that are asymptomatic**. Obviously, **symptomatic patients should undergo evaluation** with an accepted routine, usually including colonoscopy. According to the U.S. Preventive Services Task Force Screening for Colorectal Cancer: U.S. Preventive Services Task Force Recommendation Statement. External Web Site Icon AHRQ Publication 08-05124-EF-3, October 2008. Agency for Healthcare Research and Quality, Rockville:

- High-sensitivity fecal occult blood test (FOBT), which checks for hidden blood in three consecutive stool samples, should be done every year.
- Flexible sigmoidoscopy to look at the interior walls of the rectum and part of the colon should be done every 5 years with FOBT every 3 years.
- Colonoscopy to look at the interior walls of the rectum and the entire colon should be done every 10 years. Colonoscopy can be used as screening tests or as follow-up diagnostic tools when the results of another screening test are positive.
- There are more detailed guidelines for colorectal cancer endoscopic surveillance (Table 8-3).

Table 8-3: Guidelines for Colorectal Cancer Endoscopic Surveillance*

Personal History Risk	Initiate Surveillance	Interval
Following resection of single <1 cm adenoma	5–10 years postpolypectomy	If first colonoscopy is normal, resume average-risk recommendations.
Following resection of 3–10 adenomas, or ≥1 cm adenoma, or polyp with villous features or high-grade dysplasia	3 years postpolypectomy	If first surveillance colonoscopy is normal, repeat at 5 years.
Following resection of >10 adenomas	<3 years postpolypectomy	Consider evaluation for familial syndrome.
Following piecemeal removal of sessile adenoma	2–6 months postpolypectomy	Individualize.
Following curative resection for colorectal cancer	Within 3–6 months if preoperative clearing was not performed. Within 1 year postoperatively following clearance of synchronous disease.	If normal, repeat in 3 years, then if normal, every 5 years.
Inflammatory bowel disease	Within 8 years of diagnosis	Survey for dysplasia every 1–2 years.

*Endorsed by the American Cancer Society, American College of Gastroenterology, American Society of Colon and Rectal Surgeons, American Society for Gastrointestinal Endoscopy, Oncology Nursing Society, and Society of American Gastrointestinal Endoscopic Surgeons.
From Greenfield LJ, Mulholland MW, Lillemoe KD, et al, eds. *Greenfield's Surgery*, 5th ed. Philadelphia: Lippincott Williams & Wilkins; 2010.

◆ **How might this recommendation change if the patient has previously had a colon cancer removed?**

◆ One of the most productive ways to detect cancer recurrence after primary colon cancer is by **screening with carcinoembryonic antigen (CEA) measurements**. If patients with stage II or III cancer are free of disease, CEA measurement every 2–3 months for at least 2 years is worthwhile. This method detects up to 80% of recurrences. Production of CEA does not occur in up to 30% of recurrences, especially with poorly differentiated tumors or in patients who had normal CEA measurements with their primary cancer. Physical examination, which should be performed every 3–6 months, detects up to 20% of recurrences. Screening for liver function studies is also recommended.

Case 8.20 Heme-Positive Stool No. 1

A 45-year-old man is referred to you because he noted bright red blood streaks on his stool intermittently for the last 3 weeks. Otherwise, he feels fine but complains of occasional constipation. His stools have been normal caliber and brown. The history (past, family, and social) and review of symptoms are negative. On physical examination, the man's vital signs are normal. He does not appear anemic. The head, neck, chest, abdomen, extremity, and neurologic examination are all normal.

◆ **What is the appropriate diagnosis or initial management of the following findings on rectal examination or sigmoidoscopy?**

Case Variation 8.20.1. *Several hemorrhoids with evidence of recent injury*

◆ With a negative family history of colon cancer and no history of IBD or past history of colon cancer, it is likely that the source of the bleeding is hemorrhoids (Fig. 8-16). Conservative management, with sitz baths, stool softeners, and the addition of fiber to the diet, is one option. If the hemorrhoids continue to bleed despite medical management, removal in the operating room may be necessary. External hemorrhoids are surgically excised. Internal hemorrhoids can be excised or banded (Fig. 8-17). **Most surgeons still recommend colonoscopy or sigmoidoscopy to absolutely rule out colon cancer.**

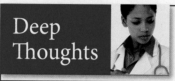

Deep Thoughts

Colorectal cancers presenting with heme-positive stools are often diagnosed late because the presence of blood in the stool is falsely attributed to hemorrhoids.

Case Variation 8.20.2. *Thrombosed hemorrhoids*

◆ Conservative management with sitz baths and stool softeners may be appropriate for thrombosed hemorrhoids. However, if individuals present with extreme pain, incision and drainage (I&D) of the hemorrhoids if thombosed may be necessary. Surgeons should be certain to excise the overlying skin and subcutaneous tissue to remove the underlying vessels. It is permissible to leave the skin open. Thrombosed hemorrhoids usually heal well after I&D, with mild analgesics and sitz baths.

Case Variation 8.20.3. *Bright red blood on the glove after rectal examination*

◆ Anoscopy or sigmoidoscopy is necessary to determine the cause of anorectal bleeding, which may be due to internal hemorrhoids, a fissure, a bleeding rectal or anal carcinoma,

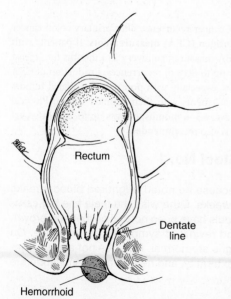

Rectum

Dentate line

Hemorrhoid

Figure 8-16: Location of external hemorrhoids. (From Chen H, Sonnenday CJ, Lillemoe KD, eds. *Manual of Common Bedside Surgical Procedures*, 2nd ed. Philadelphia: Lippincott Williams & Wilkins; 2000:163.)

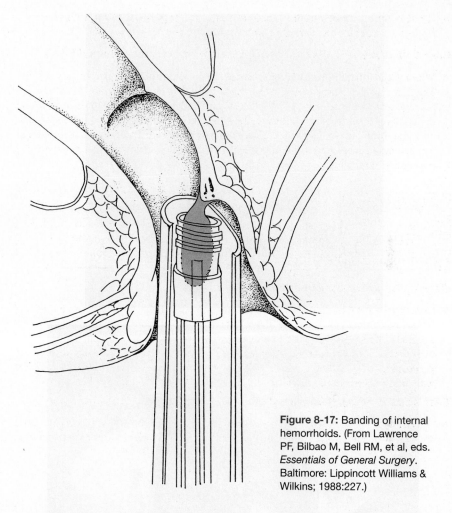

Figure 8-17: Banding of internal hemorrhoids. (From Lawrence PF, Bilbao M, Bell RM, et al, eds. *Essentials of General Surgery*. Baltimore: Lippincott Williams & Wilkins; 1988:227.)

or a polyp. If the lesion is not visualized in the anus or rectum, colonoscopy is required to ensure that a polyp or cancer is not causing the bleeding.

Case Variation 8.20.4. *A 5-cm perianal fungating mass*

◆ It is important to obtain a biopsy of this mass because it most likely represents an anal carcinoma. Transanal ultrasound may also be necessary to determine the depth of invasion and help guide your treatment strategy (Fig. 8-18).

Case 8.21 Heme-Positive Stool No. 2

A 60-year-old woman reports bright red blood on her stool. On examination, no other abnormalities are apparent. A colonoscopy finds a **polyp in her colon**.

◆ Polyps can either be pedunculated, on a stalk, or sessile, flush with the mucosa (Fig. 8-19). It is necessary to remove them because of the risk of adenocarcinoma development.

The supposed histologic progression from formation of polyps to invasive carcinoma may take up to 10 years.

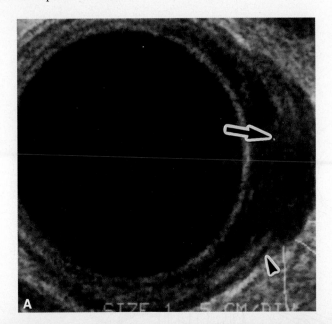

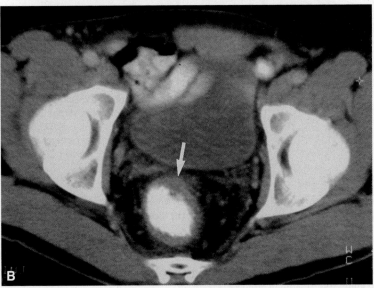

Figure 8-18: Rectal carcinoma. **A:** Endoscopic ultrasound (EUS) showing a T3 lesion with tumor extension beyond the bowel wall into the perirectal space. Arrow shows tumor in the rectal wall. **B:** CT scan showing the same patient. Arrow shows thickened rectal wall indicative of the rectal tumor. (From Wanebo HJ, ed. *Surgery for Gastrointestinal Cancer*. Philadelphia: Lippincott-Raven; 1997:175–176.)

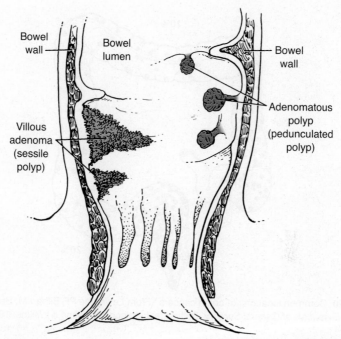

Figure 8-19: Types of polyps occurring in the colon: pedunculated polyps versus sessile polyps. (From Lawrence PF, Bilbao M, Bell RM, et al, eds. *Essentials of General Surgery*. Baltimore: Lippincott Williams & Wilkins; 1988:218.)

◆ **What is the management, prognosis, and recommended surveillance after treatment for each of the following findings?**

Case Variation 8.21.1. *A 1-cm pedunculated polyp*

◆ A **polypectomy** is appropriate, which involves placing a snare around the polyp and advancing it down the stalk. The snare is then closed as the polyp is lifted up, with the application of electrocautery to the stalk as the polyp is ensnared.

   The pathology of the lesion determines whether further resection is necessary (e.g., in the case of invasive carcinoma).

Case Variation 8.21.2. *A 5-cm pedunculated polyp*

◆ A large pedunculated polyp may require removal in a piecemeal fashion or may necessitate more than one endoscopic session for removal. These patients are at **increased risk for developing colorectal cancers** and should also have surveillance colonoscopy.

Case Variation 8.21.3. *A 4-cm flat, sessile lesion*

◆ Whether sessile polyps warrant **biopsy or attempted ensnaring** is controversial. One technique involves the injection of saline under the polyp and attempting to ensnare it in its entirety. Usually, sessile polyps less than 2 cm are possible to remove successfully, but those **greater than 2 cm** may require formal **surgical resection**.

Case Variation 8.21.4. *Severe atypia in the removed pedunculated polyp (Fig. 8-20)*

◆ Polypectomy is sufficient therapy. Close follow-up with colonoscopy is warranted.

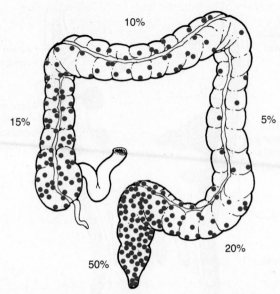

Figure 8-20: Common locations of colon cancers. (From Lawrence PF, Bilbao M, Bell RM, et al, eds. *Essentials of General Surgery*. Baltimore: Lippincott Williams & Wilkins; 1988:218.)

Case Variation 8.21.5. *Carcinoma in situ in the head of a pedunculated polyp with no extension to the stalk*

◆ **Polypectomy alone** is sufficient therapy in the case of carcinoma in situ **confined to the head** of a pedunculated polyp because **no invasion** has occurred through the muscularis mucosa. A bowel resection is not necessary. The long-term risk of lymph node metastasis is about 1–3%. Follow-up is controversial, but the general recommendations are repeat colonoscopy in 3–6 months and then at 12-month intervals.

Case Variation 8.21.6. *Carcinoma in the stalk of a pedunculated polyp*

◆ The issue of carcinoma in the stalk of the polyp is controversial. Generally, if **a margin of greater than 2 mm** is present, the cancer is **not poorly differentiated** or there is **no vascular or lymphatic invasion**. In such a case, **polypectomy** is sufficient. Otherwise, marking with a tattoo and surgical resection of that segment of bowel is necessary.

Case Variation 8.21.7. *Carcinoma in a sessile lesion*

◆ The risk of lymph node metastasis is 15% in sessile polyps with **invasive carcinoma**. The local recurrence rate following endoscopic resection is about 20% with no further resection, so bowel resection is indicated in this case. Follow-up involves repeat colonoscopy after 1 year.

Case 8.22   Heme-Positive Stool No. 3

A previously healthy 55-year-old man is referred to you for recent onset of fatigue and a 5-lb weight loss. He has no other symptoms, and history (past, family, and social) is negative. Review of symptoms is negative. On physical examination, two positive findings are evident: pale conjunctiva and black, guaiac-positive stool.

Table 8-4: **Symptoms of Left-Sided and Right-Sided Lesions**

	Right Colon (%)	Left Colon (%)	Sigmoid Colon (%)	Rectum (%)
Pain	80	70	50	5
Bowel complaints	30	50	70	80
Vomiting	30	15	3	0
Bleeding	10	10	30	70
Weight loss	50	15	20	30
Obstruction	10	20	30	3
Abscess/peritonitis	1	2	10	0
Tenesmus	0	0	0	15
Mass	70	50	40	0

◆ **What evaluation is appropriate?**

◆ The man has suspected colon cancer, particularly of the cecum or right colon because of the anemia and black stools. Identification, localization, and histology of the lesion are necessary. **Colonoscopy** is best, and it also identifies other colonic pathology such as **second lesions** or other disease processes. Colonoscopy has largely replaced barium enema. A CXR, CEA measurement, and liver function tests are warranted to check for metastatic disease. CT of the abdomen and pelvis is indicated. The current spiral CT scans are highly reliable in detecting liver lesions. Further studies are unnecessary unless organ-specific symptoms are present (Table 8-4 and Fig. 8-21).

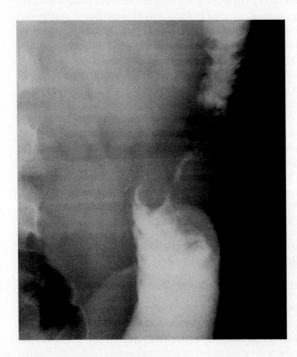

Figure 8-21: Barium enema showing an "apple core" lesion in the left colon. (From Wanebo HJ, ed. *Surgery for Gastrointestinal Cancer.* Philadelphia: Lippincott-Raven; 1997:174.)

The patient's hematocrit is low (30%), and indices demonstrate a microcytic anemia. Serum iron is decreased. Colonoscopy reveals a 5-cm exophytic mass in the cecum. The remaining studies, including CXR, CT, and liver function tests, are normal. A biopsy reveals moderately differentiated adenocarcinoma of the cecum.

◆ **What is the next step?**

◆ **Surgery** to remove the cancer is necessary. There is no need for further evaluation for the cancer, but the patient should undergo a careful medical evaluation to assess operative risk and should also receive supplemental iron preoperatively.

◆ **What would you tell the patient about his operative risk and potential complications?**

◆ The operative risk for a routine colectomy is no different from that of most abdominal procedures. Postoperative complications include the usual problems.

- Wound infection, which occurs in approximately 5%–10% of cases. The risk is higher than with a clean operation.
- A small risk of an anastomotic leak
- The need for a colostomy if an unforeseen operative problem occurs
- Involvement by tumor or injury to the ureter. This possibility warrants discussion.
- Biopsy or removal of any suspicious lesions for metastasis, particularly in the liver

The patient agrees to the surgery.

◆ **What procedures are appropriate?**

◆ A **mechanical bowel "prep," used to be standard procedure for colectomy, but evidence shows that it might not be necessary or helpful.** Some surgeons still elect to use a mechanical and/or antibiotic bowel prep most commonly using polyethylene glycol, magnesium citrate, or another potent laxative. Oral, nonabsorbed antibiotics are often given to decrease colonic bacterial levels with or without a mechanical prep, along with a single preoperative dose of a second-generation cephalosporin to diminish wound infection.

◆ A laparoscopic or open approach can be used. The initial step is a **careful assessment of the primary tumor** followed by a careful assessment for **metastasis**. Surgeons should specifically seek metastasis in the small bowel mesentery, the peritoneal surface, the diaphragm, the liver, and other locations. Even if other tumor is present, resection is still appropriate to prevent obstruction and bleeding, even though the procedure is not curative.

A partial colectomy, typically a **right or hemicolectomy**, is warranted (Fig. 8-22). In addition to removing the tumor-bearing colon, it is necessary to remove the mesenteric tissue, including the **regional lymph nodes**. Reanastomosis of the bowel involves connecting the terminal ileum to the transverse colon, a so-called ileotransverse colostomy. Closure of the rents in the mesentery prevents internal herniation and obstruction of the small bowel. Closure of the abdomen is the final step.

Suppose you have performed a right colectomy and excision of mesenteric lymph nodes. The remainder of the abdomen, including the liver, is normal.

◆ **What postoperative management is appropriate?**

◆ The patient should remain NPO on IV fluids until bowel function returns. Some surgeons would also use an NG tube. Once the patient can tolerate food, he can be discharged.

On postoperative day 2, the patient's pathology result returns; it reports moderately differentiated adenocarcinoma of the cecum, with tumor penetration through serosa. Nodes are negative.

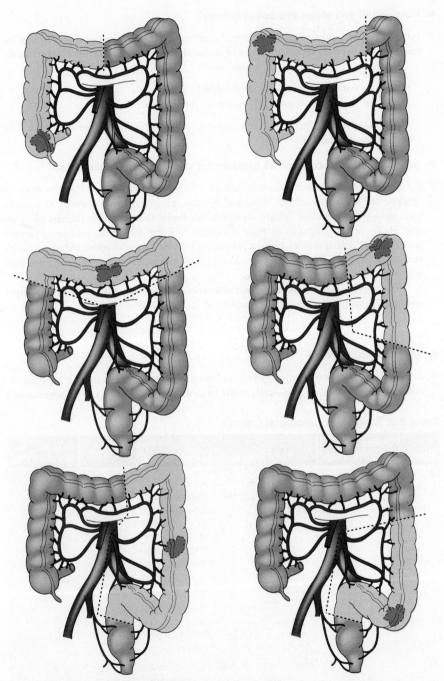

Figure 8-22: Types of colectomies performed based on location of the primary tumor. (From Greenfield LJ, Mulholland MW, Oldham KT, et al, eds. *Surgery: Scientific Principles and Practice*, 2nd ed. Philadelphia: Lippincott Williams & Wilkins; 1997:1139.)

◆ **How would you stage this colon cancer?**

◆ Staging of colon cancer, which is performed after surgical resection, is based on **depth of invasion of the primary lesion, presence of regional lymph nodes, and distant metastasis.** Two methods of staging are commonly used.

1. Dukes Astler-Collier classification (older)
2. Tumor–node–metastasis (TNM) system (more recent)

The TNM system is preferred. This tumor is a T3, N0, M0 and represents stage II or Dukes B classification (Table 8-5).

◆ **Is additional therapy such as radiation or chemotherapy warranted?**

◆ No studies have indicated that adjuvant chemotherapy has an advantage in stage II cancers. The therapy is termed "adjuvant" because it is given postoperatively to patients with no apparent residual disease. Research has found that radiation therapy plays no role. However, the prognosis in stage II cancers is worse for mucus-producing tumors and "signet" ring cell tumors, tumors presenting with bowel perforation, and tumors with venous or perineural invasion. Thus, some physicians would treat these patients with adjuvant chemotherapy.

Studies have shown that **adjuvant chemotherapy for stage III (there are multiple options)** is effective in reducing recurrence and improving survival.

The patient wants to know your plans for follow-up for recurrence of the cancer.

◆ **What do you tell him?**

◆ It is necessary to follow a patient who has undergone a curative resection for **local recurrence at the anastomosis, metastasis to the liver, distant metastasis, and occurrence of a**

Table 8-5: Staging of Colorectal Cancer

Stage	Dukes Classification	TNM Stage			Description	5-Year Survival (%)
0	—	T_{is}	N0	M0	—	—
I	A	T1 or T2	N0	M0	Tumor limited to mucosa and submucosa (T1) or deeper into bowel wall but not extending through muscularis propria (T2)	>90
II	B	T3 or T4	N0	M0	Tumor extends through full thickness of bowel wall (T3) or into adjacent structures (T4) but does not involve regional lymph nodes	60–80
III	C	Any T	N1, N2, or N3	M0	Tumor has metastasized to regional lymph nodes at various levels	20–50
IV	D	Any T	Any N	M1	Liver or other distant metastasis	<5

second primary colon cancer. Approximately 70% and 90% of recurrences become detectable by 2 and 4 years, respectively. Repeat colonoscopy at 6 months and then at 12-month intervals is necessary. More frequent monitoring of CXR, CEA, and liver function tests is essential. A rising CEA, which is 70% accurate in predicting recurrence, should prompt CT of the abdomen to examine for metastasis.

Case 8.23 Heme-Positive Stool No. 4

You see a 62-year-old woman who has heme-positive stools. You suspect colon cancer.

◆ **How would the following additional findings change the evaluation of this patient?**

Case Variation 8.23.1. *RLQ mass*

◆ A **mass palpable** in the RLQ suggests a **large tumor** that may be invading local structures such as the ureter. CT would help assess involved structures.

Case Variation 8.23.2. *Intermittent constipation and diarrhea*

◆ This common symptom of colon cancer suggests the existence of a **higher grade obstructive lesion**, which is perhaps more likely on the left side of the colon. Management may be more difficult preoperatively due to the urgency of the obstruction. Surgeons should attempt to perform a curative procedure, although the prognosis is worse for obstructive cancers.

Case Variation 8.23.3. *Crampy abdominal pain*

◆ Crampy abdominal pain also suggests intermittent obstruction. See Case Variation 8.23.2 for more information.

Case Variation 8.23.4. *Family history that is positive for colon cancer*

◆ A family history of colon cancer carries a higher risk of development of cancer. Genetic syndromes known to be associated with colon cancer include Lynch syndrome and Gardner syndrome and familial adenomatous polyposis.

Case Variation 8.23.5. *Previous colonoscopy that demonstrated multiple polyps*

◆ If the previous colonoscopy did not miss an additional lesion, it is unlikely that a new colon cancer has developed during the subsequent period. Epidemiologic data suggest that the **progression from polyp to invasive cancer** takes approximately 10 years. However, more recent data suggest another possibility: Cancer may arise from nonadenomatous tissue. The patient should still undergo repeat colonoscopy to establish a diagnosis.

Case Variation 8.23.6. *Scleral icterus*

◆ Scleral icterus could be due to a number of reasons unrelated to the tumor, but the likelihood that it is tumor-related is high. Potential tumor-related causes include **metastatic tumor replacement of the liver** and a metastasis strategically located that blocks the bile duct. An ultrasound or CT scan of the liver would help assess these possibilities.

Case Variation 8.23.7. *A younger (22 years of age) instead of an older adult (55 years)*

◆ In younger individuals, benign diagnoses such as inflammatory conditions are more likely. However, the scenario of colon cancer may still occur in young patients, and thus, a complete workup is necessary.

Case 8.24 Operative Findings in Colon Cancer No. 1

You perform a colectomy for colon cancer in a 58-year-old man.

◆ How do the following pathologic findings change the planned therapy?

Case Variation 8.24.1. Penetration of the primary tumor into the nearby abdominal wall

◆ The portion of the abdominal wall is resected as part of a more radical procedure. Involvement of adjacent structures **makes the T classification in the TNM system a T4 lesion and worsens the prognosis by 3%–5% over 5 years.**

Case Variation 8.24.2. Positive lymph nodes recognized at surgery

◆ The operation proceeds unchanged; however, the surgeon attempts to remove all involved nodes.

Case Variation 8.24.3. Positive lymph nodes recognized by the pathologist 2 days later

◆ The hemicolectomy remains the procedure of choice, and no further operative procedures are necessary. The patient has stage III disease and is eligible for adjuvant chemotherapy.

Case Variation 8.24.4. A 1-cm lesion palpable on the surface of the liver at surgery

◆ A small lesion on the liver, particularly at the edge of the liver, usually can be wedged out as a total excision. If the lesion were contiguous with vital structures such as a hepatic vein, then a biopsy of the lesion would be appropriate, with no further therapy during that operation.

Case Variation 8.24.5. An 8-cm lesion palpable on the surface of the liver at surgery

◆ Larger lesions should not be resected when discovered at the time of surgery. A major liver resection increases both the intraoperative risk of bleeding and the overall complexity and duration of the operation. Many general surgeons also are not experienced hepatic surgeons. Postoperative complications such as infection and bile leakage are possible; none of these have usually been discussed with the patient preoperatively. Most surgeons would complete the colectomy, biopsy the liver lesion, and plan resection at a later date after further evaluation.

Case Variation 8.24.6. A poorly differentiated tumor histology obtained preoperatively from the primary tumor

◆ The operative procedure is unchanged. Factors associated with a worsened prognosis include poorly differentiated tumors, especially mucin-producing and "signet cell" tumors, tumors with venous or perineural invasion, and tumors presenting with perforation.

Case Variation 8.24.7. A 2-cm nodule apparent on CXR

◆ The nodule warrants evaluation by chest CT and biopsy by percutaneous needle biopsy if suspicious for cancer. Many surgeons would include an abdominal CT to gain further information for operative planning. A metastatic lung nodule makes a curative operation very unlikely. Therefore, the colectomy does not need to be as extensive as it might be with curable cancer. However, it is still necessary to perform a colectomy to remove the primary tumor to manage it locally and prevent further blood loss or bowel obstruction.

Case 8.25 Complications of Postoperative Colectomy

Most patients who undergo an elective colectomy have an uneventful recovery in the postoperative period.

◆ **How would you manage the following situations?**

Case Variation 8.25.1. The patient becomes distended and vomits feculent material on the third postoperative day.

◆ This suggests that the patient's GI tract is not functional, which could be secondary to a persistent, postoperative ileus or a mechanical obstruction. Feculent vomiting results from bacterial overgrowth in the stomach and proximal small bowel due to failure to propel food and secretions distally. NPO feeding and IV fluids are appropriate, along with insertion of an NG tube. Evaluation of the abdomen with a physical exam and an obstructive series is necessary. The concerns are two: (1) **leakage from the anastomosis has occurred, causing a persistent ileus,** or (2) **a mechanical obstruction due to adhesions, an internal hernia, or an obstructed anastomosis.** These developments may require CT or a small bowel series to identify the problem, depending on the postoperative day and condition of the patient. The patient may require reoperation for anastomotic leakage, obstruction with ischemia, or potential ischemia.

Case Variation 8.25.2. A reddened, fluctuant area develops at the inferior aspect of the wound

◆ This suggests a **wound infection.** Management usually involves opening the involved portion of the wound down to the fascia, with inspection of the fascia to determine whether it is intact. Local wound care is sufficient for most uncomplicated wound infections.

Case Variation 8.25.3. Feculent material drains from the inferior aspect of the wound.

◆ This suggests a wound infection caused by an **anastomotic leak** that has spontaneously drained (necessitated) to the skin. **NPO feeding and IV fluids** are usually sufficient for most colon fistulas, the majority of which **will close with this therapy.** A CT scan of the abdomen determines whether there is **an undrained collection**, which needs draining either operatively or percutaneously, which is preferable. If any doubt about the **patency of the anastomosis** exists, a gentle Gastrografin enema or colonoscopy may be appropriate, although most surgeons would be very hesitant to do this early in the course of a fistula with a fresh anastomosis. A fistula with a distal obstruction due to a nonpatent anastomosis (i.e., obstructed) will not close. It requires operative revision and an ileostomy proximally to divert the fecal stream.

Case Variation 8.25.4. The patient returns to the hospital 10 days postoperatively with a temperature of 104°F and abdominal pain in the RLQ.

◆ This suggests an **abscess**, most likely in the right paracolic gutter or pelvis. Most commonly, diagnosis is by CT, and management is by percutaneous drainage. Concern regarding anastomotic leakage is also present, and the previously discussed management is appropriate (see Case Variation 8.25.3).

Case Variation 8.25.5. The patient returns in 6 months with crampy abdominal pain, decreased stool caliber, and constipation.

◆ These symptoms could represent **anastomotic recurrence** of the cancer as well as a **stricture** at the anastomosis. Strictures usually result from excessive scar formation due to inadequate blood supply to the anastomosed segments. It is also possible that a second obstructing cancer, which could have been missed at initial surgery, is causing the symptoms. **Colonoscopy** usually establishes the diagnosis.

Case 8.26   Heme-Positive Stool No. 5

A 55-year-old man presents with constipation, rectal bleeding, and a feeling of fatigue. On examination, you find a constricting hard lesion 4 cm from the anal verge. Biopsy indicates adenocarcinoma of the rectum.

◆ **What further evaluation is necessary before making a decision regarding treatment?**

◆ The following studies are necessary. **Colonoscopy** is necessary initially for visualization of the entire colon to rule out the presence of synchronous lesions. If no other lesions are found, an evaluation **determines the depth of invasion** that is warranted; this is an important prognostic sign. **Transrectal ultrasound** is useful to determine rectal wall invasion and local lymph node enlargement. **CT** or magnetic resonance imaging (MRI) is appropriate to determine **whether adjacent structures**, including the prostate, bladder, and ureters, **are involved.** CT scans may show **distant involvement** in the liver, as well as enlarged lymph nodes. A CXR and a CEA level are also warranted before surgery.

After studying this patient, you find that he has a circumferential lesion at 4 cm that is not fixed to the surrounding tissues. The transrectal ultrasound indicates that the tumor is limited to the bowel wall, and no regional or local lymph nodes are evident. The CT scan shows a normal liver and no other abnormalities. The CXR is normal. The CEA is elevated, and all other laboratory studies are normal.

◆ **What is the next step?**

◆ Resection of the tumor is warranted, assuming that the patient is an acceptable operative risk. Preoperative neoadjuvant therapy is not useful in this early-stage lesion.

◆ **What procedure is appropriate?**

◆ Most surgeons would recommend an abdominoperineal resection, which involves excision of the entire rectum with the creation of a permanent colostomy (Figs. 8-23 and 8-24). In addition, this procedure removes local lymph nodes.

◆ **The patient's tumor metastasizes to what nodal locations and other organs?**

◆ Rectal carcinomas spread by direct extension and lymphatics. Lymphatic spread parallels the superior hemorrhoidal vessels and includes the **internal iliac nodes, sacral nodes, and inferior mesenteric nodes.** Lesions less than 5 cm from the anal verge can **also spread** locally and to the **inguinal nodes,** and this should be determined preoperatively. Distal organ involvement most commonly includes the liver or adjacent structures.

◆ **What information should the patient receive about the perioperative risks and complications of abdominoperineal resection?**

◆ Several specific complications relate to abdominoperineal resection. Because the sympathetic plexus of nerves is located around the rectum, the chance of **impotence** following the procedure is high; it is estimated to be about 50%. It is essential that the patient

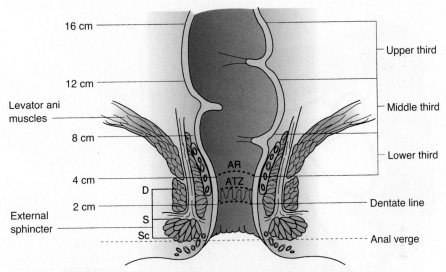

Figure 8-23: Local anatomy of the rectum as it relates to abdominoperineal resection. D, deep; S, superficial; Sc, subcutaneous; AR, anorectal ring; ATZ, anal transition zone. (From Greenfield LJ, Mulholland MW, Oldham KT, et al, eds. *Surgery: Scientific Principles and Practice*, 2nd ed. Philadelphia: Lippincott Williams & Wilkins; 1997:1140.)

be told prior to surgery about the possibility of impotence. There is also a chance that **bladder function** may be impaired following surgery. Other intraoperative risks include massive venous bleeding from the presacral space and injury to the ureter. Finally, a variety of colostomy complications, including retraction, prolapse, stricture, and obstruction, may occur.

Your patient decides to proceed with an abdominoperineal resection.

◆ **What are the essential elements of this procedure?**

◆ The basic principle of the abdominoperineal resection is removal of the entire rectum in continuity with its vascular and lymphatic supply. It is necessary to mark a colostomy site preoperatively, and the surgeon usually chooses the lower left quadrant. Placement of the patient in the lithotomy position allows both the abdominal and pelvic dissections to be performed simultaneously.

The rectum is dissected away from the surrounding tissues, attempting to avoid injury to the nerves and urinary tract. Mesenteric lymph nodes are removed with the specimen. The colon is divided at the junction of the descending colon and the sigmoid colon, and the specimen is removed. An end colostomy is performed. The perineal wound is either closed or packed with gauze.

Pathology on the specimen returns as well-differentiated adenocarcinoma of the rectum with extension into the bowel wall to the level of the muscularis propria but not involving the serosa.

◆ **What stage is this tumor (Fig. 8-25)?**

◆ This tumor is a stage I cancer.

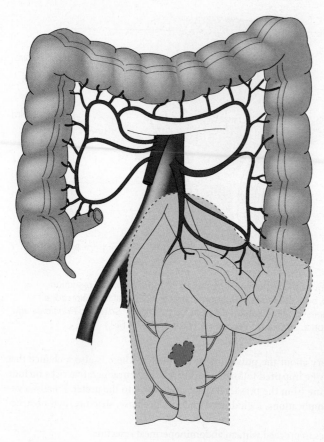

Figure 8-24: Bowel removal in abdominoperineal resection. (From Greenfield LJ, Mulholland MW, Oldham KT, et al, eds. *Surgery: Scientific Principles and Practice*, 2nd ed. Philadelphia: Lippincott Williams & Wilkins; 1997:1140.)

◆ **What other factors in this primary tumor are important in the prognosis of this patient, who has no positive lymph nodes?**

◆ A poor prognosis is associated with poor histologic differentiation of the tumor, elevated CEA level, bowel perforation, and aneuploidy.

◆ **What is the appropriate management plan for this patient once he has recovered from the surgery?**

◆ Management is similar to any patient with colon cancer.

Case 8.27 Heme-Positive Stool No. 6

You are asked to evaluate a 62-year-old man with rectal cancer.

◆ **How would the level of the lesion from the anal verge affect operative management?**

◆ It is possible to remove most rectal cancers that lie more than 5 cm proximal to the anal verge safely using an anterior approach leaving the anus and sphincter in place. If the lesion is closer to the anal verge, abdominoperineal resection is necessary because lesions within 5 cm of the anal verge have lateral margins of resection that include the anal

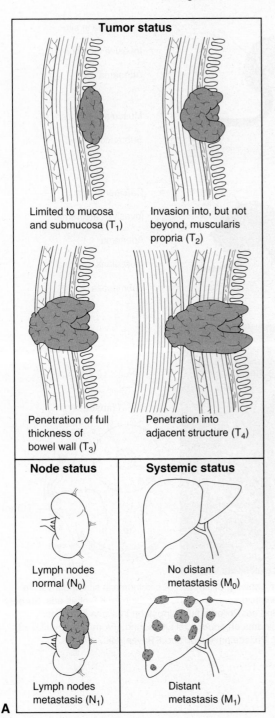

A: Staging of colon carcinoma. (*continued*)

Figure 8-25:

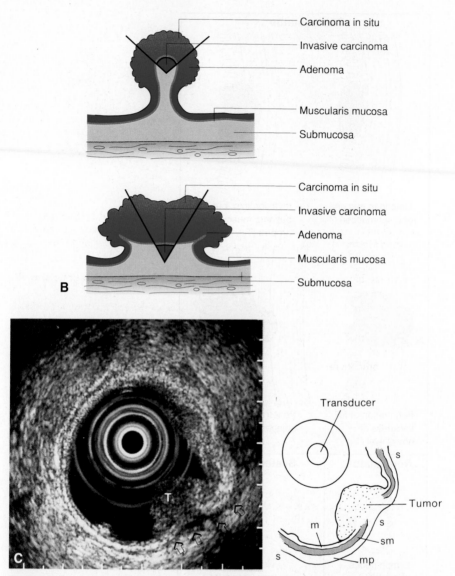

Figure 8-25: (*continued*) **B:** diagram showing distinction of carcinoma in situ and invasive malignancy of the colon. (From Greenfield LJ, Mulholland MW, Oldham KT, et al, eds. *Surgery: Scientific Principles and Practice*, 2nd ed. Philadelphia: Lippincott Williams & Wilkins; 1997:1132.) **C:** Stage T1 rectal carcinoma on endorectal ultrasound. (From Wanebo HJ, ed. *Surgery for Gastrointestinal Cancer*. Philadelphia: Lippincott-Raven; 1997:174.)

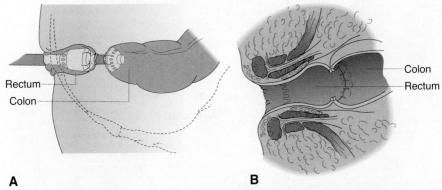

A   **B**

Figure 8-26: Low anterior bowel resection, showing **(A)** staple technique and **(B)** suture technique. (From Greenfield LJ, Mulholland MW, Oldham KT, et al, eds. *Surgery: Scientific Principles and Practice*, 2nd ed. Philadelphia: Lippincott Williams & Wilkins; 1997:1141.)

sphincter mechanism. Removal or disabling of this mechanism results in incontinence, obviously not a desirable situation.

Several additional factors that influence this practice mostly relate to the type of lesion.

QUICK CUT Local recurrence of rectal carcinoma is a common mode of failure. Therefore, ample, clear margins are mandatory at the initial procedure.

Lesions with large lateral components also require a wider margin of resection (Fig. 8-26). Thus, abdominoperineal resection is more likely for lesions larger than 5 cm. Rectal cancers that involve the regional lymph nodes (stage III) or high-risk stage II tumors also require postoperative adjuvant chemotherapy that is similar to that used with colon cancer.

◆ **When might preoperative radiation therapy be a consideration?**

◆ If lesions are large and bulky or extend outside the bowel wall into the surrounding tissue, the rate of local recurrence is higher. Thus, management usually involves **preoperative irradiation** and chemotherapy to increase resectability and decrease local recurrence.

◆ **What alternatives do patients have if they do not agree to colostomy?**

◆ The procedures previously described in this case are the standard methods for treatment of rectal cancer, but there are two additional therapeutic options.

   • One approach is **sphincter-preserving proctectomy** (Figs. 8-27 and 8-28). A rationale for this procedure relates to a change in thinking about the distal resection margin necessary to cure a patient with cancer. Previously, experts believed a 5-cm distal margin was necessary, but more recently, studies have found that a 2-cm margin is adequate for well-differentiated cancers. Additional improvements have occurred in the operative approach and with the preservation of anal continence. Combined with preoperative radiation and chemotherapy to the rectum and a temporary diverting ileostomy to allow anastomotic healing to occur, these procedures have become commonplace.
   • A second approach involves local resection of rectal tumors. In these cases, one method involves dilation of the anal sphincter and resection of the tumor. Another

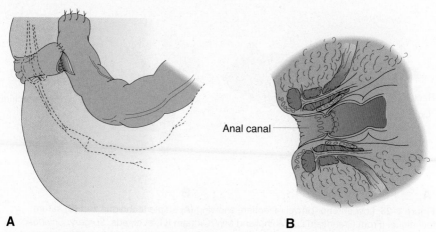

A

B

Anal canal

Figure 8-27: A: Sphincter-preserving proctectomy. **B:** Coloanal anastomosis. (From Greenfield LJ, Mulholland MW, Oldham KT, et al, eds. *Surgery: Scientific Principles and Practice*, 2nd ed. Philadelphia: Lippincott Williams & Wilkins; 1997:1141.)

method involves using a trans-sacral approach to the rectum, which allows a sleeve resection of the tumor-bearing bowel (see Fig. 8-28). Both approaches are particularly useful for small tumors in high–medical risk patients.

- Carcinomas that are less than 4 cm in diameter and involve less than 40% of the rectal wall can be resected through a transanal approach. This approach is usually reserved for T1 lesions.

◆ **How does abdominoperineal resection differ in women?**

◆ In female patients with anterior rectal wall carcinoma, removal of the posterior wall of the vagina as the anterior margin of the resection is appropriate. Surgeons should be careful not to denervate the urethra. Closure of the vagina may then occur.

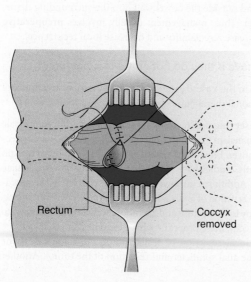

Rectum

Coccyx removed

Figure 8-28: Trans-sacral resection of a rectal cancer. (From Greenfield LJ, Mulholland MW, Oldham KT, et al, eds. *Surgery: Scientific Principles and Practice*, 2nd ed. Philadelphia. Lippincott Williams & Wilkins; 1997:1141.)

A patient undergoes a curative resection with an abdominoperineal resection.

◆ **What evaluation and management is appropriate for a new 0.5-cm lesion in the perineum?**

◆ **Biopsy** of the lesion is necessary. If the biopsy shows carcinoma, the patient should undergo a repeat CT scan, CEA level, and colonoscopy to determine the extent of the lesion and whether there are other lesions. Typically, a multidisciplinary approach using chemotherapy radiation and surgery is appropriate for treatment of a recurrence. In general, recurrent cancer has a poor prognosis.

◆ **What evaluation and management are appropriate for pelvic pain?**

◆ If this occurs in the early postoperative period, it may be secondary to **operative nerve injury or infection**. If it occurs later, it is necessary to rule out **local recurrence** of the tumor by physical examination and CT of the pelvis.

Case 8.28 Metastasis in Colorectal Cancer

You perform a curative resection for colon cancer in a 49-year-old man who has stage II cancer. You decide to follow him with serial CEA measurements and yearly colonoscopy. Initial CEA values are low and stable, and repeat colonoscopy is normal at 1 and 2 years. During the next visit, the man's CEA is now significantly elevated.

◆ **What evaluation is appropriate?**

◆ A **CXR and CT of the abdomen** to look for metastasis are warranted. A repeat **colonoscopy** may be necessary, depending on when the last one was performed.

The patient's evaluation is negative except for a new 2-cm lesion in the right lobe of the liver.

◆ **What further evaluation and management is appropriate?**

◆ The patient is a candidate for **surgical resection** if he has **no extrahepatic demonstrable metastatic** cancer, **no local recurrence** of the primary cancer, an acceptable anesthetic risk from the cardiopulmonary standpoint, and a lesion that is **in a surgically resectable location**. The more current spiral CT scans and MRI studies are reliable; they demonstrate additional hepatic metastasis in more than 80% of cases. These tests are necessary if the initial CT scan is inadequate. A CXR and colonoscopy are appropriate, but further workup is unnecessary unless the patient has additional symptoms or findings.

Typically unresectable lesions are either multiple lesions in both lobes, lesions intimate with vascular structures (e.g., hepatic veins, portal vein), lesions invading local structures (e.g., the diaphragm), or lesions occurring in cirrhotic livers. Cirrhosis increases the perioperative risk as a result of limited hepatic reserve following resection, as well as technical difficulties in transecting a fibrotic liver (see Table 7-2).

◆ **What is appropriate to tell the patient about his prognosis and the variables that affect it?**

◆ Resection of liver lesions is associated with the best survival when compared to other treatment modalities, and it should be recommended if the lesion is resectable. **Patients with solitary**

lesions that are resected have a survival as high as 33% at 5 years. The survival of individuals with two to four lesions is 15%, and unresectable lesions have a survival of close to 0%.

You decide to remove the liver lesion surgically.

◆ **What procedure and follow-up do you recommend?**

◆ It is acceptable to resect a lesion with **a formal hepatic lobectomy or segmentectomy or with a nonanatomic wedge resection, as long as a greater than 1-cm margin is obtained.** The principal reasons for unresectability intraoperatively are inability to resect the lesion due to its location, multiple lesions, or evidence for metastasis outside the liver. The major surgical risk relates to uncontrollable hemorrhage related to technical problems. With most experienced hepatic surgeons, the operative mortality is approximately 1%. Recurrence may assume the form of distant metastasis or occur at the original site of resection. CXR, serial CEA measurements, and abdominal ultrasound or CT are used to check for recurrence.

◆ **What management is appropriate for unresectable liver metastasis?**

◆ There are other options for management of unresectable lesions with local methods. Most involve some form of ablation therapy with freezing–thawing techniques (cryotherapy), injection of absolute ethanol, or destruction with radiofrequency waves **(RF ablation).** Destruction of lesions may also occur angiographically by **chemoembolization.** The hepatic artery is catheterized, and thrombotic substances such as Gelfoam are saturated with chemotherapy and injected into the region of metastasis. Most of these methods are in various stages of clinical trials.

Case 8.29 Heme-Positive Stool No. 7

A 45-year-old man presents with rectal bleeding. On examination, you find a hard lesion that involves the anal verge. Biopsy of the lesion indicates squamous cell carcinoma of the anus.

◆ **What regional nodes are most likely to be involved with metastasis?**

◆ Squamous cell carcinomas (also called epidermoid carcinoma) are the most common tumor of the anal canal. Because the symptoms are nonspecific (e.g., bleeding, drainage, pain, pruritus), the diagnosis is often delayed while the patient is treated for a benign process. The diagnosis is made by biopsy. Squamous cell carcinomas commonly metastasize to the inguinal lymph nodes, but they also metastasize to the superior rectal lymph nodes in up to 50% of patients.

◆ **What staging system is best?**

◆ The TNM system is used for staging, and treatment differs depending on the TNM stage (see Table 8-5). CT and transrectal ultrasound are warranted to determine the depth of invasion and the presence of nodal metastasis.

◆ **How would you manage the following findings?**

Case Variation 8.29.1. A 0.5-cm diameter lesion with no local extension and negative lymph nodes

◆ **Superficial small, mobile lesions warrant treatment with local excision** alone, with close follow-up to ensure that the cancer does not recur.

Table 8-6: Modified Nigro Regimen for Squamous Cell Carcinoma of the Anal Canal

Treatment	Dose	Schedule
External radiation	50 Gy to the primary carcinoma and 35–45 Gy to pelvic inguinal nodes	Start day 1 (2 Gy/day, 5 days/week for 5 weeks)
Systemic chemotherapy	Fluorouracil, 1,000 mg/m²/24 hr as a continuous infusion for 4 days	Start day 1; repeat 4-day infusion starting day 28
Mitomycin C	10–15 mg/m² as intravenous bolus	Day 1 only

From Greenfield LJ, Mulholland MW, Lillemoe KD, et al, eds. *Greenfield's Surgery*, 5th ed. Philadelphia: Lippincott Williams & Wilkins; 2010.

Case Variation 8.29.2. A 4-cm diameter lesion with no local extension and negative lymph nodes

QUICK CUT Surgery is not warranted. Treatment involves the modified Nigro protocol, which consists of chemotherapy and radiation therapy in order to eliminate the cancer.

In most cases chemoradiation treatment is successful. Abdominalperineal resection is used **only if there is biopsy-proven residual cancer.** However, even in patients with positive inguinal nodes, the modified Nigro protocol usually provides complete local control of the primary cancer (Table 8-6).

Case Variation 8.29.3. A recurrent anal carcinoma

◆ Abdominoperineal resection plays an important role in recurrent anal cancer. Perineal wound complications are common, as these patients have had radiation to the surgical field.

LOWER ABDOMINAL PAIN

Case 8.30 Left Lower Quadrant Pain No. 1

A 70-year-old woman presents to the emergency department with abdominal pain and fever that developed several hours ago. History is unremarkable, except for occasional constipation. On physical examination, she has a fever of 101°F and mild tachycardia, with a BP of 140/85 mm Hg. The abdomen is tender in the left lower quadrant (LLQ).

◆ **What is the suspected diagnosis?**

◆ **Diverticulitis** is likely in a patient with LLQ pain, tenderness, and fever. Occasionally, it is possible to palpate a mass in the LLQ.

◆ **What is the initial management?**

QUICK CUT Generally, patients with minimal symptoms or signs of inflammation may receive outpatient treatment with broad-spectrum antibiotics.

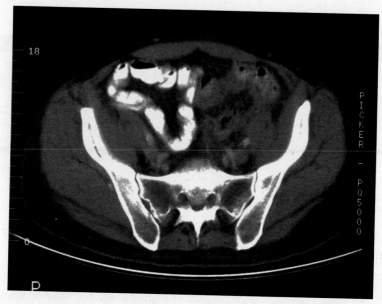

Figure 8-29: CT scan of diverticulitis, showing "fat stranding" and edema of the tissue near the inflamed colon.

Because this patient is elderly and has a fever and tachycardia, more appropriate management may be **complete bowel rest, IV hydration, and parenteral antibiotics.** If nausea or vomiting develop, NG suction may be necessary. An abdominal obstructive series is warranted to check for free air and to search for other diagnoses. A clinician may choose to perform a **CT scan to examine for inflammation, abscess, diverticula, and a thickened sigmoid bowel wall, which confirms a diagnosis of diverticulitis (Fig. 8-29).** However, CT is not mandatory in uncomplicated patients.

Another concern is that the symptoms are from a **perforated colon cancer**; signs and symptoms may be similar. The management plan should include careful, **serial abdominal examinations** to check for progression of the disease.

On this management, the patient exhibits rapid improvement and becomes hungry.

◆ **What would the management plan be now?**

◇ Management may entail a high-fiber diet, which is recommended after recovery from the initial attack. If she remains afebrile, she can be discharged. Outpatient treatment with broad-spectrum antibiotics is appropriate for 7–10 days.

◆ **What is the likelihood that this patient will have another episode of diverticulitis?**

◇ The recurrence rate is high and may be up to 40 % but can be decreased with a high fiber diet.

◆ **What long-term follow-up is necessary?**

◇ **Colonoscopy** or barium enema may be appropriate after the patient has recovered to **confirm the presence of diverticula** and the **absence of colon cancer (Fig. 8-30).**

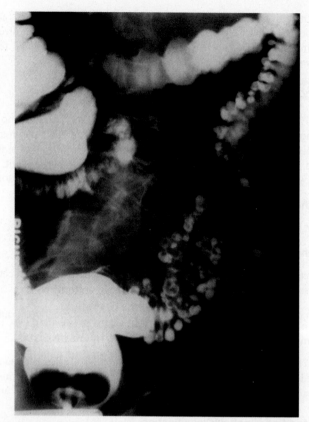

Figure 8-30: Barium enema showing multiple diverticula. (From McKenney MG, Mangonon PC, Moylan JA, eds. *Understanding Surgical Disease: The Miami Manual of Surgery*. Philadelphia: Lippincott-Raven; 1998:154.)

Case 8.31 Left Lower Quadrant Pain No. 2

The woman described in Case 8.30 returns 6 months later with a recurrence of the same problem.

◆ **How does this change the proposed management plan?**

◇ Initially, the patient should be managed in the same manner, with bowel rest, IV antibiotics, and analgesics. After the second episode of **diverticulitis, an elective resection** is usually scheduled 4–6 weeks after the inflammation has resolved. Resection is often recommended because the **risk of a significant complication** such as perforation or abscess formation increases with each recurrent episode.

◆ **What procedure is appropriate?**

◇ **Removal of the diverticula-bearing colon** (colectomy) is warranted, which means that the surgeon must have a good description of the colon and the location of the diverticula. This necessitates either preoperative or intraoperative colonoscopy. The rectum caudad to the peritoneal reflection in the pelvis is usually free of diverticula and does not need removal. In most patients, a short segment of the sigmoid colon is involved with diverticula, with the remaining bowel free of disease. With proper planning, a colonic reanastomosis (colocolostomy) is possible without the need to perform a colostomy.

Case 8.32   Left Lower Quadrant Pain No. 3

You admit a 75-year-old woman with LLQ pain, fever, and nausea who has a presumptive diagnosis of acute diverticulitis. An obstructive series is unremarkable, and the WBC count is 15,000 cells/mm³. Therapy with antibiotics, bowel rest, and IV fluids begins, with a plan to follow her clinically. Despite this treatment, the patient deteriorates, with continued pain, increasing fever, and rising WBC count.

◆ **What is the suspected problem?**

◆ The patient has a free perforation or an intra-abdominal abscess.

◆ **What is the appropriate evaluation?**

◆ CT may demonstrate abscess, perforation, or other complications of the acute inflammatory process. In addition, it may also reveal the presence of diverticula.

The CT scan demonstrates a loculated fluid collection in the pericolic gutter.

◆ **What management is appropriate?**

◆ A loculated fluid collection with a CT-guided needle insertion of a catheter into the collection is warranted. This method allows the fluid to be sampled and drained. The treatment algorithm for diverticulitis is complex and based on the Hinchey classification (Table 8-7 and Fig. 8-31).

Table 8-7: Modified Hinchey Classification

Hinchey Classification	Modified Hinchey Classification	Comments
	0 Mild clinical diverticulitis	Left lower quadrant pain, elevated white blood cells, fever, no confirmation by imaging or surgery
I Pericolic abscess or phlegmon	Ia Confined pericolic inflammation—phlegmon	
II Pelvic, intra-abdominal, or retroperitoneal abscess	II Pelvic, distant intra-abdominal, or retroperitoneal abscess	
III Generalized purulent peritonitis	III Generalized purulent peritonitis	No open communication with bowel lumen
IV Generalized fecal peritonitis	IV Fecal peritonitis Fistula colovesical/ colovaginal/coloenteric/ colocutaneous	Free perforation, open communication with bowel lumen
Obstruction	Large and/or small bowel obstruction	

From Greenfield LJ, Mulholland MW, Lillemoe KD, et al, eds. *Greenfield's Surgery*, 5th ed. Philadelphia: Lippincott Williams & Wilkins; 2010.

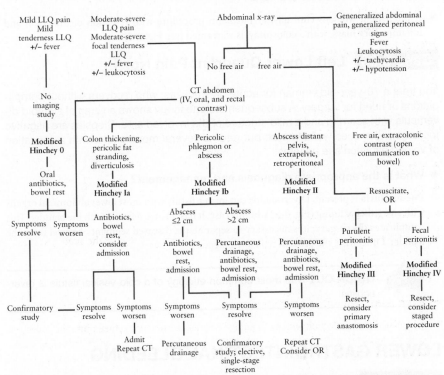

Figure 8-31: Symptoms suggestive of diverticulitis. (From Greenfield LJ, Mulholland MW, Lillemoe KD, et al, eds. *Greenfield's Surgery*, 5th ed. Philadelphia: Lippincott Williams & Wilkins; 2010.)

The drained fluid is purulent and contains gram-negative bacilli. With a catheter left in the collection, the patient improves.

◆ What is the appropriate management?

◆ It is necessary to leave the drainage catheter in place until the cavity shrinks to a small size and the drainage stops. If the patient tolerates food and remains afebrile, she can be discharged. However, many patients with a persistent ileus or functional obstruction from the edema do not tolerate food and require TPN for a period of time.

Indications for elective surgery include a single episode of complicated diverticulitis or two or more episodes of complicated diverticulitis. It is appropriate to consider surgical therapy after one episode of diverticulitis in an immunocompromised patient.

Deep Thoughts

If possible and safe, colon resection for diverticulitis should be done electively by treating the complications of diverticulitis with antibiotics, gut rest, and percutaneous drainage of abscesses to minimize complications of surgery.

◆ **How would the proposed management change if the patient did not improve with catheter drainage?**

◆ If the patient worsens clinically, a Hartmann procedure with resection of the colon and inflammatory mass, with a colostomy, is warranted (see Fig. 8-5).

Case 8.33 ◆ Left Lower Quadrant Pain No. 4

You treat a 70-year-old woman for acute diverticulitis, who recovers without complications or need for surgery. A subsequent colonoscopy shows an area of sigmoid diverticula with scarring and a mild stricture of the involved area. Biopsies are negative for tumor. She does well at home but returns several months later with a sensation of voided air when she urinates.

◆ **What is the appropriate diagnosis and management?**

◆ **Pneumaturia** is present. Diverticulitis can form a fistula with most lower abdominal organs with an epithelial lining (Fig. 8-32). In this case, it has formed a fistula with the bladder. This complicates the surgery; it is necessary to separate the diseased segment of bowel from the bladder. Otherwise, the procedure is unchanged.

 QUICK CUT The most common etiology of a colo-vesical fistula is diverticulitis.

LOWER GASTROINTESTINAL BLEEDING

Case 8.34 ◆ Massive Lower Gastrointestinal Bleeding

A 70-year-old woman who has been in good health presents to the emergency department with a 4-hour history of large amounts of bright red blood per rectum. A brief history is otherwise negative. On physical examination, her heart rate is 115 beats per minute with a BP of 105/70 mm Hg. She appears tired but alert. Her conjunctiva appears pale, and her mucous membranes are dry. Heart and lungs are normal except for a resting tachycardia. The abdomen is soft and nontender, and bright red blood per rectum is evident. She has no peripheral edema and weak but present pulses. Neurologically, she is intact.

◆ **What is the initial evaluation and management plan?**

◆ The patient's signs and symptoms, including fatigue, tachycardia, dry mucous membranes, and pale conjunctiva, are suggestive of **hypovolemia**. Like all elderly patients, this woman is particularly susceptible to volume depletion because of her higher risk of heart disease. Therefore, it is necessary to insert two large-bore IV lines and **1–2 L of lactated Ringer solution**, or 0.9 L normal saline, immediately to replace the isotonic fluid lost. She also requires placement on a monitor. Routine blood studies and a CXR are warranted. A coagulation evaluation is necessary to be certain that she has normal blood clotting, and blood for transfusion should be made available. Placement of a Foley catheter is indicated to help evaluate the adequacy of resuscitation.

 QUICK CUT Placement of an NG tube for lavage is warranted to evaluate and rule out an upper GI bleed.

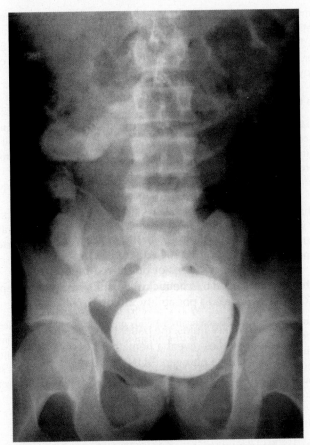

Figure 8-32: Contrast study of the bladder, showing a fistula between the colon and the bladder, a common occurrence. (From McKenney MG, Mangonon PC, Moylan JA, eds. *Understanding Surgical Disease: The Miami Manual of Surgery*. Philadelphia: Lippincott-Raven; 1998:141.)

If the lavage from the NG tube is positive for blood, an upper endoscopy is necessary. **Anoscopy** should also take place in the emergency department to examine for hemorrhoids, bleeding rectal varices, or other anorectal pathology.

Once the resuscitation is under way, it is necessary to take a more careful history and perform a more detailed physical examination to evaluate for pre-existing diseases, prior surgery, and other problems that might influence decision making. Constant **re-evaluation of the resuscitation** should be a high priority.

◆ **What are the most likely diagnoses?**

◆ The most common causes of rapid lower GI bleeding are **bleeding diverticula and vascular ectasias**. Other causes of bright red blood per rectum include Meckel diverticulum, aortoenteric fistula, ischemic colitis, IBD, hemorrhoidal disease, and rectal varices. Colonic neoplasms are also a possibility, although colon cancer rarely causes massive lower GI bleeding.

After receiving IV fluids, the patient's BP and heart rate improve, and she seems more energetic. Laboratory studies reveal a hematocrit of 38% and a mildly elevated serum Na at 148 mEq/L and a blood urea nitrogen (BUN) of 30 mg/dL. Since you initially saw her, she has had no further rectal bleeding. Her NG aspirate contains bile, and anoscopy reveals no bleeding source.

◆ **What are the next management steps?**

◆ Admission for **stabilization, observation for further GI bleeding, and diagnostic workup** is warranted. Close monitoring in an intermediate or intensive care unit is necessary. Although the initial hematocrit is 38%, it takes several hours for the hematocrit to equilibrate before it is an accurate measure of blood cell volume; it should be checked every several hours. If it continues to decrease, a blood transfusion may still be required.

The patient has remained stable overnight with a heart rate of 80 beats per minute, a normal BP with no orthostatic changes, and a hematocrit that has drifted down to 32%. No further episodes of rectal bleeding have occurred. She is currently hungry and feeling much better.

◆ **What is the likelihood that this patient will experience another episode of bleeding?**

◆ The likelihood that she will bleed again depends on the cause of the GI bleed. The **natural course of diverticular bleeds is to stop spontaneously**. Bleeding colonic diverticula have less than 25% likelihood of rebleeding, although 20% of affected patients continue to bleed and require operative intervention. Patients with vascular **ectasias stop bleeding spontaneously in about 90% of cases**, although the risk of rebleeding is approximately 25% and 46% after 1 year and 3 years, respectively.

◆ **What is the next step?**

◆ It is necessary to **determine the cause** of the GI bleed. In this case, in which the bleeding has stopped, the most valuable procedure is **colonoscopy**.

QUICK CUT Whether colonoscopy is performed during this admission or as an outpatient, it is critical to not overlook this procedure. Although colon cancer is unlikely, a missed cancer is a major oversight.

Colonoscopy may take place during hospitalization or electively after discharge. If it occurs during admission, a bowel "prep" with 4 L of polyethylene glycol solution is appropriate.

If **vascular ectasia** is evident, treatment with **coagulation** with a monopolar current is appropriate. The most significant risk is colonic perforation from colonic coagulation. Bleeding colonic **diverticula are not amenable to endoscopic treatment**, but this approach **does permit localization** of the bleeding site on occasion. Bleeding polyps may be coagulated or, in the case of pedunculated polyps, ensnared. "Tattooing" of the bleeding site involves the submucosal injection of methylene blue or India ink, which allows precise localization if operative intervention is necessary (i.e., in the case of a colonic mass or polyp).

Colonoscopy indicates multiple diverticula in the left colon and no vascular ectasia. There is no active bleeding. The woman has a stable hematocrit and is tolerating a regular diet.

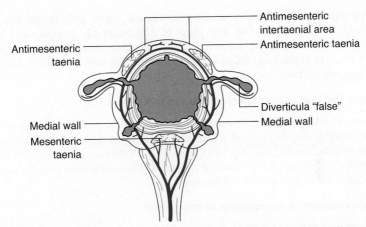

Figure 8-33: The blood supply of the colonic wall and its association with diverticula within the wall of the colon, which explains why diverticulosis has a tendency to bleed. (From McKenney MG, Mangonon PC, Moylan JA, eds. *Understanding Surgical Disease: The Miami Manual of Surgery.* Philadelphia: Lippincott-Raven; 1998:154.)

◆ What is the next step?

◆ Discharge with outpatient follow-up is appropriate. Most physicians would place the patient on **iron** and a high-fiber diet, which may lessen the chance of the development of additional diverticula.

◆ Why are diverticula associated with bleeding?

◆ Colonic diverticular bleeds result from an **underlying vasa recta artery penetrating the bowel wall** through the neck or the apex of a diverticulum and become eroded. Although most diverticula in the colon are left-sided, right-sided colonic diverticula are more apt to bleed (Fig. 8-33).

◆ What are vascular ectasias?

◆ Vascular ectasias, or **arteriovenous malformations**, are thought to arise from the degeneration of intestinal submucosal veins and overlying mucosal capillaries. As the disease progress, communications between submucosal arteries and veins form. When the mucosa erodes or becomes disrupted for some reason, massive lower GI bleeding may result.

Case 8.35 Persistent Bleeding with a Massive Lower Gastrointestinal Bleed

You admit a 68-year-old woman with bright red bleeding per rectum. The presumptive diagnosis is bleeding from a colonic diverticulum or vascular ectasia. After resuscitation and 2 units of blood, she stabilizes. Initial evaluation reveals no evidence of an upper GI bleed, no hemorrhoids, and no evidence of a coagulopathy. You plan to further evaluate the patient the next day if she remains stable. That evening, her hematocrit is 35% after transfusion.

The next morning, she begins to bleed profusely again with bright red blood per rectum. Her heart rate has also risen to 130 beats per minute, and her BP is 100/60 mm Hg. A repeat hematocrit is 24%. You again resuscitate her and administer 2 more units of packed RBCs. Although you had planned to perform a colonoscopy, it has not yet taken place.

◆ **What is the overall management plan at this point?**

◇ The patient's **rebleeding is significant** because of her **cardiovascular instability** and a very **low hematocrit despite previous transfusion**. Medical management has failed, and surgery to stop the bleeding will most likely be necessary. Colonoscopy during active bleeding is unlikely to demonstrate the bleeding cause and is associated with a significant risk of perforation due to poor visibility of the colon.

◆ **What evaluation is appropriate at this point?**

◇ Determination of the site of bleeding is essential.

 QUICK CUT With rebleeding, the options for diagnosing the cause of the GI bleed include technetium-labeled RBC scan or mesenteric angiography.

The choice between these two procedures depends on the current rate of bleeding, the instability of the patient, and the surgeon's preference.

- **Angiography** is probably better **for less stable patients** because of better monitoring and resuscitation capability in the angiography suite as well as **for those who are bleeding at a more rapid rate**. It can isolate a lesion bleeding at a rate of 0.5–1.0 mL/min or more.
- **Technetium-labeled RBC scanning** is better for **more stable patients** who are **bleeding more slowly**. It can detect bleeding at a rate of 0.1 mL/min or more. One limitation of RBC scanning is that it cannot precisely localize the site of the bleeding, making the results difficult to interpret. However, some physicians recommend always obtaining an RBC scan before an angiogram (Fig. 8-34).

An angiogram demonstrates an active bleed in the lower sigmoid area and no evidence of vascular ectasia elsewhere in the colon.

◆ **What is the management plan?**

◇ The patient has clear evidence of **continued bleeding**, has proven **cardiovascular instability**, and has now received **4 units of packed RBCs**. At no single specific point is surgery indicated, but each of these conditions is a relative indication for surgery, and the combination is certainly an indication. Many surgeons would explore most patients with lower GI bleeds once they had required **4–6 units of blood**; experience dictates that patients who have bled that much are likely to continue to bleed. A large amount of transfusion carries its own set of risks, such as transfusion reaction, coagulopathy, and infection.

   Most surgeons would take this patient **urgently to the operating room**. In fact, most surgeons would say that the decision to proceed with an angiogram included a decision to perform surgery (i.e., **the angiogram is a preoperative test**). It is critical to identify the probable bleeding site prior to proceeding to the operating room. Otherwise, the surgeon does not know which portion of the colon to remove.

You have decided that operative intervention is necessary.

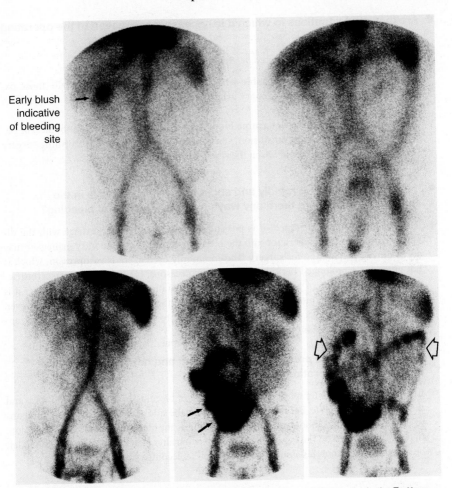

Early blush indicative of bleeding site

Figure 8-34: Red blood cell scan showing hemorrhage at the area of diverticulosis. **Bottom center:** Accumulation of blood (small arrows) in a presumed bleeding site. Blood traveling distally in the colonic lumen (large arrows).

◆ **What operation is appropriate?**

◆ Before induction of anesthesia takes place, it is necessary to be certain that resuscitation is **adequate** and the hematocrit is acceptable. Based on the location, either a **left or right hemicolectomy** to remove the bleeding source is appropriate; this is a **preoperative decision**. It is not recommended that a surgeon tries to be too precise and removes only the site of bleeding, such as a diverticulum or a particular segment of bowel; this is associated with a high rebleeding rate. It is still necessary to explore the abdomen to be certain that there is no other significant pathology. Then the planned colectomy takes place. Because of the cathartic effect of blood in the colon, most patients with massive lower GI bleeds have a sufficiently clean colon to allow performance of a **primary anastomosis**. When patients are unstable or severely malnourished, and primary anastomoses are less likely to heal, colostomy is a safer option.

◆ **Are there any situations in which it is necessary to proceed to the operating room sooner?**

◆ Certain patients should be explored *before* they require 4–6 units of blood.

- Patients who become **unstable with the bleeding** (perhaps), especially those patients with significant coronary artery disease and angina who have instability in vital signs
- Patients with **hard to determine blood types**, including unusual antibodies, or patients who desire no transfusion, such as **Jehovah's Witnesses**. Performing surgery at an earlier time would lessen the risk associated with hemorrhage.

◆ **If a patient is bleeding rapidly and subsequently hypotensive in the angiography suite, are there any ways to lessen the rate of bleeding?**

◆ If the bleeding site is identified, it is possible to control active hemorrhage with the direct infusion of a vasoconstrictor into the bleeding vessel. This temporary maneuver may occur during preparation for surgery. The commonly used agent is **vasopressin**, which is not given for a prolonged period of time for two reasons: (1) its coronary vasoconstrictor effect, and (2) 50% of patients have a recurrence of bleeding within 12 hours after it is discontinued. Another means of treatment during angiography is **embolization**. However, there is an increased risk of transmural intestinal necrosis in the large bowel, so this approach may be reserved for poor surgical candidates.

◆ **Why not bypass the preoperative angiogram and determine the site of bleeding in the operating room?**

◆ It is **very difficult** to attempt to determine the site of bleeding in the operating room, and the results are **unreliable**. Because they do not know the side of the bleeding, many surgeons would perform a total abdominal colectomy as long as the bleeding is localized to the colon. In part, this is based on the experience that rebleeding after lesser procedures (i.e., blind left or right hemicolectomy) is associated with a high rebleeding rate and high mortality.

OTHER BENIGN LOWER GASTROINTESTINAL TRACT DISORDERS

| Case 8.36 | **Syndromes of Acute Colonic Dilation and Obstruction** |

An 88-year-old woman who is receiving long-term care in a nursing home is brought to the emergency department with a history of constipation and a recent deterioration in mental status. Her BP is 100/60 mm Hg, with a heart rate of 120 beats per minute. She has abdominal distention and moans when you examine her abdomen. Rectal examination reveals no stool.

◆ **How would you evaluate this patient?**

◆ Hydration is necessary. Electrolytes, a CBC, and an abdominal obstructive radiographic series to rule out obstruction or other abdominal pathology are also warranted.

◆ How would you evaluate the following radiologic findings?

Case Variation 8.36.1. Sigmoid volvulus

◆ A sigmoid volvulus occurs most commonly in debilitated patients from nursing homes, often as a result of chronic laxative use, chronic illness, or dementia. Sigmoid volvulus develops from a clockwise twist of mobile sigmoid colon around the mesentery, leading to a closed loop obstruction. A barium enema confirms the volvulus.

> **QUICK CUT** In stable patients with no peritonitis or signs of sepsis, it is often possible to "detorse" the sigmoid colon by rigid proctosigmoidoscopy and placement of a rectal tube.

Definitive therapy is usually planned during the same hospital stay. The treatment is **either sigmoid colectomy** with diverting colostomy or resection with primary anastomosis, depending on the preoperative condition of the patient (Fig. 8-35). If endoscopic management is unsuccessful, urgent laparotomy is required. The recurrence rate is approximately 30%.

Case Variation 8.36.2. Cecal volvulus

◆ Most patients with **cecal volvulus require urgent surgical treatment (Fig. 8-36).** Attempts at detorsion with a barium enema or colonoscopy are usually not successful. Surgical options include detorsion alone, cecopexy, or right colectomy. In stable patients with viable bowel, the operation of choice is right colectomy with primary anastomosis.

Case Variation 8.36.3. Massively dilated right colon to the level of the midtransverse colon with distal colonic decompression

◆ **Acute pseudo-obstruction, or Ogilvie syndrome,** is defined **as acute massive dilation of the cecum and right colon without evidence of mechanical obstruction.** This commonly occurs in hospitalized patients in the intensive care unit who are intubated and seriously ill.

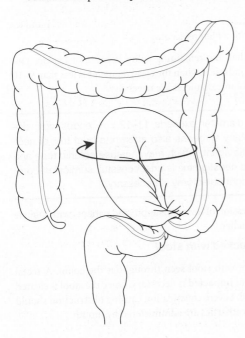

Figure 8-35: Detorsion of volvulus, which requires treatment with insertion of a rectal tube followed by elective sigmoid colectomy.

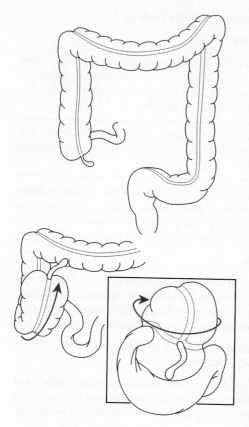

Figure 8-36: Types of torsion with cecal volvulus.

The cecum preferentially dilates more than the remaining colon because of Laplace law. Conservative, nonoperative treatment is indicated when the cecal diameter is less than 9–10 cm. Serial radiographic films to follow colonic diameter are necessary.

 QUICK CUT If the colon diameter exceeds 11–12 cm, endoscopic decompression is indicated. Many surgeons also attempt a brief trial of neostigmine, a parasympatholytic agent, which may increase colonic tone and counteract the dilation. If the neostigmine is unsuccessful, surgical decompression of the cecum or a right colectomy is necessary.

Many surgeons would perform decompression of immunosuppressed patients with Ogilvie syndrome when the colon diameter is smaller.

Case Variation 8.36.4. *Entire colon packed with stool*

◆ This finding is indicative of constipation, with stool seen throughout the colon. A rectal examination to **ensure that the stool is not impacted** is necessary. Once the stool is cleared from the vault, enemas may be performed. Severe constipation causing obstruction should always be treated from below before any cathartics are administered by mouth.

Case 8.37 Rectal Prolapse

A 65-year-old woman presents with anorectal discomfort. She says that she has trouble initiating defecation. In addition, she feels a protrusion from her rectum when she is finished moving her bowels. On examination, a patulous anus and a rectal prolapse are evident.

◆ **What management is appropriate?**

◆ Rectal prolapse, which may occur during defecation, has an unknown cause but may be related to neuromuscular deficiencies and decreased rectal sensation, particularly in the elderly (Fig. 8-37). Most patients have a patulous anus and weakened external sphincters. Numerous operations are appropriate for the management of rectal prolapse. If the prolapse is entirely internal, treatment with a high-fiber diet to normalize bowel function is warranted, and it may be possible to avoid surgery. However, **if the prolapse is external and resulting in rectal bleeding** and no other causes of lower GI bleeding are discovered, surgery may be necessary. Many operative strategies are appropriate for rectal prolapse.

- **Rectopexy**, in which the rectum is fixed to the sacrum without removing a portion of the rectum
- A low anterior resection, which removes the upper and middle portions of the rectum, along with the redundant sigmoid colon (**transabdominal rectosigmoid resection**)
- A perineal approach, which removes the prolapsed rectum and sigmoid colon with the proximal sigmoid colon anastomosed to the transitional zone 1–2 cm above the dentate line

Case 8.38 Perianal Problems

A 30-year-old man presents with rectal pain that is particularly severe during defecation. On examination, you note an ulcerated area in the anal canal that is very painful when touched.

◆ **What management is appropriate?**

◆ Anal fissures involve tears in the anoderm, which is reputedly caused by trauma from passage of hard stools but can also result from other diseases such as IBD. They are associated with pain during bowel movements and tenderness on palpation. Blood is usually found on the toilet tissue after wiping. Anal fissures are almost always located in the posterior midline. A sentinel tag may be seen at the anal verge.

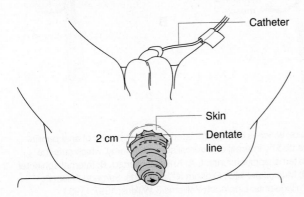

Catheter

Skin

2 cm

Dentate line

Figure 8-37: Rectal prolapse. (From Greenfield LJ, Mulholland MW, Oldham KT, et al, eds. *Surgery: Scientific Principles and Practice*, 2nd ed. Philadelphia: Lippincott Williams & Wilkins; 1997:1194.)

◆ What management is appropriate?

◆ Most anal fissures respond to **conservative treatment**, including bulk agents, stool softeners, and sitz baths. If the fissure is **deep and chronic**, lateral **sphincterotomy**, which divides a portion of the internal anal sphincter, may be necessary (Fig. 8-38). The hypothesis that reflex stimulation and spasm of the internal anal sphincter is important in pathogenesis is the basis for this procedure. More than 90% of anal fissures heal after lateral sphincterotomy. **Biopsy of suspicious, chronic fissures** to rule out anal cancer is warranted.

A patient presents with a history of **persistent perianal drainage**. On examination, a sinus tract with granulation tissue is apparent.

◆ What is the most likely diagnosis?

◆ This patient most likely has a **fistula-in-ano**, which is the residua of a previous abscess that failed to completely heal (Fig. 8-39). Instead, a chronic tract formed with an internal connection to an anal crypt and an external connection to the perianal skin.

◆ What management is appropriate?

◆ Treatment involves **unroofing** the tract, **draining** any undrained collection, and **allowing the tract to re-epithelialize**. If the tract traverses the anal sphincter, a seton or string should be placed within the tract and allowed to traverse the sphincter without making the patient incontinent.

A patient presents with severe anal pain, a tender fluctuant perianal mass, and fever.

◆ What is the likely diagnosis and appropriate management?

◆ The most likely diagnosis is **perianal abscess**, which results from an infection that occurs in anal crypts and glands that are present at the dentate line. There are four basic types

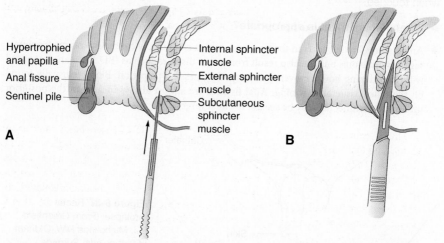

Figure 8-38: Location of anal fissure, which is often associated with hypertrophy of anal papilla and a sentinel pile. This may be treated by internal or external sphincterotomy, which cuts the internal sphincter but leaves the external sphincter intact. **A:** Knife is inserted. **B:** Internal sphincter is transected. (From Greenfield LJ, Mulholland MW, Oldham KT, et al, eds. *Surgery: Scientific Principles and Practice*, 2nd ed. Philadelphia: Lippincott Williams & Wilkins; 1997:1198.)

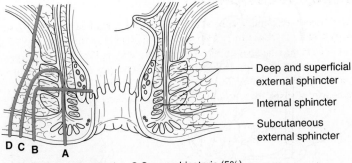

A Intersphincteric (75%)   C Suprasphincteric (5%)
B Trans-sphincteric (20%)   D Extrasphincteric (<1%)

Figure 8-39: Typical fistula-in-ano. (From McKenney MG, Mangonon PC, Moylan JA, eds. *Understanding Surgical Disease: The Miami Manual of Surgery*. Philadelphia: Lippincott-Raven; 1998:162.)

of abscess: perianal, ischioanal, intersphincteric, and supralevator. Treatment of the first two types requires drainage through a perianal incision. An intersphincteric abscess, which causes pain within the anal canal, may require drainage within the anal canal. The supralevator, a higher, more complex abscess may arise from the perianal area or higher within the abdomen; the decision regarding the site of drainage depends on its location and origin. **The primary treatment is drainage, not antibiotics.**

A patient complains of pain and drainage in his **sacrococcygeal area** of the lower back. You examine him and find an abscess in that location.

◆ **What management is appropriate?**

◆ This condition is a **pilonidal abscess**, which is an infection in a hair-containing sinus in the sacrococcygeal area. Treatment involves **unroofing** the abscess, removing all hair, and leaving the wound open to heal by secondary intention.

Case 8.39 Colostomies

A 58-year-old man is having a stoma created in the operating room the next day.

◆ **What preparation is necessary?**

◆ The patient should meet with the physician and enterostomal therapist to be educated about stomas and their care. The most common complication related to a stoma is leakage around the appliance (bag) and patient dissatisfaction due to a poor location of the stoma on the abdominal wall. A stoma should be placed where it can be cared for conveniently and not in a skin fold where leakage could occur. It is best to determine this position preoperatively, with the patient in a sitting position. Other postoperative complications include parastomal herniation, bowel obstruction abscess, and fistula formation.

Your resident asks you to describe the different types of stomas.

◆ **How would you respond?**

◆ Stomas are artificially created openings between the intestine or urinary tract and the abdominal wall. Stomas may be temporary or permanent. Most temporary stomas are created to divert

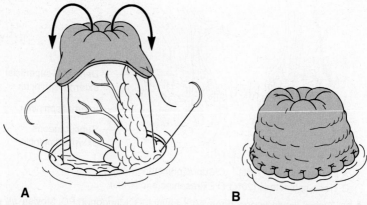

Figure 8-40: Performance of ileostomy. **A.** ileum being sewn to the skin. **B.** After completion of the ileostomy (From Greenfield LJ, Mulholland MW, Oldham KT, et al, eds. *Surgery: Scientific Principles and Practice*, 2nd ed. Philadelphia: Lippincott Williams & Wilkins; 1997:1100.)

the fecal stream while either healing of an anastomosis occurs or an inflammatory process related to GI leakage subsides. Pairs of end stomas that act as single openings ("double barrel" stomas) or loops that are brought up onto the abdominal wall and opened are temporary stomas. Loop stomas are not totally diverting and must be separated like "double barrel" stomas for complete diversion. Distal bowel stomas are termed mucous fistulas because their only contents are mucosal-derived mucus and no stool. If the distal bowel is closed and not brought to the abdominal wall but rather dropped back into the pelvis, it is termed a Hartmann pouch. This is commonly done for sigmoid resections for diverticulitis when the bowel cannot be safely reconnected. Loop stomas, cecostomies, and tube cecostomies can also be performed to decompress a distended segment of bowel temporarily such as in Ogilvie syndrome (Fig. 8-40).

◆ Permanent stomas are most commonly used in the following situations (presented in order of decreasing frequency):

- Following an abdominoperineal resection in which an end sigmoid colostomy is created
- An ileostomy following total proctocolectomy for ulcerative colitis. (However, many patients who previously underwent reconstruction with a continent ileostomy are now having ileoanal pull-through procedures. Typically, the surgeon creates a pouch or a reservoir and anastomoses it to the anus.)
- An ileal conduit draining the urinary system to the skin

Ileostomies and ileal conduits can be constructed in a fashion to make patients continent. After creation of a nipple valve, catheter insertion and drainage is periodically necessary.

Because the output from ileostomies is particularly irritating to the skin, ileostomies are designed to result in continence or protrude from the skin so that their output drops directly into the appliance (in the same manner as a spigot). Carefully applied appliances are critical to the success of ileostomies.

Both continent ileostomies and ileoanal pouches are susceptible to "pouchitis," an inflammatory process in the pouch hypothesized to be secondary to some form of bacterial overgrowth. Patients feel weak, have fever, and may have abdominal or pelvic pain and malodorous stool. Symptoms usually resolve with a course of metronidazole.

Chapter 9

Endocrine Disorders

Bruce E. Jarrell, W. Bradford Carter, Eric Strauch

Key Thoughts

1. Thyroid nodule: first steps are good history, exam for nodes and vocal cord function, fine-needle aspiration (FNA), and neck ultrasound (US).

2. Papillary carcinoma is the most common thyroid cancer and has a high cure rate.

3. Papillary and medullary carcinomas are multicentric, spread to regional lymph nodes, and are treated with total thyroidectomy.

4. Follicular thyroid carcinoma spreads through vessels, is associated with systemic metastasis, and can be treated with either a total thyroidectomy or lobectomy and isthmusectomy. Follicular carcinoma also has a high cure rate.

5. Primary hyperparathyroidism is due to adenoma and should be treated for symptomatic patients and for asymptomatic patients with a serum calcium greater than 11.5 mg/dL.

6. Secondary hyperparathyroidism is associated with renal failure, is due to hyperplasia, and is associated with low serum calcium.

7. Incidentally found adrenal masses should be observed if they are nonfunctional and less than 4 cm in size.

Case 9.1   Thyroid Nodule Found on Examination

A 29-year-old woman presents for evaluation of a thyroid nodule that her primary care physician noted on a routine examination. She is otherwise healthy. Her only significant history is two previous normal pregnancies. On physical examination, all systems appear normal except the neck. An **isolated 1-cm firm nodule** is present in the right lobe of the thyroid gland that moves when the patient swallows.

◆ **How does a patient's history and physical examination influence your evaluation?**

◆ Your greatest concern is that this nodule represents thyroid cancer, so it is important to obtain information regarding risk factors for thyroid cancer, including radiation history, family history, voice and airway, symptoms, and thyroid nodule pattern. A past history (10–25 years) of **low-dose ionizing radiation** (<2,000 rad) to the neck carries a 40% risk of thyroid cancer; the most common cancer following radiation is papillary carcinoma. Radioactive iodine ablation has not been associated with increased incidence of thyroid cancer.

◆ A **family history** of thyroid cancer is significant. Medullary thyroid cancer is inherited as an autosomal dominant trait, and testing for the existence of a point mutation of the *RET* gene in a family can establish a diagnosis. In a suspicious lesion, examination of serum calcitonin may be appropriate. Elevated values are highly suggestive of medullary carcinoma, and screening for the RET mutation is then warranted. Positive results suggest multiple endocrine neoplasia (MEN). Evaluation of affected patients for pheochromocytoma, adrenal medullary hyperplasia, and hyperparathyroidism is necessary before surgery.

> **QUICK CUT** A history of hoarseness as well as the presence of a hard, fixed nodule; dyspnea; dysphagia; cervical lymph node enlargement; and vocal cord paralysis suggest malignancy.

You perform a complete history and physical examination and find that the woman has no risk factors for thyroid cancer. On examination, the nodule is solitary and not hard or fixed. The vocal cords move normally.

◆ **What is the next step in evaluation?**

◆ Most surgeons would perform an **FNA** of the lesion (Fig. 9-1). This involves local anesthesia, aspiration of the mass using a syringe and 21–25-gauge needle, and sending the aspirate for cytology. A US of the thyroid may be performed to scan for additional, suspicious nodules and to evaluate the nodule for suspicious features. If the nodule is complex (cystic and has solid components), FNA should be performed with US guidance to biopsy the solid component.

> **QUICK CUT** FNA poses little risk and can firmly establish a diagnosis in a majority of cases.

◆ Approximately two thirds of aspirates demonstrate benign processes. Of the remaining aspirates, approximately one half demonstrate malignant cells, and one-half are indeterminate. A **cyst** necessitates complete aspiration and follow-up. If it is **large (>4 cm)** or **recurs** several times following aspiration, or if the aspirate is hemorrhagic, **removal** to eliminate the risk of malignancy (up to 15% in large cysts) is required.

FNA has become the standard of care for diagnosing thyroid nodules. Other methods of evaluation are no longer as useful. In general, **scanning** the thyroid with radioactive iodine is generally **not appropriate** in the initial evaluation of solitary thyroid nodules. "Cold" nodules have a 15% chance of being malignant, whereas "hot" nodules are rarely cancerous. **US** is sensitive for evaluating the quality of nodules and criteria for FNA; scanning for additional, suspicious, nonpalpable nodules; and discriminating cysts from nodules. US is generally **used to follow the size** or recurrence of cysts following FNA or nodular progression. US-guided FNA of suspicious thyroid nodules improves yield, with fewer nondiagnostic FNA biopsies. Thyroid function tests are also generally not necessary for evaluation of thyroid nodules unless there are symptoms of hyperthyroidism or hypothyroidism. Elevated thyroid-stimulating hormone (TSH) may be a driver of nodular development. Once a benign diagnosis is established, TSH may be monitored as part of thyroid suppression therapy with thyroxine.

You perform FNA of the nodule.

◆ **What measures would you recommend for each of the various cytology results?**

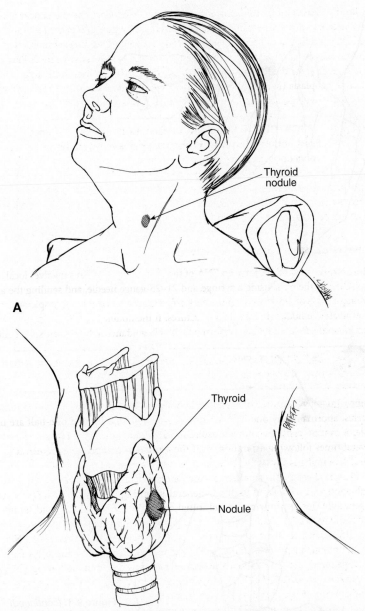

A

B

Figure 9-1: Technique of fine-needle aspiration shown in four steps. **A.** palpable thyroid nodule. **B.** Nodule location within the thyroid gland. (*continued*)

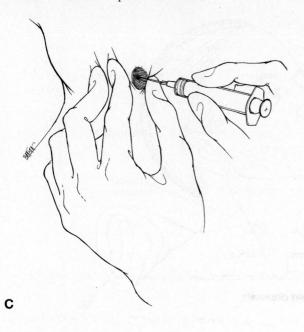

C

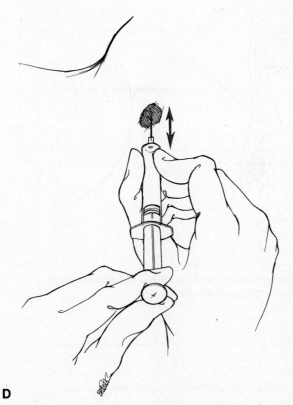

D

Figure 9-1: *(continued)*
C. Stabilization of the thyroid
nodule with one hand while the
needle is placed into the nodule
with the other hand. **D.** Aspiration
of the thyroid nodule. (From Chen
H, Sonnenday CJ, Lillemoe KD,
eds. *Manual of Common Bedside
Surgical Procedures*, 2nd ed.
Philadelphia: Lippincott Williams
& Wilkins; 2000:305–308.)

Case Variation 9.1.1. Colloid nodule

◆ This is a benign result, and there is no need for surgery to eliminate the risk of malignancy. Medical management with thyroid hormone supplementation as needed for elevated TSH and follow-up with intermittent US for nodule progression are sufficient. Surgery would be necessary only if the nodule changes significantly or for compressive symptoms or tracheal deviation.

Case Variation 9.1.2. Papillary carcinoma

◆ This is a malignant condition, and surgery is appropriate. A total thyroidectomy is generally performed due to a significant rate of multicentric disease.

Case Variation 9.1.3. Medullary carcinoma

◆ This is a highly malignant tumor, and surgery is recommended. A total thyroidectomy is performed due to a significant rate of multicentric disease. Medullary thyroid cancer spreads early to regional lymph nodes, so central lymph node dissection and careful evaluation of lateral lymph node basins is essential at the time of surgery.

Case Variation 9.1.4. Psammoma bodies

◆ These structures are a marker for papillary cancer, and a thyroidectomy is recommended.

Case Variation 9.1.5. Amyloid deposits

◆ This substance and calcitonin staining suggest medullary cancer, and a total thyroidectomy is mandatory.

Case Variation 9.1.6. Undifferentiated cells

◆ This finding indicates an anaplastic cancer, and either chemotherapy and radiation or salvage operative therapy is appropriate.

Case Variation 9.1.7. Hürthle cells

◆ The presence of sheets of Hürthle cells signifies either an adenoma or a low-grade cancer. Therefore, lobectomy is indicated. If cancer is present, a total thyroidectomy is indicated.

Case Variation 9.1.8. Follicular cells

◆ The diagnosis of follicular adenoma versus carcinoma is based on the presence or absence of capsular or vascular invasion, so a thyroid lobectomy is usually performed for diagnostic purposes.

Case Variation 9.1.9. Lymphocytic infiltrate

◆ This suggests lymphoma or chronic lymphocytic thyroiditis, which can be differentiated by flow cytometry. Lymphomas are radiosensitive, so radiation is appropriate. Thyroiditis requires no surgery and may require thyroid hormone replacement.

Results of the FNA indicate that a **malignant tumor is present,** and you decide to proceed with surgery.

◆ **You should advise your patient about what risks of surgery?**

   ◆ Any surgical procedure involves the basic risks of bleeding and infection.

 QUICK CUT Serious complications of thyroid surgery include injury to the recurrent laryngeal or the external branch of the superior laryngeal nerve as well as devascularization of all four parathyroid glands with resultant hypocalcemia.

◆ With a total thyroidectomy, the risk of injury to these nerves (0.5%–5.0%) is increased due to the bilateral dissections. A unilateral recurrent laryngeal nerve injury results in hoarseness due to vocal cord paralysis; a bilateral nerve injury causes bilateral cord paralysis and airway compromise and may require tracheostomy; and an external branch of the superior laryngeal nerve injury alters the high-pitched singing voice. Resection of the thyroid places the parathyroid glands at risk, with subsequent hypoparathyroidism, causing **hypocalcemia** and hyperphosphatemia if all four parathyroid glands are injured (Fig. 9-2).

The FNA returns with a diagnosis that requires surgery. You are now in the operating room ready to explore the patient's neck.

◆ **What decisions need to be made in the operating room regarding each of the following cancers?**

Case Variation 9.1.10. Papillary cancer

◆ The peak incidence of papillary cancer, the **most common type of thyroid cancer**, is 30–40 years. Approximately 5% of patients present with distant spread at the time of diagnosis. Patients with lesions 1 cm or less are divided into two groups: one, patients with **previous head and neck radiation**, who should undergo a **total thyroidectomy**; and two, those patients who have **not had radiation**, who can undergo a limited **thyroid lobectomy**

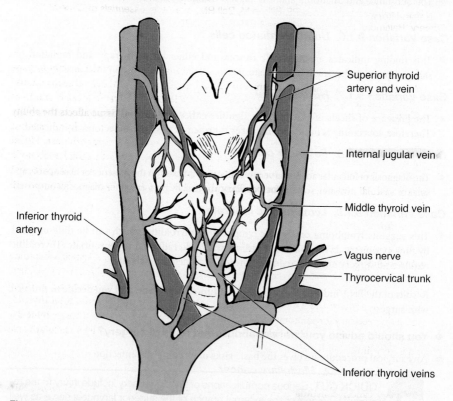

Figure 9-2: Blood supply of the thyroid. (From Jarrell BE, Carabasi RA III, Radomski JS. *NMS Surgery*, 4th ed. Philadelphia: Lippincott Williams & Wilkins; 2000:322.)

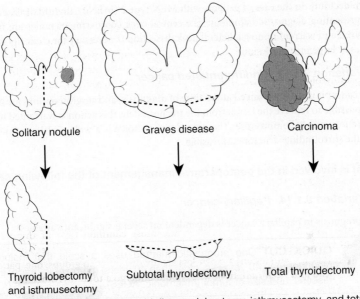

Solitary nodule   Graves disease   Carcinoma

Thyroid lobectomy and isthmusectomy   Subtotal thyroidectomy   Total thyroidectomy

Figure 9-3: Surgical resections in thyroid disease: lobectomy, isthmusectomy, and total thyroidectomy. (From Lawrence PF, Bilbao M, Bell RM, et al, eds. *Essentials of General Surgery*. Baltimore: Lippincott Williams & Wilkins; 1988:281.)

and isthmusectomy (Fig. 9-3). Due to the increased incidence of multicentricity in papillary cancer, some physicians recommend a total thyroidectomy. Many surgeons choose total thyroidectomy because it allows for the use of radioactive iodine to localize and treat local disease or distant metastases. The presence of normal thyroid tissue affects the ability for radioactive iodine to localize in the residual cancer. Further, after total thyroidectomy, thyroglobulin can be used as a tumor marker for persistent or recurrent disease. Nodal excision via a central compartment lymph node dissection or compartmental lymph node dissection should be performed for clinically positive lymph nodes. Central compartment lymph node dissection is done for papillary thyroid cancer, as up to 60% of patients will have subclinical metastases.

Case Variation 9.1.11. *Follicular cancer*

◆ Follicular cancers, which represent 15%–20% of thyroid cancers, are more prevalent in iodine-deficient areas. Peak incidence occurs about 40–50 years of age. Formal **lobectomy and isthmusectomy** is appropriate for excision of a well-circumscribed lesion that is identified as a follicular neoplasm by FNA. No additional surgery is necessary for a tumor described as a **microinvasive follicular carcinoma** (see Fig. 9-3). However, **total thyroidectomy** is necessary for microinvasive lesions greater than 4 cm or for an invasive follicular cancer greater than 1 cm. Follicular cancer has a propensity to spread by a vascular route and is very limited in lymphatic spread.

Case Variation 9.1.12. *Medullary cancer*

◆ Medullary cancer constitutes 5%–10% of all thyroid cancers. There are two forms: **80% are sporadic**, and **20% are familial** (MEN). Histologically, these tumors feature hyperplasia of C cells (parafollicular) with amyloid. Management of these tumors is based on total thyroidectomy. In the case of patients with MEN type 2 (MEN2), thyroid disease is usually the presenting diagnostic pathology. The central neck compartment nodes are frequently involved and warrant removal. Lateral neck dissection is necessary for clinically suspicious nodes or large primary lesions.

Case Variation 9.1.13. Undifferentiated cancer

◆ This cancer is usually **advanced at the time of diagnosis,** and surgical options are limited. If it is possible to remove the lesion from the trachea safely, this action is warranted to prevent future respiratory compromise. The procedure of choice is a wide excision of the thyroid and the surrounding structures, if feasible.

◆ **What is involved in the postoperative management of the following cancers?**

Case Variation 9.1.14. Papillary cancer

◆ The prognosis in papillary cancer is dependent on several significant variables.

 QUICK CUT One prognostic method uses a scale that includes age (younger than 40 years vs. older than 40 years), pathologic grade, extent of disease, and size of tumor (mnemonic: AGES).

◆ Thus, low-risk patients are young and have a well-differentiated tumor with no metastasis. Another method involves the **MACIS** scale (distant metastases, age at presentation, completeness of resection, extrathyroidal invasion, and size of mass), which considers two additional factors. **Survival in low-risk patients** is as high as **100% at 10 years,** whereas **survival in high-risk patients** is as low as **20% at 10 years.** There is an ongoing debate concerning the use of lobectomy versus total thyroidectomy based on risk stratification using the "AGES" and "MACIS" scales.

Postoperative management also usually includes TSH **suppression with thyroid hormone** and possibly **iodine-131 (^{131}I) ablation** based on risk assessment. Thyroglobulin levels (a protein only made by thyroid cells) can be used as a tumor marker for persistent or recurrent disease. Rising thyroglobulin levels warrant a search for residual disease by US or iodine scanning. Regional lymph node dissection is performed for progressive or symptomatic disease.

Case Variation 9.1.15. Follicular cancer

◆ Many of the prognostic factors in follicular cancer are similar to those in papillary cancer. In addition, the presence of **vascular invasion worsens the prognosis. Survival** is approximately **80% for favorable lesions and 60% for unfavorable lesions at 10 years.** Postoperative adjuvant therapy centers on ^{131}I ablation treatment. Ablation of the residual thyroid also allows successful monitoring for recurrent thyroid cancer, using thyroglobulin as a tumor marker.

Case Variation 9.1.16. Medullary cancer

◆ **Treatment with ^{131}I and thyroid suppression postoperatively are not useful** because the tumor arises from C cells. Some centers use external irradiation postoperatively for advanced cases, although the benefit of this therapy is unproven. Prognosis is related to the extent of disease, with an overall **survival of 80% at 10 years but less than 45% with lymph node involvement.** Patients may be monitored by measuring **serum calcitonin and carcinoembryonic antigen (CEA) levels.**

Case Variation 9.1.17. **Undifferentiated cancer**

◆ Anaplastic cancer, which constitutes only 5% of all thyroid cancers, has a peak incidence in the seventh decade. Tumors are usually large, with 50% presenting with positive nodes. Approximately 30% of patients present with distant metastasis. The lung has been the most common site of distal metastasis. The **prognosis is extremely poor.** However, **multimodality therapy** with pre- and postoperative chemotherapy and radiation treatment are typically used.

Case 9.2   Symptomatic Hypercalcemia

A 75-year-old woman presents to your office after routine laboratory tests demonstrate **a calcium level of 14 mg/dL.** A plain radiograph of the patient's hand demonstrated bone reabsorption **(osteitis fibrosa cystica).** She also complains of generalized **fatigue.**

◆ **What additional laboratory tests do you wish to order?**

◆ In the process of the evaluation of symptomatic hypercalcemia, it is necessary to measure parathyroid hormone (PTH) levels, as well as serum alkaline phosphatase and phosphate levels.

◆ **Does the woman have hyperparathyroidism?**

◆ The presence of hypercalcemia and elevated plasma PTH is diagnostic for hyperparathyroidism (Fig. 9-4). If the PTH and calcium levels are elevated, additional testing with a 24-hour urine collection for calcium excretion is necessary to rule out familial hypocalciuric hypercalcemia (FHH). Hypercalcemia and elevated PTH with normal or elevated calcium excretion over 24 hours suggest the diagnosis of **primary hyperparathyroidism** (Table 9-1).

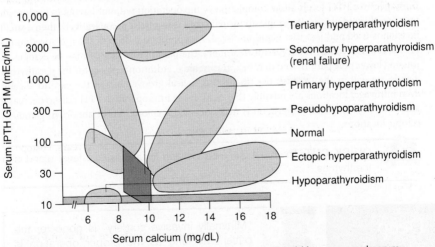

Figure 9-4: Relation between serum immunoreactive parathyroid hormone and serum calcium in patients with hypoparathyroidism; pseudohypoparathyroidism; ectopic hyperparathyroidism; and primary, secondary, and tertiary hyperparathyroidism. GP1M, guinea pig antiserum 1M. (From Greenfield LJ, Mulholland MW, Lillemoe KD, et al, eds. *Greenfield's Surgery*, 5th ed. Philadelphia: Lippincott Williams & Wilkins; 2010.)

Table 9-1: Common Presenting Symptoms of Hyperparathyroidism

Symptom	Frequency
Muscle weakness	2/3
Myalgia	1/2
Arthralgia	1/2
Nephrolithiasis	1/3
Constipation	1/3
Polyuria	1/3
Psychiatric disorders	1/7
Peptic ulcer disease	1/8

◆ **What is the most likely pathologic cause of the hyperparathyroidism?**

 QUICK CUT Parathyroid adenomas are the most common lesions leading to primary hyperparathyroidism.

◆ Parathyroid **carcinoma is present in less than 2% of cases.**

You measure her PTH and plot it on Figure 9-4 and find that she has primary hyperparathyroidism.

◆ **What is your plan at this point?**

◆ Surgical correction is the appropriate therapy. The most common studies are technetium-99m sestamibi scintography (Fig. 9-5) and US to help localize the abnormal gland or glands. Intraoperative PTH levels allow completion of the operation without having to explore all four parathyroid glands. If a single abnormal gland is localized preoperatively, then a small incision is used and just that gland removed. An appropriate drop of the measured intraoperative PTH confirms successful treatment. The parathyroid glands may be ectopic. A missing lower pole parathyroid may be intrathyroidal. Additional places for the parathyroid glands are within the thymus, the tracheoesophageal groove, and in the carotid sheath; even intravagal locations are possible (Fig. 9-6). If the intraoperative PTH fails to decrease, a traditional four-gland exploration is necessary with exploration for abnormal glands in ectopic locations.

 QUICK CUT The most common location for a missing inferior gland is in the thymus.

 Deep Thoughts "Minimally invasive surgery" is good for the patient as long as the proper operation is performed.

Persistent calcium elevation has occurred postoperatively.

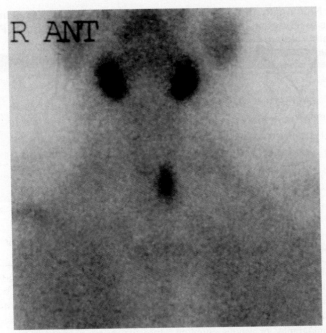

Figure 9-5: An example of a sestamibi scan, which demonstrates the parathyroid glands and helps visualize adenomas. The upper hot spots are the submaxillary salivary glands and the lower hot spot is a parathyroid adenoma.

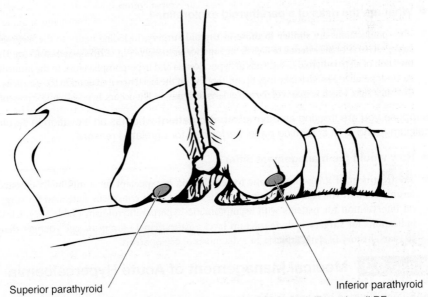

Superior parathyroid   Inferior parathyroid

Figure 9-6: Normal locations of the parathyroid glands, lateral view. (From Jarrell BE, Carabasi RA III, Radomski JS. *NMS Surgery*, 4th ed. Philadelphia: Lippincott Williams & Wilkins; 2000:323.)

Table 9-2: National Institutes of Health Consensus Development Conference's Indications for Surgical Intervention in Patients with Asymptomatic Primary Hyperparathyroidism

Indications/Contraindications
Markedly elevated serum calcium (>1.0 mg/dL above normal)
History of an episode of life-threatening hypercalcemia
Reduced creatinine clearance
Presence of one or more kidney stones detected by abdominal radiography
Markedly elevated 24-hr urinary calcium excretion
Substantially reduced bone mass as determined by direct measurement (dual-energy x-ray absorptiometry *T* score <−2.5)

From Greenfield LJ, Mulholland MW, Lillemoe KD, et al, eds. *Greenfield's Surgery*, 5th ed. Philadelphia: Lippincott Williams & Wilkins; 2010.

◆ **How would you manage this situation?**

◆ This patient has **persistent hyperparathyroidism**. First, the diagnosis of primary hyperparathyroidism must be confirmed. Urinary calcium excretion should be measured to confirm that the patient does not have FHH. Repeat technetium-99m sestamibi scintigraphy and US as well as computed tomography (CT), magnetic resonance imaging (MRI), angiography, or venous sampling. Once the "missing" gland has been localized, **re-exploration** through a neck or a lateral direct approach is necessary. In cases where a persistent intrathymic parathyroid is found, a **thymectomy** through a cervical incision or a median sternotomy is warranted. Ectopic supernumerary glands, when present, are found most commonly in the tracheoesophageal groove or mediastinum.

◆ **What are the risks of a parathyroid exploration?**

◆ The complications are **similar to those in thyroid surgery**, including injury to the recurrent laryngeal nerve or the external branch of the superior laryngeal nerve, or hypoparathyroidism. The resection of all parathyroid tissue leads to hypocalcemia and hyperphosphatemia. In the immediate postoperative period, tetany may occur. Tapping on the facial nerve adjacent to the ear elicits a Chvostek sign, which is spasm of the orbicularis oris muscle. If it occurs, hypocalcemia is present.

Suppose you are treating an **asymptomatic patient** who has an elevation in serum calcium found on a screening panel performed for unrelated reasons.

◆ **How would the management differ?**

◆ The treatment of the asymptomatic hypercalcemia is expectant for a minimally elevated serum calcium. The National Institutes of Health put out a consensus statement for surgical intervention for patients with asymptomatic hyperparathyroidism (Table 9-2): Clear indications for surgery include calcium level greater than 11.5 mg/dL, age younger than 40 years, history of renal lithiasis, or a diagnosis of osteoporosis.

Case 9.3   Medical Management of Acute Hypercalcemia

A 45-year-old man presents to the emergency department with nausea, fatigue, and weight loss, as well as drowsiness, abdominal pain, and altered mental status. He has a history of bipolar disorder and kidney stones. His **serum calcium level is 16 mEq/L.**

Table 9-3: Initial Treatment of Acute Hypercalcemia with Symptoms

1. Hydration with normal saline
2. Calcium diuresis with furosemide
3. Initiation of bisphosphonates
4. Treatment of underlying cause

◆ **What is the most likely cause of the man's disorder?**

◆ This patient is suffering from acute hypercalcemia.

 QUICK CUT Parathyroid adenoma is the most common benign cause of hypercalcemia.

Malignancy such as breast carcinoma is a common cause of hypercalcemia. It is a common diagnosis in **women with metastatic breast cancer**. Other causes of hypercalcemia include parathyroid hyperplasia, multiple myeloma, hyperthyroidism, sarcoidosis, milk alkali syndrome, vitamin A intoxication, thiazide diuretics, renal cell carcinoma, squamous cell cancer of the lung (secretes a PTH-like substance), and FHH.

◆ **What acute treatment should this man receive?**

◆ Hypercalcemia results in an osmotic diuresis in the earlier phases of the disease, which leads to a vicious cycle of alternating dehydration and worsening hypercalcemia. Therefore, the initial treatment must be rehydration with normal saline. After the patient is hydrated, furosemide, which leads to a brisk diuresis high in calcium, is necessary. Calcitonin may be used acutely to lower calcium levels. Other agents used to control hypercalcemia on an extended basis are bisphosphonates like zoledronic acid and cinacalcet (Table 9-3).

The man's calcium has returned to a near-normal level after several days of therapy. After you plot his PTH value on a nomogram, you note that it is inappropriately high for the corresponding serum calcium and is compatible with primary hyperparathyroidism.

◆ **What management strategy would you recommend?**

◆ With primary hyperparathyroidism, **neck exploration** and removal of abnormal parathyroid glands is recommended. Most commonly, a single adenoma is present, but **multiple adenomas occur about 5% or more** of the time and should be an object of search. Removal of an adenoma is curative in the vast majority of cases.

Case 9.4 | Secondary Hyperparathyroidism

You receive a consult from the renal service to consider parathyroidectomy in a 34-year-old man who is undergoing dialysis.

◆ **What is the most likely diagnosis?**

◆ Patients with chronic renal failure retain phosphate as their glomerular filtration rate decreases. Hyperphosphatemia causes hypocalcemia, which elevates serum PTH, and this syndrome is termed secondary hyperparathyroidism. Calcium absorption from the gut and vitamin D metabolism are also impaired.

◆ **How do you decide whether surgical management is warranted?**

◈ Medical management is usually appropriate in patients with chronic renal failure and secondary hyperparathyroidism. This includes controlling the hyperphosphatemia with phosphate-binding agents and dietary restriction along with calcium and vitamin D supplementation. Surgical management is indicated when **bone pain, fractures, intractable pruritus, or ectopic calcifications in the soft tissues (calcium tachyphylaxis)** are present.

> **QUICK CUT** The common operative finding in secondary hyperparathyroidism is hyperplasia of all glands.

◆ Excision of all but 50 mg of parathyroid tissue is warranted. This remaining tissue may be left in place or transplanted to a more accessible site such as the forearm. Transplantation of the tissue is useful if the patient fails to recover from the effects of secondary hyperparathyroidism after surgery and needs removal of additional parathyroid tissue. It is much simpler to find remaining tissue in the forearm rather than in the neck, where the risks of injury to nerve and other vital structures are greater.

◆ **What is the typical management?**

◈ Most patients who receive a renal transplant have a return of normal parathyroid function. Occasionally, they develop high serum calcium postoperatively; this condition is termed **tertiary hyperparathyroidism**. The parathyroid glands do not respond to the return of renal function and continue to overproduce PTH. If this condition persists for 1 year and homeostasis does not occur, a **3 1/2-gland resection** is indicated.

Occasionally, renal transplant patients develop parathyroid abnormalities.

Case 9.5 Hyperparathyroidism and Severe Hypertension in the Same Patient

The same 34-year-old man undergoes **neck exploration** surgery for primary hyperparathyroidism (see Case 9.4). During the procedure, he becomes **uncontrollably hypertensive**, with a blood pressure (BP) of 210/140 mm Hg. The operative team checks routine possibilities such as improper endotracheal tube placement, inadequate oxygenation, and inadequate level of anesthesia, but this does not demonstrate a cause.

◆ **What do you advise?**

◈ This patient may be experiencing a **catecholamine release** from an undiagnosed pheochromocytoma. It is necessary to terminate the current operation and admit the patient to the intensive care unit for further evaluation. A combination of both alpha- and beta-blockers can be used to obtain immediate control of the hypertension; it is important to achieve alpha blockade before beta blockade because unopposed alpha stimulation can be fatal.

You do this and the man's BP is controlled.

◆ **What is the next step?**

◈ It is necessary to test for the presence of a **pheochromocytoma**.

> **QUICK CUT** Pheochromocytomas are the "10%" tumor; 10% are malignant, extra-adrenal, epinephrine producers, or bilateral.

More than 90% of pheochromocytomas result in elevated levels of **urinary catechols, metanephrine, and vanillylmandelic acid or plasma fractionated metanephrines**. MRI using T2 weighted imaging may demonstrate a tumor brightness threefold greater than the liver. This is useful in the patients with additional tumor deposits of tumor in the abdomen that are intra-abdominal but extra-adrenal. For tumors that are difficult to locate, the octreotide scan often localizes the tumor (Fig. 9-7), or ^{131}I metaiodobenzylguanidine **(MIBG)** scan is used. A nuclear MIBG scan material selectively accumulates in chromaffin tissue, with a high sensitivity and even higher specificity for pheochromocytomas. After tumor localization, alpha blockade should be obtained using phenoxybenzamine for 10–14 days before surgery. Beta blockade is used in patients with persistent tachycardia or a previous heart history. Treatment is adrenalectomy either through an open or laparoscopic approach.

You establish a diagnosis of pheochromocytoma and localize it with the imaging studies.

◆ **What is the next management step?**

◆ A significant number of tumors are bilateral and extra-adrenal, and transabdominal exploration either open or laparoscopically allows the surgeon to explore these areas more extensively. However, it is important to perform the **resection** with minimal manipulation of the tumor to avoid a release of catecholamines. Extra-adrenal pheochromocytomas occur along the abdominal aorta in a distribution similar to the sympathetic chain.

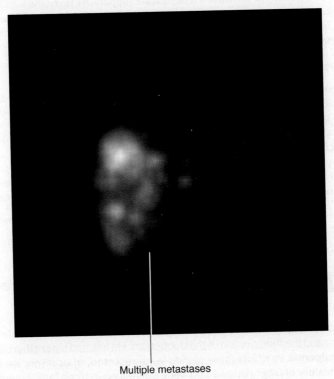

Multiple metastases

Figure 9-7: Octreotide scan, showing multiple metastases to the liver and duodenum.

Case 9.6   Acute Development of a Tender Neck Mass

A 38-year-old woman complains of a sudden onset of a swollen, tender thyroid gland. Her family physician has referred her for evaluation of this tender neck mass.

◆ **What is the most likely diagnosis?**

◇ This patient is presumably suffering from a case of painful, **subacute thyroiditis.** In the early stages of disease, patients present with hyperthyroidism due to the sudden release of thyroid hormone directly from acutely injured thyroid follicles.

 QUICK CUT The general finding associated with thyroiditis is an elevated erythrocyte sedimentation rate (ESR).

Histology is classic for giant cell granulomas around degenerating thyroid follicles.

◆ **How do you want to proceed with this patient's management?**

◇ Therapy consists of analgesics and anti-inflammatory medications. Steroids may be effective in more resistant cases. Surgery is not necessary. Thyroid function tests may be performed if the patient has symptoms of hyperthyroidism.

◆ **Is surgery appropriate in some cases of acute thyroid inflammation?**

◇ If it is believed that a patient has a bacterial infection, surgical drainage of an abscess might be appropriate. Bacterial infection is termed **acute suppurative thyroiditis.** Pathogens usually include *Streptococcus, Staphylococcus,* and *Pseudomonas.* Other rare causes are tuberculosis, aspergillosis, actinomycoses, and syphilis. The best treatment for these infections is antibiotics or antifungal agents with the drainage of any abscesses, if present.

◆ **How would you manage this patient?**

◇ Hashimoto thyroiditis is an autoimmune disease that involves the replacement of immune-damaged thyroid tissue with lymphocytes and plasma cells. These patients are most frequently **hypothyroid and often present with painless, nodular masses** in their thyroid gland. Laboratory tests reveal low thyroxine, triiodothyronine, and elevated TSH levels and elevated thyroid peroxidase antibodies.

No specific therapy for Hashimoto thyroiditis is available, but thyroid replacement is necessary if the inflammatory process leads to hypothyroidism, which is common. **Biopsy of all suspicious lesions is necessary**, and patients with **compressive symptoms of the trachea** should undergo palliative resection to relieve the obstruction.

A patient presents with a painless thyroid mass and is hypothyroid. Biopsy indicates **Hashimoto thyroiditis (chronic lymphocytic thyroiditis).**

Case 9.7   History of Hyperparathyroidism and Intractable Duodenal Ulcers

A 40-year-old man is referred to you by his gastroenterologist for **intractable ulcers** in the stomach and the third portion of the duodenum. He has had a **parathyroidectomy for hypercalcemia** in which three glands were resected. In addition, he reports a significant history of ulcer disease and neck operations in three family members.

Table 9-4: **Gastrinoma**

Parameter	Description
Symptoms	Peptic ulcer disease
	Diarrhea
	Esophagitis
Diagnostic tests	Serum gastrin measurement
	Gastric ulcer analysis
	Secretin stimulation test
Anatomic localization	Duodenum and head of pancreas (gastrinoma triangle)

◆ **How would you evaluate this patient?**

◆ First-line investigation should be to rule out a chronic *Helicobacter pylori* infection, a medically treatable source of chronic ulcer disease. It is also necessary to obtain a serum gastrin level to determine if the ulcer disease is due to hypergastrinemia (Table 9-4). If the *H. pylori* test is negative and the basal serum gastrin is over 600 pg/mL (>1,000 pg/mL is diagnostic), you suspect a **gastrinoma (Zollinger-Ellison syndrome [ZES])**. There are two forms of ZES: one is sporadic, and the other is familial and associated with MEN1. Other associated diseases in MEN1 are pituitary adenoma, parathyroid hyperplasia, and pancreatic endocrine tumors. Presenting features of pituitary neoplasms, which occur in 15%–50% of patients with MEN1, include vision symptoms (local compression) or hypersecretion (lactation). Treatment involves resection of the affected side of the pituitary (partial hypophysectomy). The pancreatic endocrine tumors include gastrinoma, insulinoma, and VIPomas. There has also been an association with bronchial carcinoids.

 QUICK CUT The diagnosis of hypergastrinemia is established by an elevated unstimulated serum gastrin level or with a positive calcium or secretin stimulation test to augment the gastrin response.

The man's gastrin level is 1,200 pg/mL.

◆ **What are the next steps in evaluation?**

◆ The presence of hypergastrinemia may result from a gastrin-secreting tumor, an incomplete previous gastric resection, or G-cell hyperplasia. Treatment includes initiation of a proton pump inhibitor (PPI) after the diagnosis of gastrinoma is confirmed. Because this patient has no previous surgery, **localization** of a gastrin-secreting tumor is performed using CT and MRI. These tumors are typically located in the head of the pancreas and within the duodenal wall to the right of the superior mesenteric vessels in the gastrinoma triangle. Other measures used to determine localization are endoscopic US scanning, angiogram, and venous sampling for gastrin (Fig. 9-8).

You establish a diagnosis of a gastrin-secreting tumor, which appears to be in close proximity to the head of the pancreas.

◆ **Would you recommend surgery?**

◆ If unresectable disease is found such as diffuse hepatic metastases, the patient should be treated with long-term PPIs. Otherwise, the patient should be offered surgical exploration

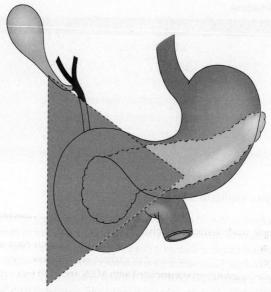

Figure 9-8: Location of gastrinomas. Most gastrinomas are found within the gastrinoma triangle. (From Greenfield LJ, Mulholland MW, Oldham KT, et al, eds. *Surgery: Scientific Principles and Practice*, 2nd ed. Philadelphia: Lippincott Williams & Wilkins; 1997:262.)

with attempt at curative resection. Sporadic gastrinomas are usually solitary and have a better prognosis after resection than those associated with MEN1, which can be multifocal.

♦ **What is the operative strategy?**

♦ **Location of the tumor and removal of as much tumor as possible** are necessary. This process includes intraoperative **endoscopy** to identify duodenal lesions, as well as intraoperative **US** to isolate the mass.

 QUICK CUT The surgeon should use surgical enucleation for gastrinoma, which preserves pancreatic mass, to remove the tumor.

However, when the mass involves or abuts a large pancreatic duct, a Whipple procedure or removal of the involved pancreas, typically a distal pancreatectomy, should be performed. Treatment of malignant or metastatic gastrinomas that are not resectable used to involve gastric resection (traditional) or highly selective vagotomy; however, PPI treatment has supplanted these surgeries. Streptozocin is the primary chemotherapeutic agent used for tumor control.

Deep Thoughts

Sometimes the treatment can lead to worse problems than the disease, and not every disease can be cured. Make sure the treatment does not lead to more morbidity then the disease.

Table 9-5: Insulinoma

Parameter	Description
Symptoms	
Neuroglycopenia causes	Confusion, personality change, coma
Catecholamine surge causes	Trembling, diaphoresis, tachycardia
Diagnostic tests	Monitored fast
	Insulin/glucose ratio
	C peptide and proinsulin blood levels
Anatomic localization	Evenly distributed throughout pancreas

◆ **How might the presentation change if the gastrinoma were an insulinoma?**

◆ **Insulinomas** are the next most frequently observed lesions. Affected patients present with the Whipple triad: fasting hypoglycemia (glucose <60 mg/dL), symptomatic hypoglycemia, and relief by administration of glucose. These patients have an elevated insulin secretion (C peptide must be measured to exclude self-administration of excess insulin) (Table 9-5). Usually, insulinomas associated with MEN are small (<1 cm) and multicentric as opposed to sporadic; 80% of these are solitary. Insulinomas have only a 10% incidence of malignancy.

◆ **What would be the operative strategy for an insulinoma?**

◆ **The operative management of insulinomas is similar to that of gastrinomas.** If the tumors are unresectable insulinomas, diazoxide, an inhibitor of insulin release, is appropriate.

Case 9.8   Medullary Carcinoma of the Thyroid

A 30-year-old woman presents with an asymptomatic mass in her thyroid. Her endocrinologist performed fine-needle biopsy, which revealed amyloid-like material and C-cell proliferation consistent with medullary carcinoma of the thyroid. On examination, her BP is significantly elevated.

◆ **What is the next management step?**

◆ This patient presumably has a **medullary thyroid cancer** associated with **MEN2**, a syndrome with autosomal dominant inheritance.

QUICK CUT In MEN2A, the constellation of pathology involves a medullary thyroid cancer, parathyroid hyperplasia, and pheochromocytoma. In MEN2B, the pattern is similar, with the exception of an associated marfanoid body habitus and ganglioneuromas but lacking pheochromocytoma.

It is necessary to obtain markers for a pheochromocytoma in the case of suspected MEN2A with hypertension. These indicators include urine catecholamines. Presenting features of pheochromocytomas include either sustained or episodic hypertension with primary complaints of frontal pounding headaches, episodic diaphoresis, palpitations, or anxiety. Bilateral occurrence is more frequent (60%–80%) than with sporadic pheochromocytoma (10%).

You evaluate the patient and find that she does not have a pheochromocytoma.

◆ **What surgical procedure is recommended?**

◆ A total thyroidectomy and removal of lymph nodes in the central compartment of the neck is appropriate. Lateral nodal compartment resection is indicated for clinically suspicious lymph nodes.

Case 9.9   Incidentally Discovered Adrenal Mass

A 50-year-old woman has an episode of acute diverticulitis. She presents to your office after having an abdominal CT scan to examine for an occult perforation. No perforation is apparent, but the scan demonstrates a 4-cm right adrenal mass (Fig. 9-9). On history and examination, she is asymptomatic and otherwise normal, with no hypertension or other findings supporting an adrenal disorder.

◆ **What is your clinical plan?**

◆ Clinical management of an **incidental adrenal mass** depend on the diameter of the lesion and whether symptoms are present. In lesions that are 5 cm or more in size, the incidence of adrenal cortical carcinoma is high, and surgery is recommended. Operative therapy usually involves a wide resection of the adrenal gland.

 QUICK CUT The consideration of metastatic disease processes such as lung cancer is also appropriate because the adrenal gland is a common site for metastasis.

In lesions less than 5 cm in size, a careful history and physical examination for obvious tumors and endocrinologic syndromes is warranted. Biochemical assessment to examine for elevated levels of catecholamines, cortisol, aldosterone with plasma renin activity, and serum potassium is also appropriate. If these tests indicate that the mass is functional, removal of the adrenal is necessary. If the lesion is nonfunctional, it is appropriate to follow the lesion with serial CT scans. If no growth occurs, observation may be sufficient, and if it enlarges, removal is necessary.

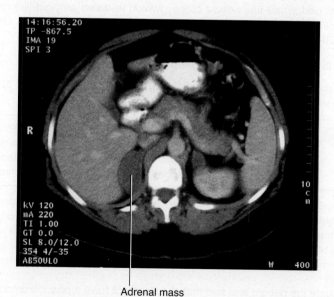

Adrenal mass

Figure 9-9: CT scan of an incidental adrenal mass.

Chapter 10

Skin and Soft Tissue Disorders and Hernias

Bruce E. Jarrell, Eric D. Strauch

Key Thoughts

1. A mole that demonstrates any of the ABCD (**a**symmetry; **b**order irregularity; **c**olor variation; **d**iameter greater than 0.6 cm, **d**ark black color) warning signs, or that is evolving in appearance, should be removed. Melanoma may occur at any site that contains skin, mucous membrane, or sites with melanocytes such as the eye. Treatment is surgical excision.

2. Thicker melanomas have a higher risk for metastasis and recurrence. Melanomas from 1 to 4 mm in thickness usually have a sentinel lymph node biopsy done also. If positive, therapeutic lymph node excision is done.

3. Sarcoma prognosis is graded by the degree of cellular atypia seen on biopsy. Best results occur when the tumor can be excised completely with negative margins.

4. Femoral hernias are less common than inguinal hernias but are associated with increased bowel strangulation.

MALIGNANT MELANOMA

Case 10.1 Evaluation of a Skin Lesion

A 42-year-old man visits you for a lesion on his left forearm. The lesion, which is not painful, has been present for several months. He believes it may be enlarging.

◆ **What aspects of the history or physical examination might be important?**

◆ A **family history of malignant melanoma** increases the risk of melanoma. Other risk factors for many skin disorders are extensive exposure to sunlight and previous dysplastic nevi or atypical moles.

Physical examination can help distinguish benign from malignant lesions. Ulceration, bleeding, and recent change in size are commonly present with malignancy. Variation in pigmentation is also a significant indicator of malignancy. **Between 5% and 10% of malignant melanomas are not pigmented**, and a significant number of basal cell carcinomas and squamous cell carcinomas are pigmented. The **ABCD rule** has been established to describe the findings suggestive of melanoma in pigmented lesions. In addition, the presence of ulceration or nodularity is a concern. A search for regional lymphadenopathy is also appropriate.

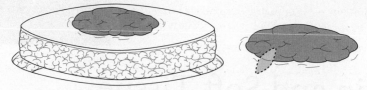

Excisional biopsy   Incisional biopsy

Figure 10-1: Excisional biopsy versus incisional biopsy. Excisional biopsy completely excises the lesion with a rim of normal tissue. It extends down to the subcutaneous tissue in order to be able to measure the depth of the lesion. Incisional biopsy excises a portion of the margin of the lesion with a segment of normal tissue.

◆ **Is excision of the lesion appropriate?**

◆ Excision of any lesion that has changed recently or has any of the listed attributes is necessary.
In **larger lesions (>2–3 cm) or lesions that are contiguous with important structures such as on the face, incisional biopsy** of full-thickness skin at the border of the lesion is warranted (Fig. 10-1). Shave biopsies should not be performed because they do not allow an adequate assessment of lesion thickness.

You decide to perform an excisional biopsy of the lesion.

◆ **What management is appropriate for each of the following pathologic conditions?**

Case Variation 10.1.1. *Benign skin lesion*

◆ No further treatment is necessary.

Case Variation 10.1.2. *Basal cell carcinoma*

◆ These lesions rarely metastasize, but they require adequate local excision **because recurrent lesions may be locally invasive.** This patient is at risk for new lesions, especially in areas of the skin exposed to sunlight. If the histologic margins are free of tumor, then no further treatment is necessary.

QUICK CUT If margins are positive, it is essential to re-excise the nevus to clear margins. The margin for large or more aggressive lesions should be 2–4 mm.

Treatment for basal cell carcinoma may also involve topical 5-fluorouracil or radiation.

Case Variation 10.1.3. *Squamous cell carcinoma*

QUICK CUT Squamous cell carcinoma is more dangerous than basal cell carcinoma because of its locally aggressive behavior and its propensity to metastasize to local lymph nodes.

◆ Squamous cell carcinoma in situ is termed Bowen disease. Local recurrence is more common with lesions 4 mm or greater in thickness, which necessitates excision with a 1-cm tumor-free margin. Lesions 10 mm or greater in thickness are more likely to be metastatic to regional lymph nodes. However, **lymph node excision** is generally recommended only for **clinically palpable nodes**, except where behavior of the primary lesion is very aggressive. Treatment with topical 5-fluorouracil or radiation is also appropriate.

Case Variation 10.1.4. *In situ melanoma*

◆ It is necessary to re-excise the lesion to a 0.5–1-cm margin of normal tissue. This approach should result in a cure.

Case Variation 10.1.5. *Dysplastic nevus*

◆ This benign neoplasm of melanocytes with areas of **atypia** may represent a transition between benign nevus and melanoma. Only adequate excision is necessary, with close examination for other suspicious lesions and routine surveillance.

Case 10.2 | Diagnosis of Malignant Melanoma in a Skin Lesion

After excision of the lesion from the forearm of the patient described in Case 10.1, pathologic findings indicate malignant melanoma.

Deep Thoughts

Protection from ultraviolet exposure can significantly decrease the risk for developing skin malignancies such as melanoma, squamous cell carcinoma, and basal cell carcinoma.

◆ **How is this lesion staged?**

◆ The current methods for staging melanoma principally relate to the depth of penetration or thickness of the lesion. The two commonly used classifications are the **Clark level and Breslow thickness** (Fig. 10-2; Table 10-1). The tumor–node–metastasis (TNM) stages correlate highly with patient survival (Fig. 10-3; Table 10-2).

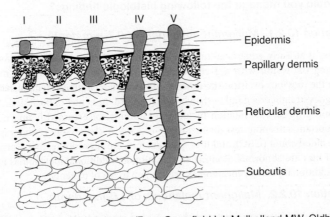

Figure 10-2: Clark levels in melanoma. (From Greenfield LJ, Mulholland MW, Oldham KT, et al, eds. *Surgery: Scientific Principles and Practice*, 2nd ed. Philadelphia: Lippincott Williams & Wilkins; 1997:2233.)

Table 10-1: Staging of Melanoma: Breslow Tumor Thickness and Clark Level

Breslow Tumor Thickness (mm)	Primary Tumor Classification	Clark Level	5-Year Survival (%)
	T0	I	>95
≤0.75	T1	II	89
0.76–1.49	T2	III	75
1.50–2.49	T3	IV	58
2.50–3.99			46
≥4.0	T4	V	25

Although there are several types of melanoma (superficial spreading, nodular, lentigo maligna, acral lentiginous), they all result in a **similar prognosis when corrected for thickness**. Nodular melanomas are another distinctive type but do not worsen prognosis when corrected for depth.

◆ **What factors in addition to histologic classification and TNM stage strongly affect survival?**

◆ The most significant finding in addition to the histologic findings and TNM stage is the presence of ulceration in the primary lesion.

 QUICK CUT Even in stage I lesions, ulcerated lesions have about a one-third reduction in survival.

Individuals with lesions located on the face or trunk have a worse prognosis than those with lesions on the extremities, and women do better than men overall.

A pathologist reviews the lesion.

◆ **How would you manage the following histologic findings?**

Case Variation 10.2.1. Malignant melanoma of 0.7-mm depth

◆ This lesion is an early, superficial finding, and **with local control, the prognosis is good. Re-excising the lesion with a 1-cm margin** should accomplish this. It is necessary to re-excise the previous excision site down to the deep fascial plane, being certain that the incision goes straight down rather than beveling toward the center of the lesion. A complete history and physical examination including examining for enlarged lymph nodes is the most important screening test for metastatic disease. A chest x-ray (radiograph) (CXR), complete blood count (CBC), and liver function tests are appropriate; they warrant follow-up only if they are abnormal. Routine examination for additional melanomas is necessary because additional primary melanomas occur in up to 5% of patients.

Case Variation 10.2.2. Malignant melanoma of 1.6-mm depth

◆ This lesion, which is more advanced, has a higher rate of local recurrence. **It warrants re-excision with a larger, 2-cm margin.** The risk of regional lymph node metastasis is approximately 40%. **If palpable nodes are present, therapeutic lymphadenectomy should**

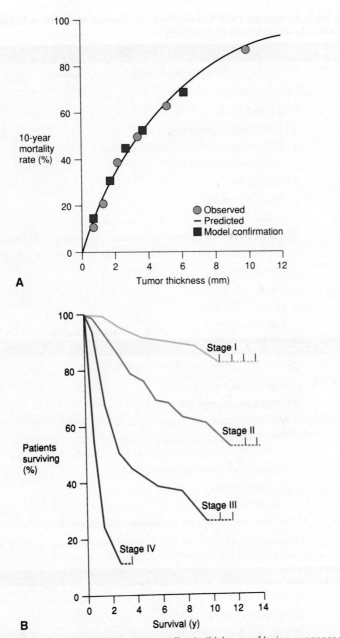

Figure 10-3: Survival in malignant melanoma according to thickness of lesion or cancer stage. **A:** Graphic relationship between melanoma tumor thickness and mortality. **B:** Survival according to American Joint Committee on Cancer staging system (see Table 10-2). (After Balch CM, Soong SJ, Shaw HM, et al. An analysis of prognostic factors in 4,000 patients with cutaneous melanoma. In: Balch CM, Milton GW, eds. *Cutaneous melanoma: Clinical Management and Treatment Results Worldwide*. Philadelphia: J.B. Lippincott; 1985:321; reprinted with permission from Greenfield LJ, Mulholland MW, Oldham KT, et al, eds. *Surgery: Scientific Principles and Practice*, 2nd ed. Philadelphia: Lippincott Williams & Wilkins; 1997:2234–2235.)

Table 10-2: American Joint Committee on Cancer Melanoma Staging System, Tumor–Node–Metastasis Definitions

Primary Tumor	
TX	Cannot be assessed (shave biopsy, regressed lesion)
T0	Unknown primary
Tis	In situ melanoma
T1	≤1-mm Breslow thickness a. Without ulceration and mitosis ≤1 mm^2 b. With ulceration or mitosis ≥1 mm^2
T2	1.01–2.00 mm a. Without ulceration b. With ulceration
T3	2.01–4.00 mm a. Without ulceration b. With ulceration
T4	>4 mm a. Without ulceration b. With ulceration
Regional Lymph Node Involvement	
NX	Cannot be assessed (previously removed)
N0	No regional node metastasis
N1	Metastasis in one regional node a. Micrometastasis (diagnosed by SLNB or elective lymph node dissection) b. Macrometastasis (clinically palpable or found on imaging studies, confirmed histologically, or gross extracapsular extension)
N2	Metastasis in two to three regional nodes a. Micrometastasis b. Macrometastasis c. In-transit or satellite metastasis without nodal metastasis
N3	Metastasis in ≥4 regional nodes, matted nodes, or in-transit or satellite metastasis with positive metastatic nodes
Distant Metastasis	
MX	Cannot be assessed
M0	No distant metastasis
M1a	Distant skin, subcutaneous, or lymph node metastasis with normal LDH
M1b	Lung metastasis with normal LDH
M1c	All other visceral metastases with a normal LDH or any distant metastases with an elevated LDH

Table 10-2: American Joint Committee on Cancer Melanoma Staging System, Tumor–Node–Metastasis Definitions *(continued)*

Stage Groupings						
	Clinical Staging*			Pathologic Staging†		
	T	N	M	T	N	M
0	Tis	N0	M0	Tis	N0	M0
IA	T1a	N0	M0	T1a	N0	M0
IB	T1b	N0	M0	T1b	N0	M0
	T2a	N0	M0	T2a	N0	M0
IIA	T2b	N	M0	T2b	N0	M0
	T3a	N0	M0	T3a	N0	M0
IIB	T3b	N0	M0	T3b	N0	M0
	T4a	N0	M0	T4a	N0	M0
IIC	T4b	N0	M0	T4b	N0	M0
		N1				
III‡	Any T	N2	M0			
		N3				
IIIA				T1–T4a	N1a	M0
				T1–T4a	N2a	M0
				T1–T4b	N1a	M0
				T1–T4b	N2a	M0
IIIB				T1–T4a	N1b	M0
				T1–T4a	N2b	M0
				T1–T4a/b	N2c	M0
				T1–T4b	N1b	M0
IIIC				T1–T4b	N2b	M0
				Any T	N3	M0
IV	Any T	Any N	Any M1	Any T	Any N	Any M1

*Clinical staging includes microstaging of the primary melanoma and clinical/radiologic evaluation for metastasis. By convention, it should be used after complete excision of the primary melanoma with clinical assessment for regional and distant metastases.
†Pathologic staging includes microstaging of the primary melanoma and pathologic information about the regional lymph nodes after partial or complete lymphadenectomy. Pathologic stage 0 or stage IA patients are the exception; they do not require pathologic evaluation of their lymph nodes.
‡There are no stage III subgroups for clinical staging.
SLNB, sentinel lymph node biopsy; LDH, lactate dehydrogenase.
From Greenfield LJ, Mulholland MW, Lillemoe KD, et al, eds. *Greenfield's Surgery*, 5e. Philadelphia: Lippincott Williams & Wilkins; 2010.

be performed. Sentinel lymph node biopsy is commonly done if lymph nodes are clinically negative in patients with melanoma 1-mm thick or greater to determine whether further therapeutic lymphadenectomy is indicated.

> **QUICK CUT** If no nodes are palpable, a sentinel lymph node biopsy is warranted. If the biopsy is positive, therapeutic lymph node dissection is indicated, even in the case of nonpalpable nodes.

Case Variation 10.2.3. *Malignant melanoma of 4.5-mm depth*

◆ This patient, who has a poor prognosis, will **most likely die from metastatic disease**. Re-excision of the lesion with a 2–3-cm margin is appropriate. In such a case, it is more likely that lymph nodes are palpable; if so, excision of the nodes is warranted because they have a tendency to erode the skin and become infected and painful. It is unlikely that an elective, or prophylactic, node dissection will be beneficial.

In addition, computed tomography (CT) of the abdomen and magnetic resonance imaging (MRI) of the brain to examine for metastasis is necessary. The patient should then enter a protocol for treatment with interferon, which has proven benefit for patients with T4 primary tumors or stage III disease.

Case 10.3   Malignant Melanoma with a Palpable Lymph Node

You remove a skin lesion from the patient in Case 10.1, and the pathologic findings indicate a Clark III malignant melanoma. After reviewing the depth of the lesion, you re-examine the patient.

◆ **How would the presence of a palpable axillary lymph node change the management plan?**

◆ The presence of axillary lymphadenopathy suggests metastatic disease, potentially stage III or IV disease. **Regional lymphadenectomy** to establish the diagnosis and to remove the involved nodes is warranted. With metastasis, there is a 75% chance of recurrence of melanoma in the next 5 years. Patients should undergo **complete staging** for the presence of distant metastasis. This usually includes CXR, liver function tests, CT of the abdomen, and MRI of the brain. Treatment with interferon may increase survival by as much as 40%.

> **QUICK CUT** Individuals with stage IV melanoma should enter a trial of therapy, usually involving immunotherapy including interleukin-2 or vaccine therapy.

Case 10.4   Malignant Melanoma with Distant Metastasis

A 46-year-old man seeks evaluation for a newly diagnosed malignant melanoma. He has a Clark III lesion and no palpable nodes. On CXR, a new lung lesion is apparent.

◆ **How does this finding alter the management plan?**

◆ A diagnosis of the lung lesion is necessary. Depending on the circumstances, it is possible to obtain this in a variety of ways, including percutaneous needle biopsy. Any distant metastasis signifies stage IV disease. Such advanced disease is usually not curable, but **systemic therapy with combination drugs** or dacarbazine may produce a response in up to one-third of patients. Some clinicians support excision of solitary lung metastasis as well as brain metastasis in melanoma when no other disease is present. Radiation therapy may relieve the pain from bone metastasis. Recently, studies have shown that complete resection combined with a polyvalent vaccine increases survival by as much as 35% at 5 years in individuals with bone metastases.

Case 10.5 Special Problems in Malignant Melanoma No. 1

A 75-year-old woman consults you because of a brownish discoloration on her cheek that has been slowly enlarging.

◆ **What management is necessary for the following lesions?**

Case Variation 10.5.1. A 5-cm irregular lentigo maligna melanoma of the cheek

◆ A lentigo maligna melanoma, which often occurs on the face, particularly in elderly individuals, tends to be **superficial** and **spreading** rather than invasive. Thus, it carries a **more favorable prognosis because of its thickness.** Management involves excision, with a narrower margin because the lesion is on the face.

Case Variation 10.5.2. A 5-cm irregular lentigo maligna (Hutchinson freckle) of the cheek

◆ A Hutchinson freckle is a large, macular, brown lesion on the cheek, which may be present for many years or decades (Fig. 10-4). This lesion is not malignant in itself, but it is typically the **precursor of lentigo malignant melanoma.** Management can involve excision and biopsy, incisional biopsy, ablation with cryotherapy or other types of ablative therapy, or observation.

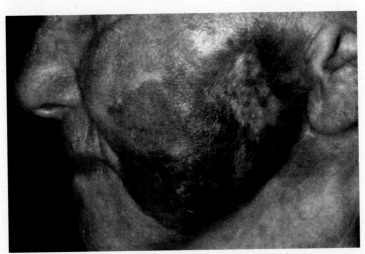

Figure 10-4: Hutchinson freckle. (From Greenfield LJ, Mulholland MW, Oldham KT, et al, eds. *Surgery: Scientific Principles and Practice*, 2nd ed. Philadelphia: Lippincott Williams & Wilkins; 1997:2232.)

Case 10.6   Special Problems in Malignant Melanoma No. 2

A 50-year-old man consults you for care of a suspected melanoma.

◆ **What management is necessary for the following lesions?**

Case Variation 10.6.1. ***A malignant melanoma of 4.2-mm depth close to the nasolabial fold***

◆ In general, the **margins of excision may be smaller on the face** when compared to peripheral lesions. This lesion must be excised in consultation with a plastic surgeon.

Case Variation 10.6.2. ***A patient with a malignant melanoma of the sole of the foot***

◆ Melanomas in this location, which are classified as acral lentiginous lesions, are more common in dark-skinned individuals. These lesions tend to be **thicker** and are associated with a **poorer prognosis.** Excision with margins appropriate for thickness is necessary.

Case Variation 10.6.3. ***A malignant melanoma of the subungual area of the index finger***

◆ Subungual melanomas are often observed due to their similarity to subungual hematomas (Fig. 10-5). Biopsy entails excision of a portion of the nail in continuity with the lesion. Re-excision following diagnosis involves **amputation at the distal interphalangeal joint.** Affected patients have a survival rate of 60%.

Case Variation 10.6.4. ***A malignant melanoma of the anus***

◆ Anal melanomas, along with other mucosal melanomas, are associated with a particularly **poor prognosis**, with mortality near 100% at 5 years. Thin lesions can be locally excised and most commonly occur at the dentate line. **Thicker lesions usually require abdominoperineal resection of the anorectum**, although wide local excision may also be performed.

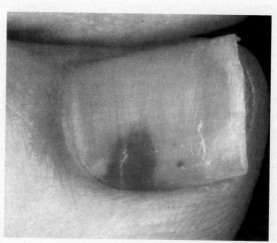

Figure 10-5: Subungual melanoma. (From Greenfield LJ, Mulholland MW, Oldham KT, et al, eds. *Surgery: Scientific Principles and Practice*, 2nd ed. Philadelphia: Lippincott Williams & Wilkins; 1997:2232.)

Abdominoperineal resection has a lower rate of local recurrence than local excision, but neither procedure produces a better patient survival rate. Regional lymph node excision is only indicated for positive inguinal nodes.

Case 10.7 Small Bowel Obstruction and History of Malignant Melanoma

A patient with a stage I malignant melanoma removed 5 years ago returns to the emergency department with abdominal distention, nausea, vomiting, and radiographic evidence of small bowel obstruction.

◆ **What management is appropriate?**

◆ Melanoma has a unique propensity to **metastasize to the peritoneal cavity** and involve the viscera; the common presentation is a small bowel obstruction. Exploration is indicated, but the prognosis is poor. Palliative treatment may be possible with solitary lesions or a resectable group of lesions, and patients may be able to leave the hospital. However, many patients succumb.

SARCOMA

Case 10.8 Sarcoma of the Lower Extremity

A 45-year-old man presents with a painless mass on his anterior thigh. The slow-growing 5-cm lesion has been present for several months.

◆ **What facts may be important in the history and physical examination?**

◆ Soft tissue sarcomas are rare neoplasms of connective tissue; clinicians diagnose approximately 6,000 new cases per year. Family history of sarcoma is uncommon, but it may increase the incidence of subsequent sarcoma. A history of therapeutic radiation (fibrosarcoma) or axillary lymphadenectomy (lymphangiosarcoma) one or two decades earlier has been associated with sarcoma development. A history of trauma with a subsequent and persistent mass can be a sarcoma misdiagnosed as a hematoma.

Physical examination is important to distinguish a sarcoma from other benign lesions such as hematoma, lipoma, fibroma, hamartoma, or hemangioma. Sarcomas occur as **firm, painless masses** that are typically larger than benign tumors. Regional adenopathy is rare (2.6%) but may be evident in several types of sarcomas (lymphangiosarcoma, epithelioid sarcoma, embryonal rhabdomyosarcoma, malignant fibrous histiocytoma, synovial cell sarcoma).

◆ **What type of biopsy or excision is appropriate?**

◆ Biopsy is directed by the size of the lesion. Excisional biopsy is indicated for masses less than 3 cm.

QUICK CUT Incisional biopsy is the initial step for sarcomas 3 cm or more. The biopsy incision should parallel the subsequent surgical incision for a definitive resection (Fig. 10-6).

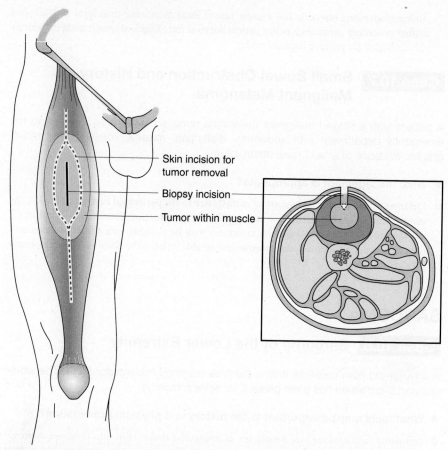

Figure 10-6: Technique for incisional biopsy of a sarcoma. (From Greenfield LJ, Mulholland MW, Oldham KT, et al, eds. *Surgery: Scientific Principles and Practice*, 2nd ed. Philadelphia: Lippincott Williams & Wilkins; 1997:2252.)

Excisional biopsies performed in lesions greater than 3 cm or perpendicular to definitive resection margins are inappropriate. The larger defect makes primary closure complex or potentially contaminates additional compartments with tumor and increases the risk for local recurrence. Core biopsy may provide accurate diagnosis in select centers, but fine-needle aspiration (FNA) provides nondiagnostic tissue and should be discouraged. In addition, frozen section biopsies of sarcoma do not lead to a reliable diagnosis.

The biopsy confirms a soft tissue sarcoma.

◆ **What pathologic features prompt concern?**

◆ Sarcomas are classified based on the tissues they mimic, not from where the tumor arises. Histologic grade is crucial for prognosis and treatment and is based on the degree of cellular atypia, amount of tumor necrosis, and the frequency of mitotic figures. Lower grade tumors, those with good prognoses, have less cellular atypia, few mitotic figures, and no necrosis. Higher grade tumors with worse prognoses have more atypia and mitosis as well as tumor necrosis. Sarcomas are usually graded as low, intermediate, or high with prognosis worsening as the grade increases.

◆ What diagnostic tests are necessary to characterize and stage the cancer?

◆ Sarcomas have a high rate of metastasis on presentation (22%); the most common sites for metastasis are the liver, lung, bone, and brain. Patients should have a metastatic workup prior to resection. A CT scan is very useful for detection of bony involvement, and an MRI scan detects involvement of adjacent soft tissue structures (e.g., muscle group definition, involvement of neurovascular bundles, and the interface between tumor and normal tissue).

Staging should be completed with the performance of abdominal–pelvic CT and plain CXR. A suspicious CXR should prompt a chest CT scan, and the presence of bone pain should prompt a bone scan (Fig. 10-7).

◆ What are the staging criteria for sarcomas?

◆ The standard TNM system is used for staging (Table 10-3).

Pathologic findings indicate that this lesion is a low-grade sarcoma. The workup is negative for metastasis.

◆ What type of resection is appropriate?

◆ Surgical therapy must balance the morbidity of the resection with the risk of local recurrence.

 QUICK CUT A basic principle in sarcoma surgery: An extensive initial resection of the primary tumor is necessary to obtain long-standing local tumor control.

Complete surgical resection including the tumor and pseudocapsule with margins is crucial for treatment of soft tissue sarcomas. Limb-sparing surgery with multimodal (surgery, chemotherapy, and radiation therapy together) as determined by location of the tumor, grade, and type is now the initial approach. Radical amputations are reserved for those who cannot undergo limb-sparing techniques.

In this case, most surgeons would perform a **wide local resection with negative margins** for two reasons: (1) it is limb-sparing and (2) it provides excellent local control (Fig. 10-8). Usually, patients have also had a previous biopsy, so the procedure also excises the previous incision and any residual hematoma en bloc without tumor spillage.

◆ How would the proposed management change if the lesion is a 15-cm–diameter, high-grade sarcoma?

◆ Large, high-grade tumors, which are associated with a worse prognosis, tend to require **more radical treatment**. Limb salvage by resection in conjunction with adjuvant or neoadjuvant chemotherapy and radiation therapy may improve patient survival or radical amputation if limb salvage is not technically feasible.

◆ What type of adjuvant therapy is appropriate?

◆ Adjuvant radiotherapy may provide an advantage in local recurrence after a wide excision for low-grade sarcomas. Radiotherapy significantly reduces the local recurrence rates of wide local excisions.

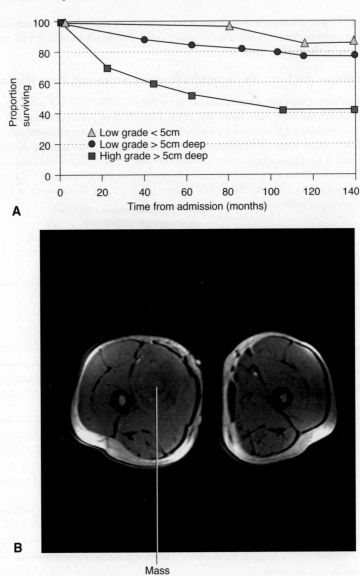

Figure 10-7: A: Kaplan-Meier survival curves. Probability of overall survival of sarcoma by stage. **B:** MRI of a thigh showing a large mass in the muscle compartment. (*continued*)

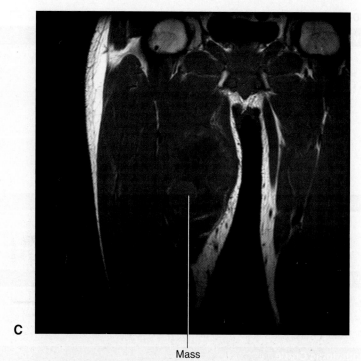

C

Mass

Figure 10-7: (*continued*) **C:** Another MRI view of sarcoma of an extremity.

 QUICK CUT Postoperative radiation therapy for limb salvage may reduce the local recurrence of high-grade sarcomas.

◆ **What new therapies are currently under investigation?**

◆ Brachytherapy, which is the application of local radiation seeds to the surgical field or residual tumor mass, can provide direct radiation therapy to the area most susceptible to local recurrence. Isolated limb perfusions of upper or lower limbs involve administration of high doses of chemotherapeutic agents (i.e., melphalan, cisplatin) or biologic modifiers (i.e., tumor necrosis factor, gamma interferon) to the extremity. These trials have produced mixed results for sarcomas.

Case 10.9 Metastatic Sarcoma to the Lung

A 52-year-old man, who has been seeing you every 3 months after excision of a low-grade sarcoma on his thigh, returns for his 1-year follow-up visit. There is no evidence of local recurrence. A CXR obtained as part of routine follow-up reveals a new, 1.5-cm mass in the right upper lobe.

◆ **What is the next step?**

◆ The finding on CXR is not unusual; **most recurrences** (80%) **occur within the first 2 years after primary resection**. After an abnormal CXR, the next step is a chest CT with contrast

Table 10-3: Staging of Soft Tissue Sarcoma—Definition of TNM

Primary Tumor (T)

Tx	Primary cannot be assessed
T0	No evidence of primary tumor
T1	Tumor limited to organ or tissue of origin and <5 cm in greatest dimension T1a superficial T1b deep
T2	Tumor >5 cm in greatest dimension T2a superficial T2b deep

Regional Lymph Nodes (N)

Nx	Regional lymph nodes cannot be assessed
N0	No regional lymph node metastasis
N1	Regional lymph node metastasis

Distant Metastasis (M)

Mx	Presence of distant metastasis cannot be assessed
M0	No distant metastasis
M1	Distant metastasis

Histopathologic Grade

Gx	Grade cannot be assessed
G1	Well differentiated
G2	Moderately differentiated
G3	Poorly differentiated
G4	Undifferentiated

Stage Grouping

Stage	G	T	N	M	Notes
IA	G1–G2	T1a or T1b	N0	M0	Low-grade (well differentiated), small, superficial, or deep
IB	G1–G2	T2a	N0	M0	Low-grade, larger, superficial
IIA	G1–G2	T2b	N0	M0	Low-grade, large, deep
IIB	G3–G4	T1a–T1b	N0	M0	High-grade (poorly differentiated), small, superficial, deep
IIC	G3–G4	T2a	N0	M0	High-grade, large, superficial
III	G3–G4	T2b	N0	M0	High-grade, large, deep
IV	Any G	Any T	N1	M0	Any metastasis
	Any G	Any T	N0	M1	

Superficial tumor is located exclusively above the superficial fascia without invasion of the fascia; deep tumor is located either exclusively beneath the superficial fascia or superficial to the fascia with invasion of or through the fascia or superficial and beneath the fascia. Retroperitoneal, mediastinal, and pelvic sarcomas are classified as deep tumors.
a, superficial; b, deep.
From American Joint Committee on Cancer. *AJCC Cancer Staging Manual*, 5th ed. Philadelphia: Lippincott-Raven; 1997.

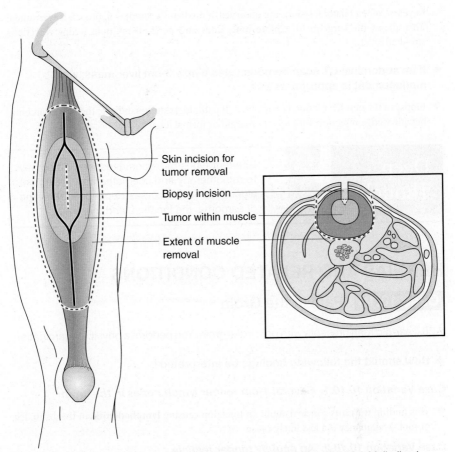

Skin incision for
tumor removal

Biopsy incision

Tumor within muscle

Extent of muscle
removal

Figure 10-8: Wide excision of lower extremity sarcoma. (From Greenfield LJ, Mulholland MW, Lillemoe KD, et al, eds. *Greenfield's Surgery*, 5th ed. Philadelphia: Lippincott Williams & Wilkins; 2010.)

to characterize the new lesion and detect any other lesions. A CT scan can diagnose lesions as small as 1 cm. Some surgeons would perform **needle biopsy** percutaneously to establish the diagnosis, whereas others would perform positron emission tomography (PET) and proceed with surgery if the PET scan is positive at the location of the lung mass.

Biopsy of the lesion indicates a sarcoma similar to the previously excised tumor.

◆ **What is the next step?**

◆ If the biopsy is positive for sarcoma, **a thoracic wedge resection** of the lesion is warranted.

QUICK CUT A recurrence of sarcoma is one of the few tumors in which excision of the pulmonary metastasis may result in a significant long-term disease-free interval (years).

Improvement in patient survival occurs even for simultaneous excision of several tumors and for the excision of multiple metachronous metastases over intervals of months to years. When bilateral lesions are observed, a median sternotomy approach is warranted. This allows the surgeon to explore both sides and perform multiple wedge resections simultaneously.

◆ **If an abdominal CT scan demonstrates a new 3-cm liver mass, what management is appropriate?**

◆ Biopsy of the new liver lesion is warranted. If pathologic studies indicate that it is a sarcoma, hepatic wedge resection with a 1-cm margin or formal lobectomy is necessary.

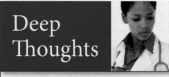

Deep Thoughts

Different types of sarcoma respond differently to radiotherapy and chemotherapy. Treatment algorithms for sarcomas depend on the type of sarcoma, the location, and the grade.

HERNIAS AND RELATED CONDITIONS

Case 10.10 Pain in the Groin

A 28-year-old man presents with pain in his groin. You perform a physical examination.

◆ **How should the following findings be interpreted?**

Case Variation 10.10.1. Several 1-cm tender lymph nodes in the groin

◆ This finding warrants concern about an infection causing **lymphadenitis** in the groin, leg, or foot. Malignancy is a less likely cause.

Case Variation 10.10.2. An acutely tender testicle

◆ If the onset of the condition is acute, it could represent **torsion of the testis**. If it is more gradual, it could be a viral orchitis or epididymitis. Torsion of the testicle, where the testicle twists around its blood supply, is a surgical emergency and the testicle must be detorted or it will necrose.

Case Variation 10.10.3. An acutely tender epididymis

◆ **Epididymitis** may result from a number of causes (e.g., infection, trauma).

Case Variation 10.10.4. A firm, tender mass in the medial portion of the groin

◆ Medial location of the mass represents a typical location for a direct inguinal hernia (Fig. 10-9).

Case Variation 10.10.5. A tender area in the lateral portion of the groin and an impulse that travels down the inguinal canal when he coughs

◆ A more lateral location and an impulse that travels down the canal suggest an indirect hernia (see Fig. 10-9).

Case Variation 10.10.6. A firm, tender mass below the inguinal ligament

◆ Location inferior to the inguinal ligament suggests a femoral hernia (see Fig. 10-9).

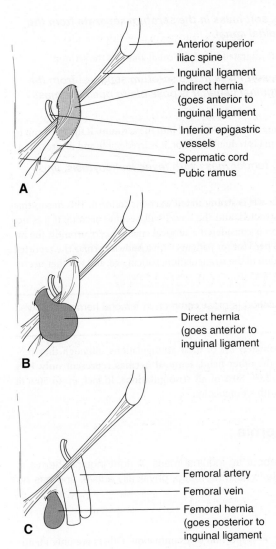

Anterior superior
iliac spine

Inguinal ligament

Indirect hernia
(goes anterior to
inguinal ligament

Inferior epigastric
vessels

Spermatic cord

Pubic ramus

A

Direct hernia
(goes anterior to
inguinal ligament

B

Femoral artery

Femoral vein

Femoral hernia
(goes posterior to
inguinal ligament

C

Figure 10-9: Different types of hernias. **A:** Indirect. **B:** Direct. **C:** Femoral. (From Fitzgibbons RJ Jr, Greenburg AG, eds. *Nyhus and Condon's Hernia*, 5th ed. Philadelphia: Lippincott Williams & Wilkins; 2002:78.)

Case Variation 10.10.7. *A firm, tender mass with nausea, vomiting, and abdominal distention (see Fig. 10-9)*

◆ A loop of intestine may be **incarcerated** or **strangulated** in the hernia. The estimated incidence of small bowel obstruction due to hernia has fallen from 50% to less than 20% since routine hernia repair has been advocated once a hernia is identified.

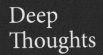

Deep
Thoughts

Incarcerated hernias are assumed to be strangulated or can become strangulated and need to be reduced or surgically repaired emergently.

Case Variation 10.10.8. **A large, soft mass in the scrotum separate from the testicle with fullness in the inguinal canal.**

◆ Most likely, a segment of bowel has migrated down the canal and into the scrotum.

Case Variation 10.10.9. **A large, soft mass in the scrotum separate from the testicle with a fullness in the inguinal canal. It is possible to push the mass back into the abdomen.**

◆ This is most likely an indirect hernia that has extended into the scrotum. If the mass can be pushed into the abdomen, the hernia is reducible. If not, it is irreducible and incarcerated.

Case Variation 10.10.10. **A firm, tender mass with fever, leukocytosis, and acidosis**

◆ The possibility that a **segment of bowel is strangulated** warrants concern. This means that the blood supply has become obstructed, and the bowel will become necrotic if it is not reduced immediately. This situation is considered a surgical emergency. Currently, the incidence of strangulation is 1%–3% per year for patients with a known hernia. The reported mortality, which is related to duration of the strangulation, patient age, and whether necrosis is present, is as high as 12%.

 QUICK CUT Strangulation is most common in femoral hernias, followed by indirect hernias.

Direct hernias account for approximately 3% of these strangulations, although they represent 30% of groin hernias. On the other hand, **femoral hernias represent only 10% of groin hernias but account for 33%–50% of all strangulations.** In fact, up to 50% of femoral hernias initially manifest with strangulation.

Case 10.11   Inguinal Hernia

A 55-year-old man consults you about an inguinal mass. A right inguinal hernia is present on routine examination. He is asymptomatic, physically active, and has no other medical problems.

◆ **How is a hernia detected?**

◆ Many hernias are readily apparent on inspection or examination. Others are only identified by a maneuver that accentuates the defect, most commonly by inserting a finger in the cephalad portion of the scrotum and up along the inguinal canal region. If the patient coughs or the intra-abdominal pressure otherwise increases, the examiner feels an impulse or segment of tissue travel down the canal and touches the fingertip.

Performance of this maneuver indicates that the patient has a hernia.

◆ **What is the difference between a direct hernia and an indirect hernia?**

◆ An **indirect hernia**, which usually has an intact posterior surface called the floor of the canal, **originates at the internal ring** and traverses down the inguinal canal. A **direct hernia**, a weakness in the floor of the canal, **originates medially to the inferior epigastric vessels**. The surgical approach and repair of both types of hernias is similar in adults.

This appears to be a direct hernia.

◆ **What is the next step in the patient's evaluation?**

◆ An assessment of the patient's general physical condition, a review of his history, and a minimal set of laboratory studies are necessary.

 QUICK CUT Occasionally, hernia development is associated with other conditions that might increase abdominal pressure such as obesity; chronic obstructive pulmonary disease (COPD); ascites; benign prostatic hypertrophy, which causes bladder outlet obstruction; and colon or rectal obstruction resulting from tumors, constipation, and similar disorders. All these conditions require further evaluation before surgery.

Most of the listed conditions have signs or symptoms that could be detected with a complete history and physical examination. Smoking tobacco is associated with an increased incidence of hernias.

No additional history or physical findings indicative of other diseases are evident.

◆ **Is surgical repair of the hernia recommended?**

◆ If the physical condition of the patient is acceptable, repair of the hernia is appropriate.

 QUICK CUT The risk of intestinal strangulation of the hernia is the most compelling reason for hernia repair.

This risk varies with the type of hernia; hernias with a narrow neck pose a higher risk. Femoral hernias are particularly prone to strangulation (Fig. 10-10). Other significant reasons for repair include local pain, enlargement, inability to lift, and patient preference.

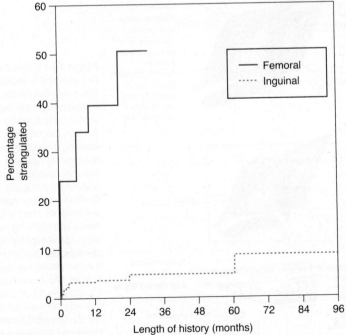

Figure 10-10: Cumulative incidence of strangulation with inguinal and femoral hernias.

♦ **What are the surgical options for hernia repair and their advantages?**

♦ The basic surgical options for a direct or indirect hernia are open and laparoscopic repair.

OPEN REPAIRS

♦ **Bassini repair** involves a reconstruction of the posterior inguinal canal, with a suturing of a superior abdominal wall layer (internal oblique muscle, transversus abdominal muscle, and **transversalis fascia**) to an inferior location on **the inguinal ligament** and iliopubic tract (Fig. 10-11).

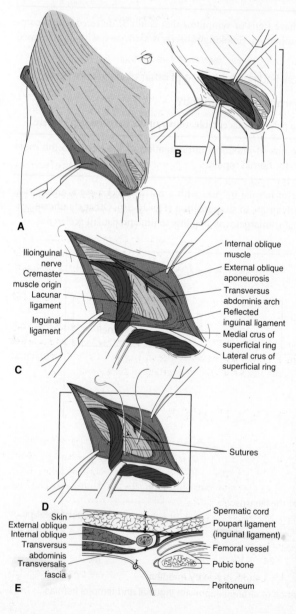

A

B

Ilioinguinal nerve
Cremaster muscle origin
Lacunar ligament
Inguinal ligament

Internal oblique muscle
External oblique aponeurosis
Transversus abdominis arch
Reflected inguinal ligament
Medial crus of superficial ring
Lateral crus of superficial ring

C

D

Sutures

Skin
External oblique
Internal oblique
Transversus abdominis
Transversalis fascia

E

Spermatic cord
Poupart ligament (inguinal ligament)
Femoral vessel
Pubic bone
Peritoneum

Figure 10-11: Bassini repair. **A:** Parasagittal section through the groin. The hernia (through a weakness in the transversalis fascia) is repaired by suturing the transversalis fascia to the shelving (reflecting) edge of the inguinal ligament. **B:** The external oblique aponeurosis and external ring are opened. **C:** The spermatic cord is elevated. **D:** The transversalis fascia and shelving (reflecting) edge of the inguinal ligament are exposed. **E:** Suturing of the two structures together follows. (Redrawn from Fitzgibbons RJ Jr, Greenburg AG, eds. *Nyhus and Condon's Hernia*, 5th ed. Philadelphia: Lippincott Williams & Wilkins; 2002:36, 69.)

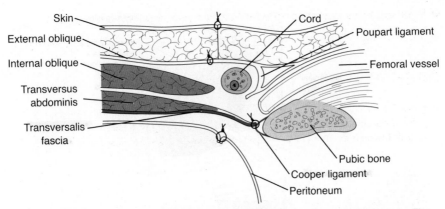

Figure 10-12: Cooper ligament or McVay repair. Parasagittal section through the groin. The hernia (through a weakness in the transversalis fascia) is repaired by suturing the transversalis fascia to Cooper ligament, which is a portion of the periosteum of the pubic bone. The exposure is similar to that shown for the Bassini repair but with deeper dissection to expose the pubic ramus with Cooper ligament. (Redrawn from Fitzgibbons RJ Jr, Greenburg AG, eds. *Nyhus and Condon's Hernia*, 5th ed. Philadelphia: Lippincott Williams & Wilkins; 2002:36.)

Bassini repair was a widely practiced procedure, but as tension free repairs have reported lower recurrence rates, this repair has lost favor.

◆ **Cooper ligament repair** is similar to Bassini repair except that the inferior sutures are placed into Cooper ligament, which is the **periosteum of the pubic ramus** (Fig. 10-12). This approach is better for femoral hernias and attenuated inguinal ligaments.

 QUICK CUT Most hernia repairs attach the transversalis fascia to either the inguinal ligament or the periosteum of the pubic ramus to the inguinal ligament.

◆ **Shouldice repair,** another widely practiced procedure, involves attaching a reinforced transversalis fascia to the inguinal ligament in multiple layers.
◆ **Lichtenstein repair** uses **prosthetic mesh** to approximate the superior abdominal wall structures to the inguinal ligament (Fig. 10-13). The **use of mesh avoids creating tension on the fascial structures**, which is believed to lessen postoperative pain and recurrence. **This procedure has become popular with a high percentage of surgeons.**

LAPAROSCOPIC PROCEDURES

◆ Laparoscopic procedures are acceptable and effective and have gained wide acceptance.
Transabdominal preperitoneal repair involves attachment of mesh to the floor of the inguinal canal from the preperitoneal space (i.e., from within the abdominal cavity) but in a preperitoneal location (Fig. 10-14). Its major complications are general anesthesia and the risk of abdominal adhesion at the laparoscopic sites.
Totally extraperitoneal repair entails inflation of a balloon in the preperitoneal plane to expose the inguinal floor. Once exposed, the floor can be laparoscopically repaired using a prosthetic mesh to cover the defect.

The patient wants to know the potential complications of the procedure and his chance for cure.

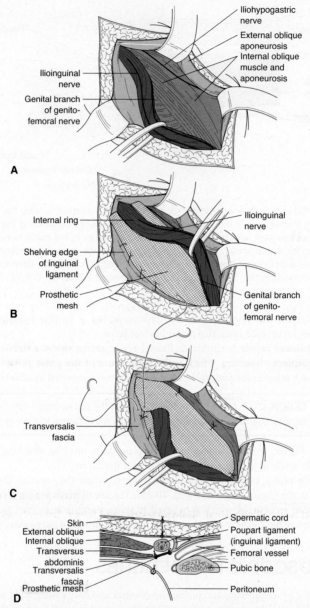

Figure 10-13: Lichtenstein repair. **A:** The hernia (through a weakness in the transversalis fascia) is repaired by a piece of mesh sutured to the transversalis fascia and shelving edge of the inguinal ligament. **B:** The spermatic cord together with its cremasteric covering, external spermatic vessels, and genital nerve is raised, and the cremasteric fibers are cut transversely or longitudinally at the level of the internal ring. **C:** The spermatic cord is placed between the two tails of the mesh. **D:** The lower edges of the two tails are sutured to the inguinal ligament for creation of a new internal ring made of mesh. (Redrawn from Fitzgibbons RJ Jr, Greenburg AG, eds. *Nyhus and Condon's Hernia*, 5th ed. Philadelphia: Lippincott Williams & Wilkins; 2002:36, 151, 153.)

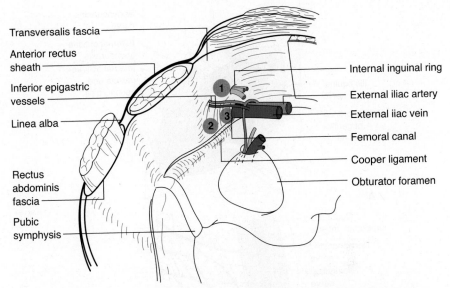

Transversalis fascia

Anterior rectus sheath

Inferior epigastric vessels

Linea alba

Rectus abdominis fascia

Pubic symphysis

Internal inguinal ring

External iliac artery

External iiac vein

Femoral canal

Cooper ligament

Obturator foramen

Figure 10-14: Laparoscopic repair of inguinal hernia. A view of the posterior aspect of the inguinal region. No. *1* is the site of an indirect inguinal hernia, which is lateral to the inferior epigastric vessels, traveling down the inguinal canal. No. *2* is the site of a direct inguinal hernia, which is medial to the inferior epigastric vessels, traveling directly through the posterior wall of the inguinal canal. No. *3* is the site of a femoral hernia, which is deep to the inguinal ligament, traveling through the femoral canal. All three types of hernia result from defects in the transversalis fascia. There are several approaches to hernias in these locations using a laparoscope. Repairs generally involve the use of onlay mesh graphs, mesh plugs, and stapling devices. (From Greenfield LJ, Mulholland MW, Oldham KT, et al, eds. *Surgery: Scientific Principles and Practice*, 2nd ed. Philadelphia: Lippincott Williams & Wilkins; 1997:1222.)

◆ **How do you respond?**

◆ The principal complications of hernia repair are injuries to nerves, bleeding, the intestine, or the vas deferens and the blood vessels to the testicles. Injury to the genital branch of **genitofemoral nerve, ilioinguinal, iliohypogastric, and lateral femoral cutaneous nerves** may occur, resulting in sensory defects (Fig. 10-15). The rate of recurrence, which varies according to the type of procedure and the experience of the surgeon, is 1%–10%. Other problems such as testicular atrophy, edema, and ischemia are rare. Wound infection and wound hematoma occur in less than 1% of cases.

Successful repair of the patient's hernia using the Lichtenstein method has occurred.

◆ **What instructions should the patient receive regarding short- and long-term follow-up?**

◆ The patient should **avoid lifting for the first 6 weeks** after hernia surgery. By that time, the wound should have regained 75%–90% of its final strength. Gradual progression to full lifting is then possible. Most surgeons would see the patient in the office 1 week and 6 weeks postsurgery to monitor healing of the incision. Patients who have any wound complications or questions about hernia recurrence should return to the office.

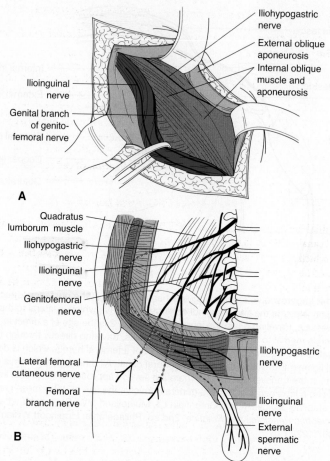

Figure 10-15: A: Distribution of the nerves of the inguinal region. **B:** The nerves seen from a hernia incision. The nerves exposed during repair are the most commonly injured, causing sensory defects in their distribution. (Redrawn from Fitzgibbons RJ Jr, Greenburg AG, eds. *Nyhus and Condon's Hernia*, 5th ed. Philadelphia: Lippincott Williams & Wilkins; 2002:39, 151.)

Case 10.12 Additional Hernia-Related Problems

A 32-year-old man has an inguinal hernia. You are repairing the hernia and are almost ready to make your incision. Your resident asks you to describe the surgical landmarks of the inguinal canal.

◆ **What structures would you identify?**

◆ The most important structures to identify and preserve while repairing the hernia are the ilioinguinal nerve and spermatic cord. Obviously, knowledge of the internal and external rings and general anatomy are important.

   Your resident asks you to briefly describe the difference between the following hernias.

◆ **What is your response?**

Case Variation 10.12.1. An adult and a pediatric inguinal hernia

◆ Pediatric hernias rarely involve a defect in the floor of the inguinal canal; thus, they are indirect inguinal hernias.

 QUICK CUT Pediatric hernias differ from adult hernias in that pediatric hernias usually represent a persistent patent processus vaginalis.

There is a direct communication between the peritoneal cavity and inguinal canal and scrotum in hernias in children, which are usually intermittent and are detected by the child's mother. There is a **high incidence of bilaterality**, and many surgeons repair both sides simultaneously. Repair is usually limited to a **high ligation of the sac** with no abdominal wall repair because no abdominal wall defect is present (Fig. 10-16).

Case Variation 10.12.2. An inguinal and femoral hernia

◆ An **inguinal hernia** is a defect in the abdominal wall allowing structures to pass down the inguinal canal, or through the floor of the inguinal canal, toward the scrotum. The **femoral hernia**, which is more common in women, **typically produces a mass below the inguinal ligament**. The hernia passes into the upper thigh through a space bounded anteriorly by the iliopubic tract (reflection of the inguinal ligament), posteriorly by Cooper ligament (pubic ramus) periosteum, medially by the pubic tubercle and its ligamentous attachments, and laterally by the femoral vein. Repair of a femoral hernia involves closing the femoral space with either mesh or a Cooper ligament (McVay) repair (Fig. 10-17).

You are repairing an inguinal hernia.

◆ **In addition to nerves, what other structures can be intimate with the hernia and therefore injured in the repair?**

◆ Hernias, so-called sliding hernias, may involve other structures that form part of a wall of a hernia (Fig. 10-18). Sliding hernias most commonly occur in indirect hernias. **The most common forms involve the bladder, cecum, or sigmoid colon.** The protrusion of a portion of the intestine wall into the hernia sac results in a Richter hernia. The protrusion of a

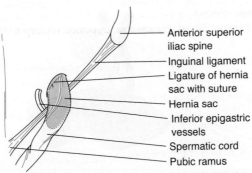

Anterior superior
iliac spine
Inguinal ligament
Ligature of hernia
sac with suture
Hernia sac
Inferior epigastric
vessels
Spermatic cord
Pubic ramus

Figure 10-16: Pediatric hernias, which are characterized by a patent processus vaginalis with a communication between the peritoneal cavity and the inguinal canal, are repaired by "high" ligation of the sac at the point where it just enters the peritoneal cavity. There is no defect in the floor of the inguinal canal; no repair is necessary there. (Redrawn from Fitzgibbons RJ Jr, Greenburg AG, eds. *Nyhus and Condon's Hernia*, 5th ed. Philadelphia: Lippincott Williams & Wilkins; 2002:78.)

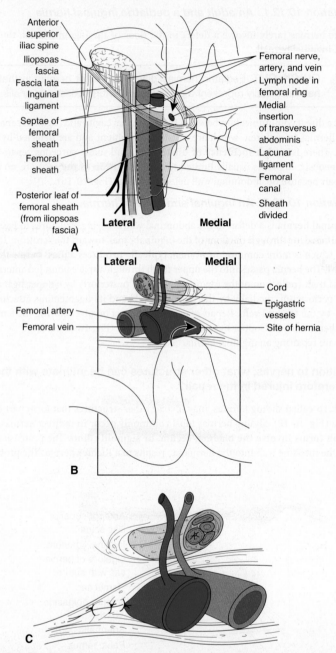

Figure 10-17: A: The femoral sheath and its associated structures. The anterior leaf of the sheath is continuous with the transversalis fascia of the anterior abdominal wall, and the posterior sheath is derived from the iliacus fascia (a portion of the transversalis fascia). Arrow in A and B indicate site of hernia. **B:** Femoral hernias enter the femoral canal, which lies just medial to the femoral vein within its sheath. **C:** A crucial, transitional suture that includes connective tissue investing the femoral vein is necessary to obliterate the defect completely. (*continued*)

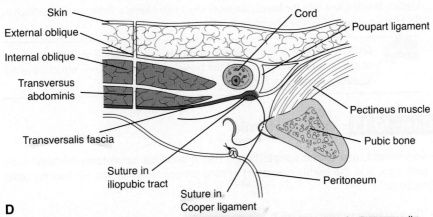

Skin
External oblique
Internal oblique
Transversus abdominis
Transversalis fascia
Suture in iliopubic tract
Cord
Poupart ligament
Pectineus muscle
Pubic bone
Peritoneum
Suture in Cooper ligament

D

Figure 10-17: (*continued*) **D:** Repair of a femoral hernia involves suturing the transversalis fascia/femoral sheath to Cooper ligament, similar to a Cooper ligament repair. (From Fitzgibbons RJ Jr, Greenburg AG, eds. *Nyhus and Condon's Hernia*, 5th ed. Philadelphia: Lippincott Williams & Wilkins; 2002:68, 191, 194.)

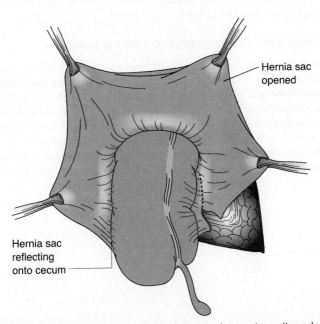

Hernia sac opened

Hernia sac reflecting onto cecum

Figure 10-18: Sliding hernia. The visceral peritoneum covering a retroperitoneal organ is also part of the wall of the hernia sac. The organ must be dissected away from the sac and returned to the peritoneal cavity, after which the hernia is repaired using standard methods. (From Greenfield LJ, Mulholland MW, Oldham KT, et al, eds. *Surgery: Scientific Principles and Practice*, 2nd ed. Philadelphia: Lippincott Williams & Wilkins; 1997:1219.)

Meckel diverticulum into the hernia sac results in a Littré hernia. Other structures such as the ovary and appendix may also occur in a hernia.

 QUICK CUT It is important to recognize the presence of a sliding hernia at the time of surgery so that the bowel or other contained structure is not injured during the repair.

Case 10.13   Ventral Hernia

A 46-year-old man with a ventral hernia had a previous laparotomy for adhesions 1 year ago, and the hernia has been getting progressively larger. He has no other symptoms.

◆ **Do you recommend repair?**

◆ Hernia repair is generally recommended because there is a risk of bowel incarceration and strangulation, which is greater for defects with a narrow neck. Progressive enlargement of the defect, making later repair more difficult, is also a possibility. Hernia repair might not be appropriate if the patient's medical condition is poor and the operative risk is excessive. However, repair is definitely warranted if a previous episode of bowel obstruction or other major complication related to the hernia has occurred.

◆ **How involved a procedure is repair of a ventral hernia?**

◆ Some ventral hernias are simple and easy to repair with primary closure. Larger or recurrent hernias may be very difficult to repair because of **inadequate tissue strength, insufficient tissue, infection,** or **poor nutrition.** Prosthetic mesh, which is sometimes required for closure, carries the risk of infection. In addition, most ventral hernias require entry into the peritoneal cavity and dissection of the bowel off the posterior surface of the hernia sac. This is associated with the risk of bowel injury as well as the probability of postoperative ileus, abdominal distention, and pulmonary complications such as atelectasis. The laparoscopic approach is now often used for ventral hernia repairs when technically feasible.

Chapter 11

Breast Disorders

Bruce E. Jarrell, Emily Bellavance, Michelle Townsend-Watts,
Katherine Tkaczuk, Eric D. Strauch

Key Thoughts

1. Because breast cancer is so common, self-examinations and screening mammography are important elements for early detection.

2. Screening mammography reduces breast cancer mortality by 30% in patients older than age 50 years.

3. One or more first-degree relatives who have had breast cancer is the most common increased risk factor.

4. Strong family history of breast cancer (multiple family members) or diagnosis of breast cancer at a young age may be associated with genetic mutations including deleterious mutations in BRCA1 and BRCA2. The presence of these mutations may affect the treatment choices made by the patient.

5. It is imperative to confirm that the correct suspicious lesion was biopsied, particularly if the biopsy is negative. This can be accomplished by physical exam, specimen radiography, intraoperative ultrasound, or postoperative radiologic evaluation.

6. Ten percent to 20% of lesions diagnosed as ductal carcinoma in situ have an infiltrative component at excision. Thus, complete excision of diseased tissue with negative margins is important.

7. Lobular carcinoma in situ is associated with (i.e., is a marker for) an increased risk of breast cancer, both invasive ductal and lobular, in both breasts.

8. Survival rates are the same for patients treated with aggressive resection (mastectomy) versus breast conservation (lumpectomy and radiation). Radiation therapy after lumpectomy greatly reduces the chance of local recurrence.

9. Tumors often drain to particular nodes first, called the *sentinel nodes.* In breast cancer, this is most commonly in the axilla and can be detected by the injection of dye or radiotracer into the lymphatics. If this node is negative for tumor, then the remaining axillary nodes are negative. This technique has saved many patients the morbidity of an axillary lymph node dissection.

10. Systemic adjuvant therapy for positive axillary nodes decreases the risk of recurrence of breast cancer by up to 30%.

11. Local advanced breast cancer and inflammatory breast cancer require multimodal therapy including induction chemotherapy, surgical resection, and postoperative radiation therapy.

12. Stage for stage, survival for men with breast cancer is similar to that of women.

13. A bloody nipple discharge is most commonly from an intraductal papilloma and is locally excised.

Case 11.1 Screening for Breast Cancer

A 42-year-old woman comes to you for routine evaluation. Her past history is significant for no previous visits to a physician. She asks your advice regarding prevention and early detection of breast cancer. Physical examination reveals no breast or axillary abnormalities.

◆ **What management advice should you give this woman?**

◆ Breast cancer affects one in eight women at some point in their lives. Most physicians recommend breast self-examination, as well as breast examination by a physician once yearly. Traditionally, screening mammogram starts at age 40 years. Screening recommendations are outlined in Table 11-1.

The woman asks what factors increase her risk of breast cancer.

◆ **What do you tell her?**

◆ Research has demonstrated that breast cancer has hereditary patterns.

 QUICK CUT The most common factor that increases the risk of breast cancer is having one or more first-degree relatives who have had breast cancer.

Inherited breast cancer can be associated with identifiable genetic mutations including deleterious mutations in the BRCA1 and BRCA2. BRCA1 and BRCA2 are also associated with ovarian cancer.

Other conditions place women at a high risk for breast cancer (Table 11-2). Based on a careful history revealing a first-degree relative with breast cancer, you decide that this patient is at increased risk for breast cancer.

Table 11-1: Recommended Screening Level

Woman's Risk Level	Mammography	Magnetic Resonance Imaging (MRI)*
Normal	Annual starting at age 40 years	
Lobar carcinoma in situ Atypical ductal hyperplasia Atypical lobular hyperplasia	Annual after diagnosis	
Personal history of breast cancer	Annual after diagnosis	
BRCA+; multiple first-degree and second-degree relatives; bilateral in first-degree premenopausal relative; breast/ovarian cancer family history	Annual starting 10 years younger than youngest relative but not younger than 25 years	Annual
Hodgkin lymphoma treated with mantle radiation	Annual starting 8 years after treatment	Annual

*MRI and mammogram should be scheduled 6 months apart to screen patient twice yearly, as cancers in these patients may be rapidly growing.
From DeVita VT Jr, Lawrence TS, Rosenberg SA, et al, eds. *DeVita, Hellman, and Rosenberg's Cancer: Principles and Practice of Oncology*, 9th ed. Baltimore: Lippincott Williams & Wilkins; 2011.

Table 11-2: Risk Factors for Breast Cancer

Factor	High Risk	Low Risk
Relative Risk More Than 4×		
Age	Older	Younger
History of cancer in one breast	Yes	No
Family history of premenopausal or bilateral breast cancer	Yes	No
Relative Risk 2–4×		
Any first-degree relative with breast cancer	Yes	No
History of primary cancer of ovary or endometrium	Yes	No
Age at first full-term pregnancy	Older than 30 years	Younger than 20 years
Oophorectomy	No	Yes
Body habitus, postmenopausal	Obese	Thin
Relative Risk 1–2×		
Age at menarche (younger than 12 years)	Early	Late
Age at menopause (older than 55 years)	Late	Early

Adapted with permission from Kelsey JL, Gannon MD. The epidemiology of breast cancer. *CA Cancer J Clin*. 1991;41(31):146–165.

◆ **How might this change your advice and management?**

◆ Increased risk should prompt both a more frequent surveillance for any abnormalities and a higher degree of suspicion for any given finding. Based on degree of risk, experts have developed general guidelines for necessary screening.

The woman wants to know how screening tests will improve her chances of survival if she is affected by breast cancer.

◆ **What do you tell her?**

◆ Several studies have demonstrated that **annual mammography detects lesions when they are smaller, before they are evident on physical examination.** This benefit appears to be strongest in women between 50 and 64 years of age. The American Medical Association has extended this to women between the ages of 40 and 50 years. Most screening studies for breast cancer are associated with a mortality reduction of 30% or more in women older than 50 years of age.

Mammographic screening should begin **earlier if there is a strong family history.** In women with first-degree relatives who have had breast cancer, some physicians would recommend beginning annual mammography 10 years before the age of the relative at diagnosis of the cancer. Women with greater than 20% lifetime risk of developing breast cancer should also be screened with annual breast magnetic resonance imaging (MRI). Mammograms are reliable; however, **it is never appropriate to delay biopsy of a clinically suspicious lesion just because a mammogram is negative.**

◆ **What risks do mammograms pose?**

◆ The primary risks associated with mammography are radiation exposure and false-negative results. The radiation exposure for most modern mammograms is 0.1–0.3 rad per study. For comparison, radiation exposure from chest radiography is 0.05 rad per study. Experts believe that the radiation from a mammogram is very low. The best estimates indicate that perhaps one death secondary to breast cancer per million women per year occurs as a result of radiation exposure. Mammograms have a false-negative rate of about 7%–20%. This rate may be higher in younger women and women with more glandular and less fatty, atrophic tissue. Mammography appears to be more accurate in older women whose glandular breast tissue has become atrophic and replaced with fat.

Case 11.2   Evaluation of a Mammographic Abnormality

A 60-year-old woman is referred by her primary physician for an abnormality on her routine mammogram. She has a negative history for breast cancer. She is G_3P_3, and since undergoing a hysterectomy 20 years ago, she has been taking estrogen replacement therapy. The mammogram shows a solid 1.5-cm mass in the upper outer quadrant. The surgeon to whom the patient is referred confirms that no masses are palpable in the breast. The axillary, supraclavicular, and cervical areas are negative for lymph nodes.

◆ **What are the various types of mammographic abnormalities?**

◆ Mammographic abnormalities can generally be classified as combinations of the following entities:

1. **Masses**
2. **Asymmetries**
3. **Microcalcifications**

◆ When an abnormality is found on screening, additional imaging is usually appropriate. The interpretation receives the Breast Imaging Reporting and Database System (BI-RADS) category 0 ("needs additional evaluation") designations. For microcalcifications, spot magnification mammographic views are usually necessary (Table 11-3 and Fig. 11-1). For masses and asymmetry, it is often necessary to supplement additional mammographic views with ultrasound to obtain a final assessment. Asymmetry or asymmetric densities can result from operative procedures, previous radiation therapy, previous infections, normal variation, other local processes, and cancer.

Table 11-3: Mammography Categories According to the Breast Imaging Reporting and Database System

Category	Interpretation
0	Needs additional evaluation
1	Normal
2	Benign findings, recommend routine screening
3	Probably benign, recommend short initial (6-month) follow-up
4	Suspicious, biopsy should be considered
5	Highly suggestive of malignancy

From the American College of Radiology. *ACR BI-RADS Atlas.* 5th ed. Reston, VA: American College of Radiology; 2014.

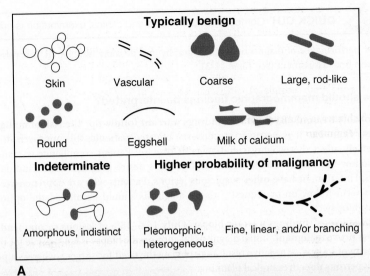

A

Figure 11-1. **A:** Diagram showing the morphology of typically benign calcifications and those with a higher probability of malignancy. **B:** A mammogram showing a spiculated mass in the breast that is positive for infiltrating ductal carcinoma.

> **QUICK CUT** Comparison to old films and clinical examination is critical.

After performance of diagnostic mammography and possibly ultrasound, it is possible to make a final assessment (see Table 11-3).

◆ **How should mammographic findings be interpreted?**

◆ **"Probably benign" (BI-RADS 3) findings warrant follow-up. The risk of malignancy is less than 2%.** It is necessary to observe affected patients; this approach does not adversely affect the prognosis and stage of disease. Patient compliance is mandatory for follow-up. Biopsy may be essential if patients desire pregnancy, are candidates for transplantation, or have other suspicious lesions. Patients who are apprehensive about short-term follow-up or request a tissue diagnosis should be offered the option of a breast biopsy.

　　"Suspicious" findings warrant biopsy. Only 15%–35% of lesions recommended for biopsy prove malignant. Initial diagnosis by core-needle biopsy is appropriate for the vast majority of lesions. A negative result may obviate the need for surgery, whereas a positive result permits directive surgical planning.

Case 11.3　Evaluation of Mammographic Microcalcifications

A 44-year-old woman has a screening mammogram, which shows a 1-cm area of pleomorphic microcalcifications, with no associated mass. These findings are suspicious for ductal carcinoma in situ. Breast examination is normal, with no palpable abnormalities.

◆ **What is the next step?**

◆ Because there are no palpable abnormalities, the radiologist would typically perform a **diagnostic mammogram**, which allows for additional views and magnification, if indicated. Ultrasound may be useful for suspicious calcifications; it can detect an occult mass in up to one third of patients. After further evaluation, the radiologist would recommend either a stereotactic-guided core-needle biopsy (Fig. 11-2) or, if the lesion is visible on ultrasound, an ultrasound-guided core biopsy. Multiple cores can be taken with an 11-gauge to 14-gauge needle. **Fine-needle aspiration (FNA) is not the preferred technique** to use for biopsy in this case because it often produces a nondiagnostic specimen. **Needle localization and open surgical biopsy may be preferable if a lesion cannot be biopsied with imaging either because of location of the lesion in the breast, breast morphology, or patient habitus** (Fig. 11-3). Image-guided biopsy results that are not concordant (not consistent with the imaging findings) or nondiagnostic should be biopsied surgically.

　　In needle localization and open surgical biopsy, a clinician puts a needle into the mammographically or sonographically demonstrated lesion under radiologic guidance and leaves it in place while the patient is transported to the operating room. Using the needle as a guide, a surgeon excises the lesion. A radiologist and the surgeon must then evaluate the specimen (specimen radiography) to ensure that the lesion has been removed. Ultrasound can be used intraoperatively to localize ultrasound-detected lesions as well.

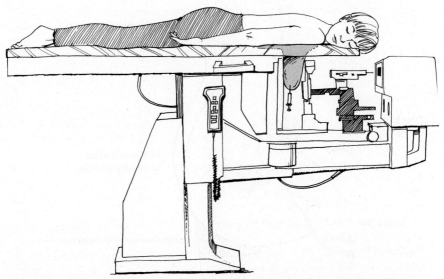

Figure 11-2: Stereotactic breast biopsy. The patient is positioned on a table that allows precise imaging of the breast lesion and image-guided biopsy of the lesion. (From Silen W. *Atlas of Techniques in Breast Surgery.* Philadelphia: Lippincott-Raven; 1996:50.)

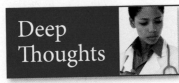

Deep Thoughts

No matter how the biopsy is obtained, it is imperative that the appropriate tissue is biopsied.

Case 11.4 Biopsy Results in Lesions Visible on Mammography

A 40-year-old woman has her first mammogram, which reveals amorphous calcifications in one breast. She then has stereotactic core biopsy.

◆ **What evaluation and management are appropriate for the following pathologic findings?**

Case Variation 11.4.1. *Ductal carcinoma in situ (DCIS)*

◆ DCIS usually manifests as incidental microcalcifications on mammography, although 5% of patients may present with a breast mass. **Surgery is necessary** (see Fig. 11-3). Even when the best technique is used for core biopsy, **10%–20% of lesions diagnosed as DCIS have an infiltrative component at excision**. Thus, careful examination and complete excision of diseased tissue is important. If lesions are incompletely excised or untreated, the 10-year risk of invasive carcinoma is 30% or more. The risk of contralateral invasive carcinoma is 5% or less over a 10-year period. In general, invasive carcinoma is more likely in larger lesions rather than smaller ones.

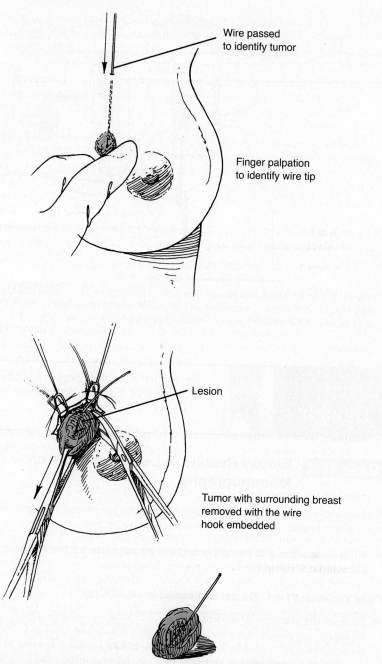

Figure 11-3: Needle localization and biopsy in a lesion that is not palpable. Under radiographic imaging, the lesion is identified and a wire with a hook is placed into the lesion to fix the wire within the lesion. The patient then goes to the operating room, where the lesion and the wire are surgically excised. A radiograph of the removed lesion and wire is then taken to be certain that the appropriate lesion has been obtained. (From Silen W. *Atlas of Techniques in Breast Surgery*. Philadelphia: Lippincott-Raven; 1996:52, 55.)

DCIS can be multifocal. DCIS has several histologic patterns, including comedo, micropapillary, and cribriform. The **comedo pattern has a higher malignant potential, with up to 30% containing invasive carcinoma**. Axillary metastasis is present in 4% of patients with the comedo variant but rare in those with other histologic patterns.

QUICK CUT Simple mastectomy with or without reconstruction is the current gold standard for diffuse and multicentric DCIS.

◆ Wide excision (partial mastectomy) and radiotherapy is a preferred alternative for smaller lesions, although some patients with an isolated focus of DCIS may still opt for a mastectomy without radiation, which is an equally effective treatment. **If wide excision is performed, it is important to document pathology-free margins in the specimen.** Local recurrence rate of DCIS is decreased by one half with wide excision and radiation. Adjuvant radiation treatment is the standard of care with breast conservation treatment for DCIS. **Nodal dissection is not necessary** because nodal metastases are rare except for the comedo variant. In the comedo case, axillary node sampling (by sentinel node approach) may be appropriate.

Case Variation 11.4.2. Lobular carcinoma in situ (LCIS)

◆ LCIS is usually an incidental finding at histopathology (Fig. 11-4). Patients rarely present with a mass, and LCIS may not be apparent on mammography. When found adjacent to a benign mass, **surveillance is appropriate. LCIS confers an increased risk of breast cancer in both breasts. Excision of LCIS is controversial because the chance of finding invasive cancer or DCIS with excision is variable in the literature (4%–25%). Pleomorphic LCIS should be excised.**

Treatment for LCIS is excision or **close observation**, with examination and mammography every 6 months for at least the next 2 years. Patient may take estrogen-blocking medication to decrease their risk of developing breast cancer in the future.

Case Variation 11.4.3. Sclerosing adenosis

◆ Sclerosing adenosis usually manifests as clustered microcalcifications on mammography. It may appear similar to invasive tubular carcinoma histopathologically (see Fig. 11-4). The associated cancer risk may be slightly higher (approximately 1.5–2×). Routine follow-up is appropriate after a diagnosis of sclerosing adenosis on core biopsy, provided there is agreement with the mammographic appearance of the targeted lesion (concordance).

Case Variation 11.4.4. Atypical ductal hyperplasia

◆ Atypical hyperplasia of the ducts or lobules may be seen in breast lesions. This condition is similar in appearance to DCIS, and the two entities are often interspersed (see Fig. 11-4). The **associated risk of cancer is four to five times higher**. When core biopsy results demonstrate atypical ductal hyperplasia, **needle localization and excision are appropriate**. From 15% to 30% of cases prove malignant, depending on the volume of tissue initially sampled. The relative risk for invasive carcinoma can be determined on the basis of histologic examination (Table 11-4). Patients with a diagnosis of atypical ductal hyperplasia should be offered risk reduction with estrogen-blocking medications.

Case 11.5 Management of a Woman with a Palpable Breast Mass

A 60-year-old woman presents with a right breast mass that was palpated by her primary care physician. She denies any breast-related symptoms, and she has

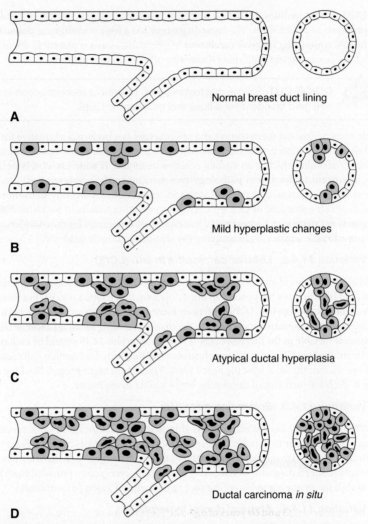

Figure 11-4: Progression of breast duct lining from normal to carcinoma in situ. A: Normal. B: Mild hyperplastic changes. C: Atypical ductal hyperplasia. D: Ductal carcinoma in situ. In the normal duct, there are two layers of cells with a myoepithelial outer layer and an epithelial layer on the inside. In the usual hyperplastic lesion, there is hyperplasia of the inner lining. With atypical ductal hyperplasia, there is secondary bridging and additional hypertrophy of the epithelial layer. In carcinoma in situ, there is marked proliferation with carcinoma limited by the basal lamina.

never had other medical problems. Her past history is significant for the following conditions:

- Menarche, age 12 years; G_2P_2, ages 23 and 25 years; menopause, age 50 years
- Family history that is negative for cancer
- Social history that is negative for alcohol and tobacco use but positive for daily caffeine use

Physical examination is normal except for the right breast, which reveals a 1.5-cm nontender mass in the upper outer quadrant that is freely movable but firm. No axillary or supraclavicular adenopathy is evident.

Table 11-4: Relative Risk for Invasive Breast Carcinoma Based on Histologic Examination

No increased risk (no proliferative disease)
Apocrine change
Ductal ectasia
Mild epithelial hyperplasia of usual type
Slightly increased risk (1.5–2×)
Hyperplasia of usual type, moderate or florid
Sclerosing adenosis, papilloma
Moderately increased risk (4–5×) (atypical hyperplasia or borderline lesions)
Atypical ductal hyperplasia and atypical lobular hyperplasia
High risk (8–10×) (carcinoma in situ)
Lobular carcinoma in situ and ductal carcinoma in situ

From Greenfield LJ, Mulholland MW, Oldham KT, et al, eds. *Surgery: Scientific Principles and Practice,* 2nd ed. Philadelphia: Lippincott Williams & Wilkins; 1997.

◆ **What management plan is appropriate?**

◆ The diagnosis is most likely carcinoma. The patient should undergo the following procedures:

1. A **mammogram** to better characterize the affected breast and its lesion(s) as well as to examine the contralateral breast for synchronous lesions
2. A **biopsy if the mass feels solid**; this procedure establishes the diagnosis in 97% of cases. A core biopsy is appropriate under image guidance. FNA for cytology, which is generally not sufficient to establish a diagnosis in 20% of cases, cannot distinguish in situ from infiltrating carcinomas.

◆ **How would the management plan change in the following women with similar physical findings?**

Case Variation 11.5.1. A 40-year-old menstruating woman

◆ **In women between 35 and 60 years of age, such breast masses are cancerous until proven otherwise.** There is no difference in the workup in the 35–60-year age group.

Case Variation 11.5.2. A 28-year-old woman

◆ **Management may differ for patients younger than 30 years of age because younger women have a higher incidence of benign lesions and a higher risk of radiation from mammography.** However, a suspicion of carcinoma is always appropriate, even in young patients. An ultrasound study and mammogram is appropriate in women older than 25 years. If the lesion were a simple cyst, then observation or simple aspiration would be the treatment, assuming the mass completely disappeared following aspiration. If the lesion were solid and typical of a fibroadenoma, a core biopsy is appropriate to confirm the diagnosis. The patient has the option for surgical removal of the fibroadenoma or observation.

Observation may be indicated for selected young women in whom nodularity or breast lumps appears physiologic. A physician may observe patients for one or two menstrual cycles and then follow them if there is no change in physical findings. It is important to note that this is acceptable standard of care only in low-risk women of young age (younger than 30 years). In older women or women at increased risk for breast cancer, definitive diagnosis is necessary. Ultrasound is warranted for evaluation of masses that develop in pregnant young women, and close follow-up is necessary. **Core-needle biopsy is appropriate if the mass persists, enlarges, or appears suspicious because the risk of cancer is significant.**

Case 11.6   Management of a Woman with "Lumpy" Breasts

A 35-year-old woman has tender breasts before her menstrual periods. She complains of "lumpy" breasts.

◆ **What evaluation and management are appropriate?**

◆ **Fibrocystic breasts,** the most common cause of this patient's condition, is a pathologic diagnosis that includes cysts, fibrosis, sclerosing adenosis, apocrine change, and hyperplasia. This disorder is uncommon before adolescence or after menopause. Usually bilateral, it is characterized by lumpy breasts and premenstrual tenderness. Possible causes include increased sensitivity to estrogen or decreased progesterone activity.

Mammography may be warranted to evaluate fibrocystic breasts. If a discrete, painful cyst is present, treatment involves cyst aspiration as long as the cyst completely disappears. Some physicians would also recommend elimination of caffeine from the diet and supplemental vitamin E. Follow-up in 3–6 months is also appropriate. If a mass is present and the diagnosis is unclear, a biopsy is necessary. **Fibrocystic breast disease is not associated with an increased risk of cancer, but cancer risk increases if hyperplastic epithelium demonstrates atypia on biopsy of fibrocystic lesions.**

Case 11.7   Management of a Breast Mass in a Young Woman

A 20-year-old woman presents with a mass in her breast. The mass is 1.5 cm in diameter, and it is firm, rubbery, nontender, and freely movable. The opposite breast and axillae are normal.

◆ **What evaluation and management are appropriate?**

◆ **Fibroadenoma** is the most common breast tumor in women younger than 25 years of age. This benign lesion, which is more common in African Americans, is a firm, rubbery, painless, movable, well-circumscribed lesion. Biopsy establishes diagnosis. Observation may be appropriate for small lesions, but many patients desire excision. Removal of larger lesions is necessary.

◆ **The lesion is 14 cm in diameter. How would the management plan change?**

◆ A **phyllodes tumor** (cystosarcoma phyllodes, giant cell fibroadenomas), a large, bulky mass of variable malignant potential with occasional ulceration of the overlying skin, is the suspected diagnosis. Factors that determine malignancy are **(1) tumor behavior** and **(2) an increased number of mitoses** per high-power field compared with benign phyllodes tumors (on histology). Treatment is local excision with generous margins that are pathologically free of disease. Fibroadenomas may also infarct and acutely enlarge, creating a similar picture.

Case 11.8   Management of a Woman with Nipple Discharge

A 34-year-old woman sees you because of nipple discharge. She has been healthy and had two uneventful pregnancies; the rest of her history is unremarkable.

On physical examination, the breasts have no masses or tenderness. A small drop of blood is noticeable on the right nipple.

◆ **What management is appropriate?**

◆ In nonlactating women, nonmilky nipple discharge is surgically significant and warrants investigation. **Important variables include whether the discharge is uni- or bilateral, contains blood, and involves single or multiple ducts and whether it is spontaneous or requires stimulation. It is essential to determine whether a mass is present and whether a mammographic or sonographic abnormality exists.** If a mass is palpable or a mammographic or sonographic abnormality is apparent, patients should be evaluated as described in previous cases (see Cases 11.2 and 11.3). If no mass is apparent, bloody nipple discharge is usually treated with a duct exploration and surgical excision of the abnormal duct. The **most common cause of bloody discharge is an intraductal papilloma** that can produce bloody or serosanguineous discharge.

The presence of a clear discharge from a single duct may also be a sign of cancer and should be evaluated the same as bloody nipple discharge. However, clear nipple discharge from multiple ducts is usually related to fibrocystic disease (cystic mastopathy) in younger women or subareolar duct ectasia in older women. Observation is warranted.

QUICK CUT Bloody discharge from a single duct requires surgical biopsy.

After cannulating the duct to identify the lesion, the surgeon excises the duct and ductal system. These lesions may have a small increased risk for carcinoma. Bloody discharge, particularly in older women, does carry a **risk of** carcinoma **(4%–13% in most studies)**. Because these cancers are usually occult and often appear as early intraductal lesions, affected patients should undergo the following measures:

1. **Mammography** to examine for other breast abnormalities
2. **Close examination** of the area around the discharge to identify a single duct that is the source of the bloody discharge

A ductogram, which places radiographic dye into the duct with a small catheter, is a method for further definition of the duct. Alternatively, probing with a small (lacrimal duct) probe may be useful. This allows location of the duct and defines the extent of the process within the breast. Once localized, the area should be **surgically excised** (Fig. 11-5). The usual diagnosis is intraductal papilloma.

Case 11.9 Staging and Prognosis in Infiltrating Ductal Carcinoma

A 57-year-old woman undergoes core-needle biopsy of a breast mass. The pathologic diagnosis returns infiltrating ductal carcinoma of the breast.

◆ **What is involved in staging this cancer?**

◆ The first steps in staging the cancer with the system involve determination of the extent of the local tumor, involvement of regional lymph nodes, and possibility of distant spread (Table 11-5). **Mammography is necessary to assess for other lesions in the same breast and opposite breast.** Cancer staging is based on the tumor–node–metastasis (TNM) classification system (see Table 11-5).

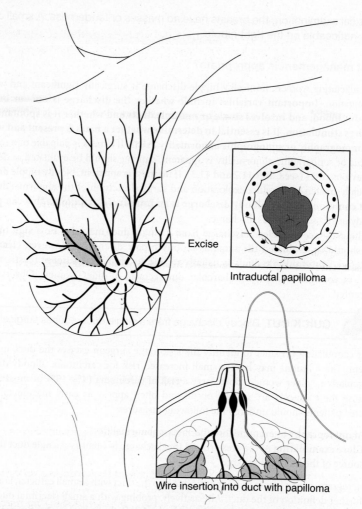

Excise

Intraductal papilloma

Wire insertion into duct with papilloma

Figure 11-5: Intraductal papilloma. As seen in cross-section, the ductal system is radially oriented and communicates with the nipple. A fine probe is placed in the duct that has blood oozing from it, and the probe is then used as a guide for excision of that ductal system. (Redrawn from Silen W. *Atlas of Techniques in Breast Surgery*. Philadelphia: Lippincott-Raven; 1996:14; Greenfield LJ, Mulholland MW, Oldham KT, et al, eds. *Surgery: Scientific Principles and Practice*, 2nd ed. Philadelphia: Lippincott Williams & Wilkins; 1997:1374.)

 QUICK CUT Clinical staging using the TNM system is more important than histopathology of the primary lesion in determining prognosis.

Prognosis is worse in the following circumstances: when axillary lymph nodes contain metastases, when the number of nodes involved with tumor exceeds four, when the primary tumor is large, and when distant metastases are present. Local disease relates to the size of the primary tumor and direct extension to the chest wall or skin (Table 11-6).

Table 11-5: **TNM Classification of Breast Cancer**

T	Tumor Size	N	Node Metastasis	M	Distant Metastasis
T0	In situ	N0	None	M0	None
T1	≤2 cm	Nmi	Microscopic <2 mm	M1	Any
T2	>2 cm to ≤5 cm	N1	Mobile in level I and II axilla		
T3	>5 cm	N2	Fixed in level I and II axilla		
T4	Direct extension to chest wall/skin	N3	Level III axillary, internal mammary, supraclavicular		

Distant metastasis is assessed by several modalities. As a routine part of staging, all patients except those with stage 0 cancer should have a chest radiograph (CXR) to detect lung metastases, as well as liver enzyme measurements to detect liver metastasis. If patients have bone pain or complain of bone-related symptoms or have neurologic signs or symptoms, it is necessary to obtain a bone scan or computed tomography (CT) scan of the head, respectively. If liver enzymes, alkaline phosphatase, or total bilirubin are abnormal, a CT scan of the abdomen is appropriate.

◆ **Are any other factors important in prognosis?**

◆ Several other factors relating to patient characteristics, lesion pathology, and molecular studies are important in prognosis. Certain histologic types as well as molecular factors also have prognostic implications (Table 11-7).

Case 11.10 Some Clinical Factors that Affect Prognosis

A 49-year-old woman presents with a breast mass. You are examining the affected breast.

◆ **How would the following clinical findings affect the woman's prognosis?**

Case Variation 11.10.1. Red edematous breast with an underlying mass

◆ This finding is typical of an **inflammatory carcinoma**, which has a worse prognosis than the usual infiltrating ductal carcinoma.

Case Variation 11.10.2. Edema of the skin overlying the mass

◆ This condition is also called **peau d'orange** because it appears similar to the surface of an orange. The associated tumor invasion of local dermal lymphatics worsens the prognosis.

Table 11-6: **Staging of Breast Cancer**

Stage 0	In situ disease	M0
Stage 1	T1N0, T0–T1Nmi	M0
Stage 2	T2N0, T3N0, T1N1, T2N1	M0
Stage 3	T3N1, any T4, any N2, any N3	M0
Stage 4	Any T any N	M

Table 11-7: Prognostic Indicators in Breast Cancer

Favorable Histologic Types
Tubular carcinoma
Papillary carcinoma   )
Mucinous (colloid) carcinoma
Paget disease of the breast
Less Favorable Histologic Types
Infiltrating ductal carcinoma (most common type)
Infiltrating lobular carcinoma (often multicentric or bilateral)
Medullary carcinoma
Better prognosis than in invasive ductal carcinoma but worse than in lobular carcinoma
Inflammatory carcinoma
Very poor prognosis
Estrogen and Progesterone Receptors
Presence of receptors
Better prognosis
DNA Ploidy
Aneuploid tumors (tumors with an abnormal amount of DNA per cell)
Worse prognosis than diploid tumors, in which metastasis may be slower and drug-resistant mutations may be less common
High S-Phase (Synthetic Phase of Mitosis) Fraction
Ki-67, a nuclear protein associated with mitosis, correlates with S-phase fraction and mitotic index.
Worse prognosis; tumors have a higher proliferative component.
HER-2/neu oncogene (also known as erb-2, related to epidermal growth factor receptor)
Worse prognosis; increased expression of gene product is associated with shorter relapse time and decreased survival rate in node-positive patients.

Case Variation 11.10.3. Extensive edema of the breast

◆ This finding, which is similar to peau d'orange, implies an inflammatory carcinoma. Breast edema may also be present secondary to nodal invasion and blockage of the axillary lymphatics. Note that any of these findings (see Case Variations 11.10.1 and 11.10.2) could also be compatible with cellulitis or abscess of the breast, and it is necessary to interpret them in terms of the individual patient. However, they are all highly likely to represent cancer.

Case Variation 11.10.4. Retraction of the skin overlying the mass

◆ This finding suggests invasion of the breast support structures and lymphatics with tumor. It worsens the prognosis.

Case Variation 11.10.5. Retraction of the nipple

◆ This finding is similar to skin retraction (see Case Variation 11.10.4). However, superficial cancers close to the nipple may cause nipple retraction and still be an early stage cancer.

Case Variation 11.10.6. Two previous aspirations of fluid from the cystic mass but rapid recurrence of the mass

◆ It is necessary to excise cysts that have been aspirated but recur to rule out cancer. Prognosis depends on pathology.

Case Variation 11.10.7. A 1.5-cm mass fixed to the deeper tissues

◆ Fixation to the chest wall indicates invasion of structures outside the breast. This finding worsens the prognosis.

Case Variation 11.10.8. A lymph node palpable in the supraclavicular area

◆ A node in this location represents **stage III disease**. First-line treatment should be systemic.

Case Variation 11.10.9. A hard, fixed lymph node in the ipsilateral axilla

◆ This finding suggests the presence of a matted group of nodes with metastases, which would give the patient a node-positive N2 status.

Case Variation 11.10.10. A soft lymph node in the ipsilateral axilla

◆ This could be an inflammatory node or a metastasis.

Case Variation 11.10.11. Small nodules on the skin of the breast

◆ These may be satellite nodules of carcinoma on the skin. Biopsy is warranted. A diagnosis of cancer worsens the prognosis.

Case Variation 11.10.12. Arm edema

◆ This finding suggests obstruction of the axillary lymphatics and worsens the prognosis.

Case 11.11 Management of a Woman with a Nipple Lesion

A 61-year-old woman presents with a crusty lesion in the nipple of her right breast. You are examining this nipple lesion.

◆ **What evaluation and management are appropriate?**

◆ A chronic eczematoid lesion of the nipple **may be benign**, but it is necessary to rule out the possibility of **Paget disease** of the breast. Ninety-five percent of patients with Paget disease have an underlying pathology, either as infiltrating ductal carcinoma or DCIS. Examination for a subareolar mass and a mammogram are essential. If a mass is present, then it should be evaluated as for any mass with biopsy. **Associated masses are present in approximately 50% of cases; these patients should undergo a central excision (partial mastectomy which includes the nipple and areola) followed by radiation or mastectomy.** If no mass is present, a biopsy of the nipple lesion is appropriate. The presence of Paget cells prompts a high suspicion for cancer and should be treated with a central partial mastectomy and radiation or mastectomy.

◆ **How would finding a subareolar mass affect management?**

◆ Evaluation of a subareolar mass is similar to any other mass (see Case 11.3).

Case 11.12 Surgical Management of Breast Cancer

You are making rounds with the attending surgeon who asks what you think are the important surgical principles in the management of breast cancer.

◆ **How would you answer?**

◆ In breast cancer, it is essential to **establish a diagnosis to determine whether the regional nodes or distant sites are involved with metastasis**. The diagnostic procedures are discussed in other cases and will not be further described (see Cases 11.2, 11.3, and 11.5). In dealing with the primary tumor, it is important to remember that the remaining breast tissue and contralateral breast also require careful evaluation. The incidence rate of multifocal and multicentric disease (as many as 60% of cases) and bilateral processes (as many as 9% of cases) is significant, and recognition of this is critical.

Wide excision with radiation therapy may suffice for a localized tumor if a good cosmetic result and adequate margins can be achieved. A mastectomy is usually recommended for a multicentric tumor or larger tumors. Sampling of axillary nodes with a sentinel node biopsy is necessary for accurate staging; clinical examination alone is not sufficient. Histologic status of level I and II axillary nodes and number of nodes involved are still the best markers of disease behavior and ultimate outcome. There is a linear decrease in survival with an increase in number of nodes involved, with more than 10 being a very poor prognostic indicator. Even more importantly, studies have clearly demonstrated that systemic adjuvant therapy given to patients with involved axillary nodes decreases the risk of recurrence of breast cancer by up to 30%.

The attending surgeon asks you to describe the basic anatomy of the breast.

◆ **What important structures would you identify?**

◆ Between 15 and 20 radially arranged lobes, each of which has 20–40 lobules, make up each breast. A duct, which converges on the nipple, provides the drainage for each lobe. The arterial supply is primarily from the internal mammary (60%) and lateral thoracic arteries (30%). Venous return is primarily via the axillary and internal mammary veins. Lymphatic drainage is principally to the axillary lymph node chain, which is divided into three levels, based on relationship to the pectoralis minor muscle (Fig. 11-6).

The attending surgeon then asks you to describe the commonly performed surgical procedures used to remove a breast cancer.

◆ **How would you describe these surgical methods?**

◆ The **modified radical mastectomy** is the removal of the breast tissue, nipple–areolar complex, and axillary lymph nodes, sparing the pectoralis major muscle (Fig. 11-7A–E). Radiation therapy is not usually used with the modified procedure. However, local radiation therapy following mastectomy is indicated for patients who have tumors greater than 5 cm in diameter that involve the margin of resection or that invade the pectoral fascia or muscle. Axillary radiation may be indicated for patients with more than three lymph nodes involved.

The **radical mastectomy** (Halsted procedure) is largely of historical significance. The surgeon removes breast tissue, nipple–areolar complex skin, pectoralis major and pectoralis minor muscles, and axillary lymph nodes. Radical mastectomies are rarely performed today; early studies found no difference in survival when patients were treated with modified radical mastectomy as compared to radical mastectomy.

The **simple mastectomy** involves the removal of breast tissue, nipple–areolar complex, and skin.

The **skin-sparing mastectomy** involves the removal of breast tissue, the nipple–areolar complex with preservation of as much overlying skin as possible. This procedure is used for patients undergoing immediate reconstruction.

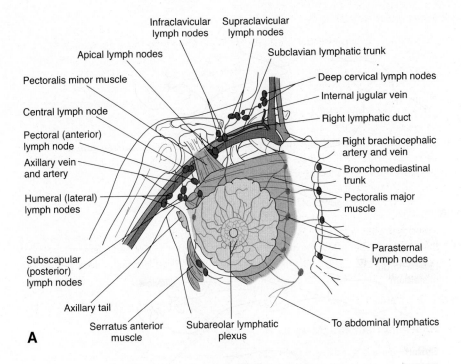

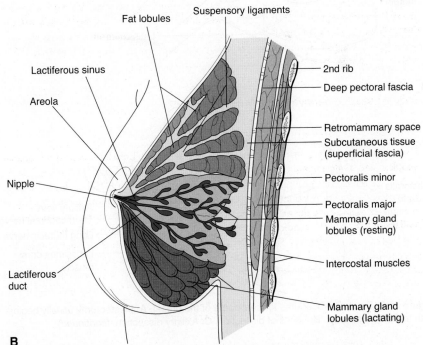

Figure 11-6: Anatomy of the breast. (From Moore KL, Agur AM. *Essential Clinical Anatomy*. Baltimore: Lippincott Williams & Wilkins; 1995:35–36.)

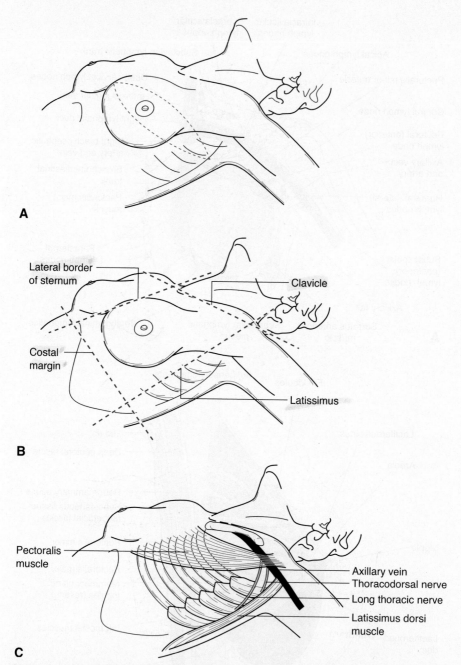

Figure 11-7: Surgical procedures for carcinoma of the breast. **A:** Mastectomy usually begins with transverse incision. **B:** Limits of dissection. **C:** Axillary dissection. (*continued*)

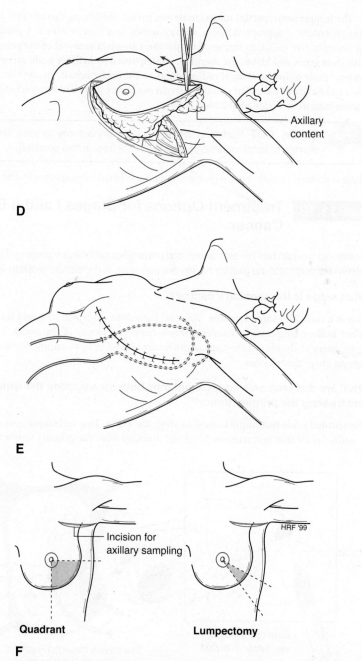

D

E

Incision for
axillary sampling

HRF '99

Quadrant   **Lumpectomy**

F

Figure 11-7: (*continued*) **D:** Breast removed from chest wall, medially from the axillae. Pectoralis fascia is taken, and the pectoralis muscle is left. **E:** Drains are placed beneath the skin flaps, and tissue is closed over chest wall. **F:** Partial mastectomy procedures, which preserve the breast mound. Axillary nodes should be sampled. (From Lawrence PF, Bilbao M, Bell RM, et al, eds. *Essentials of General Surgery*. Baltimore: Lippincott Williams & Wilkins; 1988:277.)

The **lumpectomy/partial mastectomy** is a breast-conserving therapy (see Fig. 11-7F). This procedure is appropriate for a solitary tumor in a patient who is a good candidate for postoperative radiation therapy. **Lumpectomy involves removal of the primary lesion with clear gross and histologic margins, accompanied by axillary node sampling with a sentinel node biopsy and local radiotherapy to the entire breast.** In addition, it may involve irradiation of the axillary nodes, internal mammary nodes, and supraclavicular nodes if more than three nodes are positive.

> **QUICK CUT** Radiation therapy after lumpectomy greatly reduces the chance of local recurrence (see Fig. 11-9 later in this chapter).

There is no survival difference with mastectomy compared to lumpectomy with radiation.

Case 11.13 Treatment Options for Stages I and II Breast Cancer

A 60-year-old woman has breast cancer and undergoes preliminary staging. The lesion is 1.5 cm in diameter, and no axillary nodes are palpable. A metastatic workup is negative.

✦ **What stage is this woman's cancer?**

✦ **This is a clinically stage I cancer.** The final pathologic stage will be based on the results of her axillary lymph node histology, which requires a biopsy of the nodes. Therefore, it is necessary to decide which surgical procedure will be used to sample the nodes and to remove the primary tumor.

✦ **What are this woman's surgical options, both for sampling the lymph nodes and treating the primary tumor?**

✦ The **sentinel node technique is used to stage the axilla. This technique** assumes there is a sentinel node that first receives lymphatic drainage from the primary tumor (Fig. 11-8).

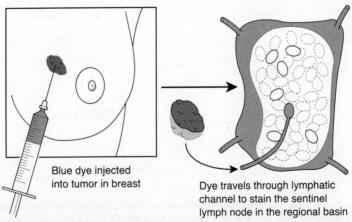

Blue dye injected
into tumor in breast

Dye travels through lymphatic
channel to stain the sentinel
lymph node in the regional basin

Figure 11-8: Sentinel node biopsy. A blue dye or a radionuclide tracer is injected around a tumor in the breast, and it moves to the axilla to the sentinel lymph node. This node, which can be identified surgically by either a radiodetector or a change in the color of the node to blue, is then removed and sampled carefully for evidence of tumor.

If this node is negative for tumor, then the remaining axillary nodes are negative (>90% of cases); if this node is positive, further metastases may exist.

Sentinel node evaluation is performed by injecting a blue vital dye (isosulfan blue) and/or technetium-99m (^{99m}Tc)-labeled sulfur colloid (a radiotracer) in the breast. The surgeon then waits for the dye or tracer to travel to the axilla. Incision and inspection of the axilla follow. The vital dye stains the lymph node blue, allowing the surgeon to identify and remove this node, the sentinel node. A handheld gamma probe identifies the node that has concentrated the radiotracer.

Treatment of the primary tumor typically involves either mastectomy (often including immediate reconstruction) or partial mastectomy with postoperative irradiation.

◆ **How do the data relating to the efficacy of mastectomy and lumpectomy with radiation therapy compare?**

◆ Several studies have compared mastectomy to breast conservation or partial mastectomy with radiation. These studies demonstrate that survival results are similar for partial mastectomy with radiation compared with modified radical mastectomy for stages I and II disease. In addition, radiation therapy after lumpectomy greatly reduces the chance of local recurrence as seen in the National Surgical Adjuvant Breast Project (NSABP) Protocol (Fig. 11-9). **In conclusion, variation in the surgical treatment of local and regional disease for stage I and II patients is not important in determining their survival.**

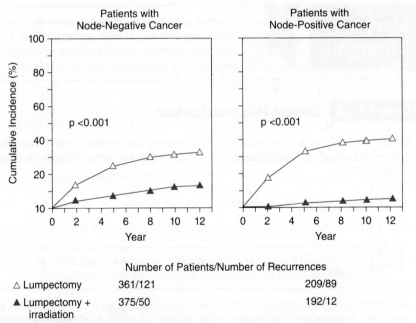

Number of Patients/Number of Recurrences

△ Lumpectomy	361/121	209/89
▲ Lumpectomy + irradiation	375/50	192/12

Figure 11-9: Life table analysis showing the incidence of recurrence of breast tumor in 1,137 patients. Radiation combined with lumpectomy effectively lowers the incidence of local recurrence. **Radiation has no effect on patient survival.** (From Greenfield LJ, Mulholland MW, Oldham KT, et al, eds. *Surgery: Scientific Principles and Practice*, 2nd ed. Philadelphia: Lippincott Williams & Wilkins; 1997:576. After Fisher B, Anderson S, Redmond CK, et al. Reanalysis and results after 12 years of follow-up in a randomized clinical trial comparing total mastectomy with lumpectomy with or without irradiation in the treatment of breast cancer. *N Engl J Med.* 1995;333:1456–1461.)

◆ **What technical considerations and patient issues are important in deciding whether mastectomy or partial mastectomy with radiation should be performed?**

◆ The most important objective in treatment of the primary tumor is complete eradication of the primary tumor. This means that it is essential to obtain adequate tumor-free tissue margins. The surgeon must assess this possibility and the final cosmetic result. In patients with small breasts and large tumors, lumpectomy may not offer a good cosmetic result. Sometimes, plastic surgery procedures can be performed at the same time as a partial mastectomy in a patient when there is a concern about the potential cosmetic results. These procedures can include a contralateral balancing procedure (breast reduction on the noncancerous side) and tissue rearrangement in the breast undergoing the resection to improve cosmesis.

Another important consideration when discussing surgical options with patients is whether or not the patient is a candidate for radiation therapy. Patients with connective tissue disease or prior radiation to the chest or breasts may not be candidates for radiation therapy and should have mastectomies.

Breast cancer support groups are effective in helping women with newly diagnosed breast cancer decide which treatment option is best for them. Patients can talk to women who have had the various procedures to learn about the pros and cons firsthand.

Deep
Thoughts

Breasts and breast surgery evoke an emotional response and this emotion must be factored into how patients decide which procedures and treatments they will undertake.

Case 11.14   Breast Reconstruction

A 38-year-old woman is scheduled for a mastectomy and sentinel node biopsy. She is concerned about her appearance and would like to know her options for breast reconstruction.

◆ **What options should you offer?**

◆ Most patients undergoing a mastectomy are candidates for immediate breast reconstruction.

QUICK CUT Immediate reconstruction allows the exact defect to be duplicated and replaced and leads to excellent cosmetic results.

Depending on patient preference, the amount of skin and breast remaining, and the patient's size, reconstruction techniques involve silicone gel, saline-filled prostheses, or vascularized flaps (Fig. 11-10). Some patients undergo placement of a temporary prosthesis (tissue expander) followed by final reconstruction at a later date when the cancer treatment is complete. Flaps are not as successful in obese patients or smokers.

Most mastectomies performed today are curative for in situ cancers and stage I and II cancers; therefore, they are amenable to reconstruction. **Relative contraindications are primary lesions involving the chest wall, extensive local or regional disease, or stage III or IV cancer.**

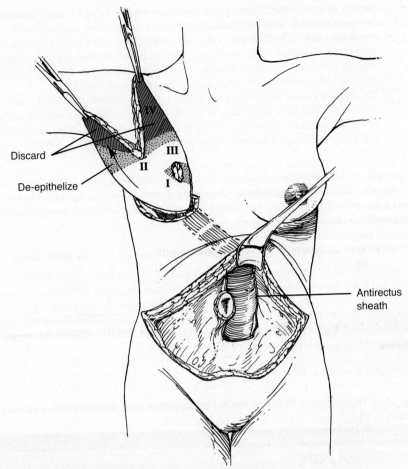

Figure 11-10: Transverse rectus abdominis myocutaneous flap. A large segment of skin, subcutaneous tissue, and muscle is isolated and swung on its vascular pedestal to reconstruct the breast. Nipple and areolar reconstruction is done typically at a later date. (From Silen W. *Atlas of Techniques in Breast Surgery*. Philadelphia: Lippincott-Raven; 1996:131.)

Case 11.15   Medical Management of Breast Cancer

You have successfully removed the primary breast cancer from a 58-year-old woman, and you have sampled her axillary nodes. You determine the stage of her cancer. Having recovered from the procedure, she asks you about long-term medical therapy.

◆ **What are her management options?**

- For **stages 0 and I cancers with small (<1 cm) tumors** (no positive nodes), lumpectomy, axillary sampling, and radiation therapy is acceptable treatment. Hormonal therapy is appropriate for estrogen receptor–positive pathology. Chemotherapy for hormone receptor–negative smaller stage I cancer is sometimes recommended.

- For **stage I cancer with larger (1–2 cm) tumors** (no positive nodes), treatment is lumpectomy, sentinel node biopsy, and postoperative radiation therapy. Adjuvant therapy is beneficial in most patients. The choice of therapy is based on estrogen receptor status, menopausal status, and the patient's overall health.
- For **stage II cancer** (larger primary lesions or node-positive disease), the surgical treatment is the same as for stage I. In patients with nodal metastasis, the axillary nodes are surgically removed (axillary dissection). Adjuvant therapy is beneficial; it is based on estrogen receptor status, menopausal status, and the patient's overall health.

Generally, some combination of radiation therapy, chemotherapy, and hormonal treatment is effective (Table 11-8). Chemotherapy is appropriate for adjuvant therapy or palliation for metastatic or recurrent disease. However, it is more toxic than hormonal therapy and may be poorly tolerated in elderly patients.

◆ **What follow-up surveillance is recommended?**

◆ Patients with breast cancer should see their physicians at least twice a year. Patients who have had lumpectomy with radiation should undergo mammography of the affected breast every 6 months for 2 years, followed by yearly mammograms. The prognosis for women with early-stage breast cancer is excellent and for those with stage I disease with an overall 5-year survival of greater than 95% for localized disease and greater than 80% for regional disease (cancer has spread to the lymph nodes).

Table 11-8: Nonsurgical Therapy for Node-Negative and Node-Positive Breast Disease

Node-Negative Disease	Treatment
Postmenopausal women	
ER-positive	Hormonal therapy (aromatase inhibitor)
ER-negative	Chemotherapy depending on tumor pathology and patient performance status
Premenopausal women	
ER-positive	Adjuvant tamoxifen ± chemotherapy
ER-negative	Adjuvant chemotherapy and individual risk assessment
Node-Positive Disease	**Treatment**
Premenopausal women	
ER-negative	Chemotherapy
ER-positive	Chemotherapy followed by tamoxifen for 5 years
Postmenopausal women	
ER-negative	Chemotherapy (benefit for patients older than 70 years of age is not clear)
ER-positive	Aromatase inhibitor and chemotherapy

ER, estrogen receptor.

Case 11.16 Treatment of Stages III and IV Breast Cancer

A 63-year-old woman presents with a 6-cm breast mass that has been diagnosed as infiltrating ductal carcinoma of the breast. She has clinically positive, matted lymph nodes in the ipsilateral axilla.

◆ **What evaluation and management steps are appropriate?**

◆ **Staging** is necessary. The cancer is stage III if there is no distant metastasis or stage IV if there is distant metastasis. Many centers would recommend the patient receive **neoadjuvant therapy, which is chemotherapy given before surgical therapy of the local disease in an attempt to reduce the tumor size.**

  • For **stage III cancer** (>5-cm lesions, fixed nodes, or inflammatory lesions), it is necessary to consult an oncologist before surgery because preoperative (neoadjuvant) chemotherapy can be beneficial.

  • For **stage IV cancer** (distant metastases), palliative chemotherapy is appropriate. Palliative radiation can also play a role in select cases. Surgery is reserved only for local control of the primary tumor for palliation.

These management methods allow a rapid assessment of the tumor response, with the potential to change chemotherapy regimens as necessary. Two to four cycles of chemotherapy are appropriate. Pre- and post-treatment MRI of the breasts is used to assess the size and extent of the tumor accurately and plan for surgery. Patients then undergo surgery followed by further radiation therapy. Some patients may receive further chemotherapy depending on the tumor response. If metastatic disease is present, palliation with radiation and chemotherapy is given, and no surgical procedure is performed unless the primary tumor is painful or infected.

Case 11.17 Breast Mass with Cellulitis and Edema

A 38-year-old woman presents with a 3-month history of a progressively enlarging breast mass. At the time she sees you, she has a 6- × 7-cm fixed mass, with erythema and edema on the upper, outer aspect of her right breast. Clinically, her axilla is positive with enlarged, firm lymph nodes.

◆ **What is the suspected diagnosis?**

◆ This patient may have an inflammatory carcinoma of the breast. The diagnosis of inflammatory cancer is a clinical diagnosis based on signs of inflammation, in the setting of a breast cancer, on physical exam.

◆ **What histologic features are typical of this condition?**

◆ The histopathology shows **cancer cells invading dermal lymphatics and vessels** with a large inflammatory component.

A surgeon confirms the physical findings and obtains a punch biopsy of the mass. Pathology reveals inflammatory carcinoma. Estrogen and progesterone receptors are negative.

◆ **What is the recommended treatment?**

◆ **Multimodality treatment** is appropriate, and evaluation by a medical oncologist and radiation oncologist is necessary. A **staging workup**, including a complete blood count (CBC), liver enzymes, alkaline phosphatase, calcium, total bilirubin, CT scan of the chest, a bone scan, and a CT scan of the liver, is warranted. Patients would first receive chemotherapy to reduce the primary tumor size and treat any possible distant micrometastasis. **If the cancer responds to chemotherapy, four to six more cycles are appropriate.** The treatment then involves modified radical mastectomy, adjuvant chemotherapy, hormonal therapy (for estrogen receptor–positive patients), and radiation therapy to the chest and regional lymph node basins. More chemotherapy may follow. If the cancer does not shrink with chemotherapy, local treatment with surgery or radiation therapy may be required at an earlier stage to control the local disease of the breast before there is any more chemotherapy.

Case 11.18   Events that Occur Later in Patients with Breast Cancer

A 55-year-old woman has a modified radical mastectomy for a stage II carcinoma of the breast.

◆ **What evaluation and management are appropriate for the following events that occur later in the woman's life?**

Case Variation 11.18.1. A small, 0.5-cm nodule in the suture line 5 years after surgery

◆ This is a **local recurrence** until proven otherwise. A biopsy is indicated.

> **QUICK CUT** It is necessary to perform a biopsy, either a surgical biopsy or a core-needle biopsy, of any abnormality occurring in a mastectomy surgical site to rule out cancer.

If the lesion is cancerous, the patient should be staged to assess for metastatic disease. Local excision is warranted in the absence of distant metastasis if the patient has had a previous mastectomy. After a previous lumpectomy and radiation therapy, a mastectomy is usually appropriate.

Case Variation 11.18.2. A mammographic abnormality in the opposite breast

◆ This may be a **new primary cancer**. Evaluation of this mammographic abnormality should proceed like any other.

Case Variation 11.18.3. Elevated liver function studies

◆ Evaluation for a **metastasis to the liver** is appropriate. Most physicians would recommend a contrast-enhanced CT scan of the abdomen. MRI with gadolinium (Gd) enhancement may be necessary in patients with poor renal function.

Case Variation 11.18.4. A fracture of the femur

◆ A **pathologic fracture** secondary to a bony metastasis should be a concern. Orthopedic repair is necessary, with local cancer control with irradiation postoperatively. This controls the cancer but does not appear to inhibit fracture union.

Case Variation 11.18.5. Decreased sensation and motor function in the right leg that is new in onset

◆ This occurrence is an emergency. An **extradural metastasis to the spine** that may be impinging on the spinal cord is a concern. Localized back pain is an earlier presenting symptom. Diagnosis of cord compression necessitates an MRI scan. Steroids, cord decompression, and radiation therapy are then warranted.

Case Variation 11.18.6. ***New-onset seizures with focal findings***

◆ This presentation should prompt concern about a possible **metastasis to the brain**. A CT scan or MRI study would determine the diagnosis. Urgent therapy with steroids is indicated to reduce the intracranial pressure followed by surgery (if indicated) or irradiation.

Case Variation 11.18.7. ***Presentation to the emergency department with coma or confusion and with no focal findings***

◆ **Acute hypercalcemia** due to bony metastasis and parathormone-related peptide is one of the many possible diagnoses.

 QUICK CUT The development of coma in any patient with a history of breast cancer should lead to the suspicion of hypercalcemia.

Case 11.19 Breast Problems in Pregnancy and the Peripartum Period

A 28-year-old woman who is 3 weeks postpartum after a normal delivery presents with a painful right breast. She is currently breastfeeding and has a low-grade fever. Examination reveals a very firm, red, tender, indurated breast mass. The axilla is mildly tender; some shotty nodes are palpable. The opposite breast is normal.

◆ **What evaluation and management are appropriate?**

◆ **Mastitis** (cellulitis) of the breast related to breastfeeding is the suspected diagnosis. It most likely is secondary to skin breaks in the nipple, allowing bacteria to enter. Examination of the breast for the usual signs of infection, including abscess formation, is warranted. The usual treatment is **warm compresses** and **antibiotics** to cover staphylococcal and streptococcal organisms. Most physicians would recommend continuing breastfeeding or use of a breast pump to allow milk "let-down."

◆ **How would management change if an area of fluctuance is present in the tender inflamed area?**

◆ The presence of an **abscess** should be a concern. If definitely present, aspiration or open **surgical drainage** is indicated. If doubt exists about the diagnosis of abscess, it may be necessary to probe and aspirate the suspected area with a needle or identify under ultrasound guidance followed by drainage (Fig. 11-11).

At the patient's initial visit, you decide that she has cellulitis with no abscess and decide to treat her with antibiotics. You follow her closely but she fails to improve even after a change in antibiotics. At 3 weeks, the breast is still tender with a very firm, inflamed mass.

◆ **Would the management plan change?**

◆ Several weeks of antibiotic therapy with no resulting improvement should place the original diagnosis in question. The patient's condition may represent inflammatory carcinoma, not a simple cellulitis. A **biopsy** of the lesion that includes a segment of skin to examine for carcinoma and possibly dermal lymphatic involvement is warranted.

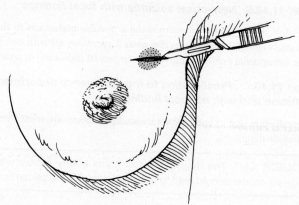

Figure 11-11: Drainage of a breast abscess. The area of fluctuance is palpated, and an incision is made with a scalpel to drain the abscess. Generally, needle drainage is insufficient to accomplish adequate drainage. (From Silen W. *Atlas of Techniques in Breast Surgery*. Philadelphia: Lippincott-Raven; 1996:43.)

◆ **If the woman were pregnant (first, second, or third trimester) and had a 2-cm breast lesion, how would the management plan change?**

◆ Breast cancer may occur in pregnancy.

 QUICK CUT The prognosis, which is based on the stage of breast cancer at diagnosis, is similar for both pregnant and nonpregnant women.

◆ Ultrasound and biopsy are necessary for the investigation of suspicious masses. Treatment plans are identical to those of nonpregnant women but are affected by trimester. Radiation treatment is contraindicated during pregnancy. Chemotherapy can be given during pregnancy after the first trimester. A sentinel node biopsy can be performed during pregnancy with radiotracer. Vital blue dye is contraindicated during pregnancy.

For **stage I and II disease**, a mastectomy or lumpectomy is safe, with an approximate 1% risk of spontaneous abortion. With lumpectomy, the remaining breast must still be irradiated after delivery. With mastectomy, irradiation is not necessary. Physicians believe that delaying radiation therapy until after delivery is safe for most patients in their third trimester. However, **lumpectomy is often discouraged in earlier pregnancy because of the need for radiation**. Certain chemotherapy regimens are safe in the second or third trimester, and therefore, both adjuvant and neoadjuvant chemotherapy can be used to treat pregnant patients.

For **stage III and IV disease**, rapid treatment with chemotherapy is essential.

Case 11.20   Breast Cancer in Patients of Advanced Age and Decreased Function

A 92-year-old woman with moderately advanced Alzheimer disease presents with a breast mass. The mass is 3 cm in diameter and is hard but freely movable within the breast. The opposite breast is normal, and no axillary nodes are palpable. She lives in a nursing home.

◆ **What options should you present to the woman's family?**

◆ If the patient has moderate or greater disability, it is acceptable to do less than in a younger or healthier individual. This usually means a family meeting to discuss the options, which range from:

1. Observation with no diagnosis
2. Needle biopsy followed by diagnosis and observation
3. Needle biopsy followed by diagnosis and lumpectomy or simple mastectomy
4. If the cancer is estrogen or progesterone receptor–positive, the patient may be treated with hormonal therapy alone.
5. Complete staging and traditional treatment (i.e., similar to a younger patient)

Case 11.21   Breast Mass in a Man

A 42-year-old man presents with a 1-cm–diameter hard nodule beneath his right nipple. It is not painful but relatively fixed to the surrounding tissue. The left breast is normal, and no axillary adenopathy is palpable.

◆ **What evaluation and management are appropriate?**

◆ It is necessary to obtain a bilateral mammogram, which can help differentiate gynecomastia from cancer. Treatment is typically with **mastectomy. However, it is important to offer a partial mastectomy with postoperative radiotherapy, as some men will choose this option.**

◆ **What should you tell the man about his prognosis?**

◆ Although breast cancer in men is rare, it does develop, typically after 60 years of age. **Stage for stage, survival for men is similar to that of women.** However, men tend to have hormone receptor–positive cancers.

Case 11.22   Gynecomastia

A 15-year-old boy is brought to see you by his mother about breast enlargement in the left breast. He is pubertal and his friends are making fun of him.

◆ **What is the appropriate management?**

◆ Gynecomastia, which is hypertrophy of breast tissue in men, occurs most commonly in adolescents and in adults at 40–50 years of age. The condition **usually spontaneously regresses** in adolescents.

◆ **How would the proposed management plans change in the following patients?**

Case Variation 11.22.1. *A 6-year-old girl with a firm 1-cm unilateral breast mass*

◆ This condition most likely represents a **breast bud** with premature or asymmetric development. Observation with parental reassurance is necessary. Excision or biopsy is contraindicated because this would diminish or stop development of that breast by removing the breast tissue.

Case Variation 11.22.2. *A 50-year-old man*

◆ In older men, breast hypertrophy is commonly associated with **medications**, including diuretics, estrogens, isoniazid, marijuana, digoxin, and alcohol abuse. Imaging with mammography and ultrasound can be helpful in diagnosing gynecomastia versus a breast mass.

Chapter 12

Trauma, Burns, and Sepsis

Bruce E. Jarrell, Thomas Scalea, Molly Buzdon

Key Thoughts

1. Primary survey: airway, breathing, and circulation (ABCs)

2. Simple pneumothorax usually presents with dyspnea and is not emergent, whereas a tension pneumothorax presents with hypotension and hypoxia and requires emergent decompression.

3. Hypovolemia is the most common cause of hypotension in trauma and is treated with fluid resuscitation. However, tension pneumothorax and cardiac tamponade cause hypotension, are not associated with hypovolemia, and are not treated with fluid resuscitation. They should be considered early during resuscitation.

4. Hemodynamically unstable patients should not go to the computed tomography (CT) scanner.

5. Closed head injuries usually are associated with hypertension, not hypotension. A key to optimal management is maintaining good oxygenation and tissue perfusion.

6. Abdominal hemorrhage often requires a laparotomy for control, whereas pelvic fracture with hemorrhage is evaluated angiographically and often treated with embolization and fracture stabilization.

7. Hypothermia is associated with coagulopathy and resultant bleeding after trauma.

8. Early sepsis causes third-space fluid losses and is treated by fluid resuscitation, antibiotics, and infectious source control.

9. Total parenteral nutrition (TPN) should be reserved for surgical patients who have inability to tolerate oral feedings and who have preoperative malnutrition, severe catabolic states, or prolonged gastrointestinal (GI) dysfunction states. TPN is associated with a significant risk for generalized sepsis secondary to catheter sepsis. Where possible, enteral feedings are preferred.

Case 12.1   Primary and Secondary Assessment of Injuries

A 24-year-old man who was in an automobile crash is brought to the emergency department.

◆ **How should the evaluation proceed?**

◆ The American College of Surgeons recommends that clinicians follow an established sequence for evaluation of most trauma patients. This order of priorities is based on the relative risk of death; individuals with the most serious life-threatening problems should receive treatment before those with less severe problems (Table 12-1). These initial priorities make up the **primary survey** for trauma patients. Most clinicians reassess patients again before proceeding to the **secondary survey** (see Table 12-1).

Table 12-1: Priorities in Trauma Evaluation

The advanced trauma life support (ATLS) course administered by the American College of Surgeons recommends that a physician or emergency medical technician perform an initial evaluation using the "ABCDE" mnemonic.

Airway

Breathing (ventilation)

Circulation

Disability (neurologic deficit)

Environment; expose patient (i.e., remove all clothing)

Initial assessment, including an "AMPLE" history

Allergies

Medications

Previous illnesses

Last meal

Events surrounding injury

Physicians should remember to protect themselves with a gown, gloves, eye protection, and mask when evaluating trauma patients.

Diagnosis of immediately life-threatening injuries, followed by rapid treatment

Reassessment of the patient's status

Diagnosis of other significant injuries, including examination of back, axillae, perineum, and rectum

Definitive treatment, including surgery, prophylactic antibiotics, and tetanus prophylaxis

QUICK CUT Continual reassessment is necessary during trauma surveys, looking for cardiovascular instability and other significant changes, particularly neurologic changes.

Case 12.2   Initial Airway Management

You are responsible for evaluating the airway of the patient in Case 12.1.

◆ **How is the initial airway evaluation performed?**

◆ Initially, it is necessary to **determine whether the airway is clear or obstructed**.

QUICK CUT If a patient can talk, the airway is patent, at least at that particular moment. Signs of airway obstruction include stridor, hoarseness, and evidence of increased airway resistance such as respiratory retractions (retraction of the soft tissues between the ribs during inspiration) and use of accessory respiratory muscles.

Visual examination of the oropharynx is appropriate in patients with altered consciousness. The presence of a gag reflex indicates that the upper airway is most likely clear. The absence of a gag reflex means that the physician should inspect the airway digitally for

Table 12-2: **Glasgow Coma Scale**

Feature	Points
Eye-Opening Response (4 points maximum)	
Spontaneous eye opening	4
Opens eyes to speech	3
Opens eyes to painful stimuli	2
No eye opening	1
Verbal Response (5 points maximum)	
Oriented (e.g., knows name, age)	5
Confused conversation	4
Inappropriate words	3
Incomprehensible sounds	2
No verbal response	1
Motor Response (6 points maximum)	
Obeys commands	6
Localizes painful stimuli (moves purposefully toward stimulus)	5
Withdraws from painful stimulus	4
Decorticate posture (abnormal flexion)	3
Decerebrate posture (extensor response)	2
No movement	1

"No response" in any category receives a score of 1; thus, the lowest possible score is 3. It must be noted if the patient has an endotracheal tube, in which case, the patient is given 1 point with the designation "T" following the GCS value. A score of 8 or less is generally used to designate coma and carries a poor prognosis for recovery provided that the patient is stable.

foreign bodies, being certain to protect the finger from being bitten. Injuries to the neck such as direct, blunt trauma, or penetrating trauma can penetrate or transect the larynx or trachea. These injuries require prompt recognition and either intubation, cricothyroidotomy, or tracheostomy.

Blunt trauma may also cause **laryngeal edema**, which may be mild when the patient is first admitted to the emergency department but become worse in the next few minutes or hours. Hoarseness, a change in voice, or stridor are clues to this condition. If laryngeal edema is suspected, intubation is necessary before airway obstruction occurs.

◆ **What are other indications for intubation?**

◆ Other indications include inadequate respiratory effort, severely depressed mental status, a Glasgow Coma Score of eight or less, inability to protect the airway, and severely compromised respiratory mechanics (e.g., as with multiple rib fractures) (Table 12-2).

Case 12.3　Initial Pulmonary Management

You clear the airway of the patient in Case 12.1. On evaluation of the lungs, decreased breath sounds in the right chest are audible. The patient has a blood pressure (BP) of 120/80 mm Hg and a heart rate of 75 beats per minute. You talk to the patient, who appears to be in no distress and well-oxygenated but mildly short of breath.

◆ **What is the next step?**

◆ The patient is stable, so an orderly evaluation of the lungs is appropriate. At this time, a chest radiograph (x-ray) (CXR) and pulse oximetry are also necessary.

  A moderately sized pneumothorax is apparent on the right side on CXR (Fig. 12-1).

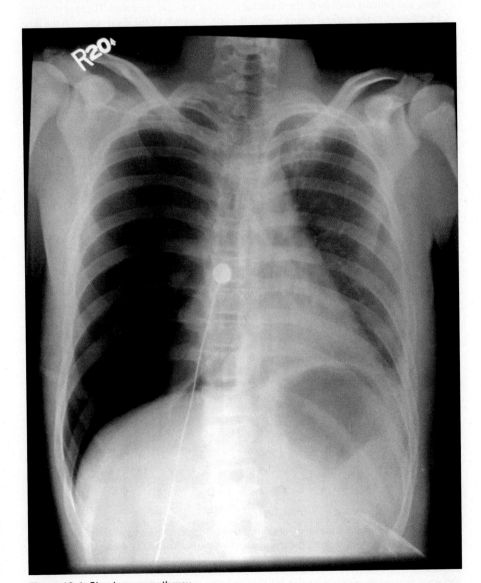

Figure 12-1: Simple pneumothorax.

◆ What is the next step?

◆ A simple pneumothorax usually occurs due to a rib fracture that lacerates the visceral pleura and underlying lung parenchyma. In trauma patients, treatment is **insertion of a large-diameter chest tube** (Fig. 12-2). It is important to **insert a finger** into the pleural space prior to inserting the tube to be certain that it is in the correct space. (It is possible to enter the peritoneal cavity by mistake, thus making the chest tube ineffective.)

Other conditions may complicate this situation. A traumatic diaphragmatic hernia may be present, allowing other structures such as the stomach, spleen, intestine, or other abdominal organs to intrude into the pleural space. In this instance, a chest tube will not reinflate the lung, and patients must go to the operating room for repair of the defect. The lung may also be adherent to the parietal pleura with adhesions. Insertion of the chest tube into the lung parenchyma is obviously injurious and would not resolve the pneumothorax. In this situation, it is important to direct the tube toward the posterior apical aspect of the pleural space.

◆ What management is appropriate for a patient with a chest tube?

◆ You would place a water seal with suction to allow reinflation of the lung. Serial CXRs are necessary. Removal of the tube may occur **when the lung is fully inflated and no further**

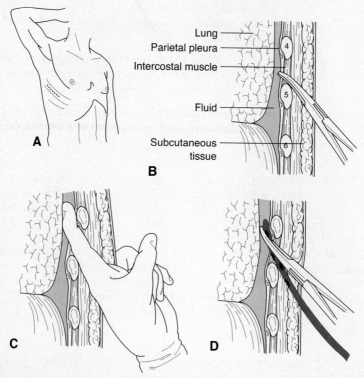

Figure 12-2: Treatment of a pneumothorax involves insertion of a chest tube. The tube is connected to an underwater seal drainage system to allow fluid and air to escape from the pleural space but not enter the space; thus, the lung remains expanded. **A:** Location for insertion of chest tube. **B:** Insertion of hemostat into pleural space. **C:** Palpation of pleural space to be certain no vital structures are adherent and likely to be injured. **D:** Insertion of the chest tube.

air leak is apparent. It is important to be certain that there are no air leaks in the tubing system and no leak at the point where the tube enters the chest wall.

◆ **How does the proposed management change in the following situations?**

Case Variation 12.3.1. Further examination indicates a laceration on the chest wall that penetrates through to the lung and "sucks" air as it moves in and out during respiration.

◆ This is termed a **sucking chest wound**. It should be sealed with an occlusive dressing, and a chest tube should be inserted at a different location.

Case Variation 12.3.2. After insertion of the chest tube and repeating the CXR, the lung does not fully inflate.

◆ The chest tube is either in the **wrong location or not functioning** properly. Tubes can be erroneously inserted into the subcutaneous tissues, have air leaks at their connections, or "clot off" (i.e., become occluded with debris). Management depends on the exact problem but includes repositioning or replacement of the tube or insertion of a second tube. The lung should rapidly expand with a correctly inserted chest tube.

Case Variation 12.3.3. After insertion of a chest tube, a large amount of air continues to leak into the chest tube over the next 6 hours, and the lung remains only partially inflated.

◆ This indicates that there may be a **major airway injury with disruption of a bronchus** or the trachea (Fig. 12-3). This condition, which is sometimes apparent on bronchoscopy, requires a thoracotomy and partial lung resection to repair the injury.

Case Variation 12.3.4. A very small pneumothorax is apparent on CXR. Your resident asks you if simple observation and no insertion of a chest tube will be effective.

QUICK CUT Observation of a small, uncomplicated pneumothorax is appropriate if it is not enlarging, if there is no free fluid in the pleural space (i.e., a hemothorax), and if the patient is asymptomatic and has no other significant injuries, especially chest injuries.

◆ Insertion of a chest tube is necessary regardless of the size of the pneumothorax or symptoms if the patient has an injury such as a fractured femur that necessitates general anesthesia in the operating room. General anesthesia, endotracheal intubation, and **assisted ventilation place the tracheobronchial tree at a positive pressure** of 20–40 mm Hg, which increases the risk of converting a small pneumothorax into a larger or even tension pneumothorax.

Case 12.4 Initial Management of Pneumothorax in a Patient with Hypotension

You clear the airway of the patient in Case 12.1. Absent breath sounds in the right chest are notable. The patient has a BP of 80/60 mm Hg. Distended neck veins are present.

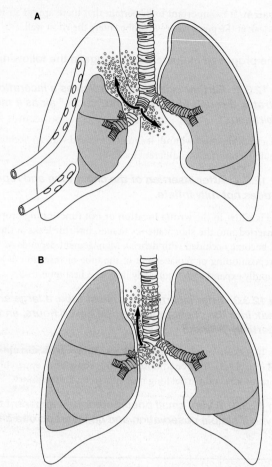

Figure 12-3: Ruptured bronchus demonstrating **(A)** pneumothorax with intrapleural rupture and **(B)** pneumomediastinum with extrapleural rupture. A ruptured bronchus, which causes persistent air leakage and pneumothorax, usually requires lung resection for repair. (From Greenfield LJ, Mulholland MW, Oldham KT, et al, eds. *Surgery: Scientific Principles and Practice*, 2nd ed. Philadelphia: Lippincott Williams & Wilkins; 1997:327.)

◆ **What management is appropriate?**

QUICK CUT With hypotension and absent breath sounds, the suspected problem is a tension pneumothorax.

◆ The usual etiology of this entity is a lung laceration that acts like a one-way valve, allowing air to enter the pleural space but preventing it from escaping, thus creating a progressively increasing positive pressure in the pleural space. As this pressure reaches venous pressure, venous return and cardiac output fall, and hypotension results and neck vein distention occurs. If immediate insertion of a chest tube is not possible, **needle aspiration** of the left chest is necessary. With a diagnosis of tension pneumothorax, the patient should experience **immediate improvement in BP**. Tube thoracostomy should immediately follow needle aspiration.

Tension pneumothorax is a clinical diagnosis (Fig. 12-4). It is necessary to perform the needle aspiration and thoracostomy prior to the CXR because the CXR takes time to complete. **Time is of the essence** in patients with hypotension.

Case 12.5 Initial Management of Hypotension and Neck Vein Distention with Normal Breath Sounds

A 42-year-old man who was in a motor vehicle crash comes to the emergency department, where you clear his airway. He has intact, normal breath sounds bilaterally and appears to be ventilating and oxygenating well. Initial assessment of the cardiovascular system reveals hypotension with a BP of 80/60 mm Hg, a heart rate of 110 beats per minute, and distended neck veins.

◆ **What is the next step?**

◆ A tension pneumothorax is the most common cause of hypotension and distended neck veins in trauma patients. However, intact breath sounds mean that it is less likely

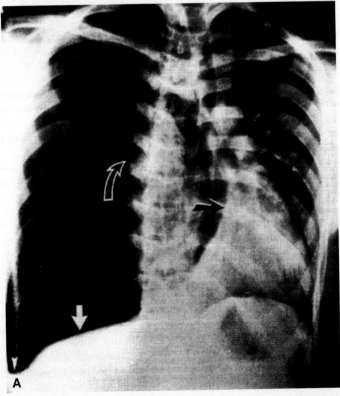

Figure 12-4: A: When air progressively accumulates in the pleural space of a patient with a pneumothorax, a tension pneumothorax develops. As the pressure increases in the pleural space, the mediastinum and trachea shift away from the pneumothorax and venous return is impaired with resultant jugular venous distention and decreased cardiac output. (From Schulman HS, Samuels TH. The radiology of blunt chest trauma. *J Can Assoc Radiol.* 1983;34:204.) *(continued)*

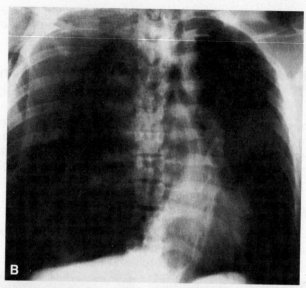

Figure 12-4: *(continued)* **B:** Right-sided tension pneumothorax with left shift of the mediastinum. (From Greenfield LJ, Mulholland MW, Oldham KT, et al, eds. *Surgery: Scientific Principles and Practice*, 2nd ed. Philadelphia: Lippincott Williams & Wilkins; 1997:324.)

that this patient has a significant pneumothorax and therefore a tension pneumothorax. **Hypotension with distended neck veins may also be secondary to cardiac tamponade. A cardiac ultrasound can be performed to make the diagnosis of cardiac tamponade as long as it can be done immediately; an emergent pericardiocentesis can be performed under ultrasound guidance.**

 QUICK CUT Emergent pericardiocentesis or pericardial ultrasound examination, if immediately available in the trauma resuscitation unit, is necessary.

If pericardial tamponade is the diagnosis, the patient should become normotensive quickly after drainage. An open procedure using a subxiphoid approach is best, although some surgeons prefer needle aspiration (Fig. 12-5). Even small amounts of blood in the pericardium (<50 mL) can limit venous inflow to the heart and cause hypotension.

After initial drainage, the **patient should go to the operating room** for a pericardial window and examination of the pericardial contents to stop the source of bleeding. Blood in the pericardium can come from various sources including myocardial, aortic, and pericardial lacerations, all of which are serious, life-threatening injuries. Other signs of pericardial tamponade such as muffled heart sounds, pulsus paradoxus (a decrease in systolic BP of more than 10 mm Hg on inspiration), or a Kussmaul sign (an increase in central venous pressure [CVP] during inspiration in a spontaneously breathing patient) are usually not readily detectable in trauma patients.

If no tamponade is present, it is possible that the patient has had a myocardial contusion. This does not usually cause cardiac failure but rather arrhythmias. It is suspected with acute electrocardiographic (ECG) changes and confirmed with cardiac enzyme analysis and cardiac imaging.

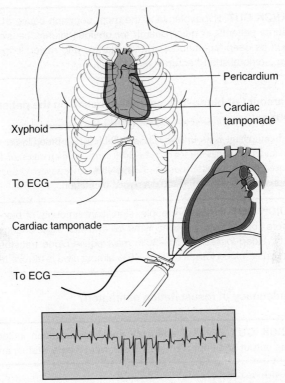

Figure 12-5: Pericardial tamponade may be diagnosed by pericardiocentesis using a subxiphoid approach. If pericardial blood is aspirated and the patient's hemodynamics improve, the patient should be taken to surgery for control of bleeding in the pericardium. (From Greenfield LJ, Mulholland MW, Oldham KT, et al, eds. *Surgery: Scientific Principles and Practice*, 2nd ed. Philadelphia: Lippincott Williams & Wilkins; 1997:1579.)

Rarely, patients with pre-existing cardiac disease have a cardiac event such as a myocardial infarction (MI) while driving, which results in driver error and the accident. In this case, primary cardiac failure could be the cause of these findings.

Case 12.6 Initial Management of Hypotension with Normal Breath Sounds and No Neck Vein Distention

A 28-year-old man is brought to the emergency department following a motorcycle accident. After you clear his airway, you intubate him after you note respiratory distress. Normal, bilateral breath sounds are present, and neck veins absent with a BP of 90/60 mm Hg and a heart rate of 125 beats per minute.

◆ **What are the appropriate steps in the initial resuscitation?**

◆ Two large-bore intravenous (IV) lines (preferably in the upper extremities) should be inserted followed by rapid infusion of at least 1–2 L of normal saline. Assessment of the response to fluids is appropriate, and further fluids must be given until the patient's BP and pulse improve.

QUICK CUT Hypovolemia is the most common cause of hypotension in trauma patients. A quick search for obvious injuries causing hemorrhage, such as deep lacerations; arterial injuries; and major, long bone fractures (e.g., femoral shaft fractures) is essential.

◆ **How is the amount of blood loss estimated based on the patient's initial presentation?**

◆ The degree of hemorrhage is grouped by classes (Table 12-3). Blood losses of less than 15% cause few physiologic changes; losses of 15%–30% cause mild changes, including tachycardia and increased pulse pressure. Losses of 30%–40% cause severe changes in vital signs including hypotension, tachycardia, and decreased mentation.

QUICK CUT In healthy people, significant amounts of blood must be lost before compensatory mechanisms fail and vital signs change. Patients who suffer blood losses of 15%–30% may require blood transfusion, and those who suffer blood losses of 30%–40% almost always require transfusion.

◆ **How is the adequacy of resuscitation estimated?**

QUICK CUT Signs of adequate initial resuscitation include acceptable urine output and improvement in heart rate, mental status, and BP.

Table 12-3: Classification of Estimated Fluid and Blood Shock in Adults: Requirements Based on Initial Presentation*

	Class I	Class II	Class III	Class IV
Blood loss (mL)	≤750	750–1,500	1,500–2,000	
Blood loss (% BV)	≤15	15–30	30–40	
Heart rate (beats per minute)	<100	>100	>120	
Blood pressure	Normal	Normal	↓	↓
Pulse pressure	Normal or ↑	↓	↓	↓
Capillary refill	Normal	Positive	Positive	Positive
Respiratory rate (breaths per minute)	14–20	20–30	30–40	>35
Urine (mL/hr)	≥30	20–30	5–15	Negligible
Mental status	Slightly anxious	Mildly anxious	Anxious/confused	Confused/lethargic
Fluid replacement (3:1 rule)	Crystalloid	Crystalloid	Crystalloid + blood	Crystalloid + blood

*For a 70-kg man.
BV, blood volume.
From Greenfield LJ, Mulholland MW, Oldham KT, et al, eds. *Surgery: Scientific Principles and Practice*, 2nd ed. Philadelphia: Lippincott Williams & Wilkins; 1997:287.

Other physiologic changes are also useful in monitoring adequacy of perfusion. These include correction of anaerobic metabolism as measured by correction of **lactic acidosis** and normalization of **venous oxygen saturation.**

Fluid resuscitation begins, and a urinary catheter is placed to monitor the patient's urine output. The patient has a right femoral fracture, with a large, swollen thigh.

◆ **What additional management is necessary?**

◆ Femoral fractures can be associated with **blood loss** into the tissues of several **liters.** To prevent ongoing hemorrhage, it is necessary to **stabilize the fracture.** Transfusion may be necessary. A major vascular injury may also be present and warrants investigation.

Hypotension continues despite rapid fluid and blood replacement.

◆ **Is it necessary to have a central venous catheter or pulmonary artery catheter to manage this patient properly?**

QUICK CUT When a patient continues to remain hypotensive and unstable despite adequate fluid resuscitation, the most important priority is a search for the underlying cause. Urgent laparotomy or thoracotomy may be indicated.

Deep Thoughts

There are limited places where a patient can hemorrhage resulting in hypovolemic shock. These include the thorax and mediastinum; the abdomen, retroperitoneum, and pelvis; the thighs; and externally.

◆ **Invasive monitoring only delays definitive therapy.** Many surgeons insert a central line into the severely traumatized patient at the time of initial resuscitation. If this procedure can be performed rapidly, it is very useful in unstable or hypotensive patients because a central line allows a large-bore catheter to be used for resuscitation. If a pneumothorax is present, many surgeons would insert the line on the same side because pneumothorax is a complication of central line insertion.

Case Variation 12.6.1. Significant hypotension continues despite resuscitation, no thoracic injury, and no obvious major long bone or soft tissue injuries.

◆ **What are the most likely causes of the hypotension?**

◆ Suspected causes are either an intra-abdominal injury or a pelvic fracture with a major vascular disruption.

Case Variation 12.6.2. Significant hypotension continues despite resuscitation, no thoracic injury, and no obvious major long bone or soft tissue injuries but in the presence of a closed head injury.

◆ **Is the closed head injury a likely cause of the hypotension in addition to a possible abdominal or pelvic injury?**

QUICK CUT A closed head injury typically does not cause hypotension as a result of the Cushing reflex.

◆ The Cushing reflex presumably occurs due to brain swelling and resultant brain ischemia. The ischemic brain sends a sympathetic nervous system message to the peripheral circulation to vasoconstrict, which maintains a normal or increased BP and thus regulates perfusion to the brain. **Bradycardia** also results because the vagus nerves are unaffected by this message and respond to the increased BP with parasympathetic stimulation to the heart, causing the decreased heart rate.

Case Variation 12.6.3. Suppose the patient is a pregnant woman in her third trimester.

◆ **What hemodynamic effects of pregnancy might be important considerations?**

◆ Heart rate increases throughout pregnancy, with increases of more than 20 beats per minute in the third trimester. Thus, an increase in pulse rate in a pregnant woman may not indicate hypovolemia. Uterine compression on the vena cava may reduce blood return to the heart, causing hypotension. Therefore, evaluation of the pregnant woman should take place when she is on her left side.

In addition, plasma volume increases during the third trimester, with a smaller increase in red blood cell (RBC) volume, causing a decrease in hematocrit. In late pregnancy, a hematocrit of 31%–35% is normal.

Case Variation 12.6.4. Suppose you were starting to put in the urinary catheter and you noticed blood at the urethral meatus.

◆ **What is the next step?**

◆ Blood on the urethral meatus indicates possible **urethral injury**. Other reasons to suspect urethral injury on secondary survey include a high-riding prostate gland on rectal examination or a penile or scrotal hematoma. Before placing a catheter in any male trauma patient, it is necessary to perform a rectal examination to search for a prostatic injury. Attempts to place a urinary bladder catheter are contraindicated because the catheter may complete a partially transected urethra and worsen the trauma. A **retrograde cystourethrogram** is used to determine whether an injury is present. Insertion of a suprapubic catheter is appropriate if an injury has occurred.

Case 12.7 Initial Cervical Spine Management

An 18-year-old man who was in a motor vehicle crash is brought to the emergency department. You are responsible for evaluating the patient's cervical spine.

◆ **What management is appropriate in the following situations?**

Case Variation 12.7.1. The patient is awake and alert.

◆ **Cervical spine precautions** include neck immobilization with a collar or a board, as used by paramedics. If no stabilization is in place, it is necessary to maintain **in-line cervical stabilization** until the neck has been stabilized by one of these methods.

QUICK CUT The next step is palpation of the neck along the posterior aspect to detect tenderness, deformity, or other abnormalities. In addition, a rapid assessment of the basic motor and sensory function of the arms and legs is necessary.

A simple way to perform this assessment involves asking the patient to move his fingers and toes and to tell you if he can feel you touch them. In addition, a **lateral cervical spine** radiograph to examine for obvious bony abnormalities is necessary (Fig. 12-6). If the initial evaluation is negative, a radiologist should view the cervical spine series, including anterior and oblique views, and be convinced that no abnormalities exist. A CT scan of the cervical spine can also be performed to look for a fracture particularly if the patient needs a CT scan of another area such as the head. The cervical spine precautions may be discontinued at that time only if the patient can be adequately examined clinically.

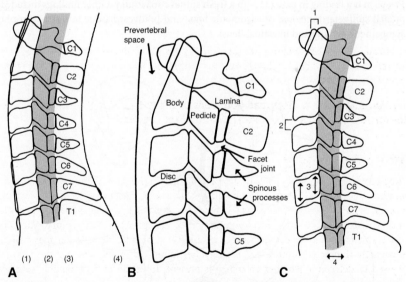

Figure 12-6: A: On lateral radiography, the seven cervical vertebrae plus the top of the body of T1 should be visible. **B:** Injuries are suspected if a bony structure is fractured or crushed. Other indications of injury include misalignment of the vertebrae, fluid in the prevertebral space, "step-offs" from one vertebra to another, fracture of the odontoid, and misalignment of the facet joints. **C:** Number *1* shows the proper alignment of C1 and C2, number *2* shows normal disk space and vertebral alignment, number *3* shows normal vertebral body structure and forces in a shearing fracture, and number *4* shows normal canal for spinal cord. (From Wilson RF, ed. *Handbook of Trauma: Pitfalls and Pearls*. Philadelphia: Lippincott Williams & Wilkins; 1999:8.)

Case Variation 12.7.2. **The patient is comatose.**

✦ An examiner **cannot clear the cervical spine** in a patient who is comatose, disoriented, or combative. Therefore, the precautions must continue until the patient's condition improves. Some surgeons obtain a magnetic resonance imaging (MRI) scan of the cervical spine in the comatose patient, and if no abnormalities exist, clear the patient.

Case Variation 12.7.3. **The patient has loss of neurologic function below the neck.**

✦ Negative radiographs do not rule out an injury, particularly if neurologic symptoms or neck tenderness is present.

 QUICK CUT If neurologic deficits, radiologic abnormalities, or cervical spine tenderness are present, then a cervical spine injury should be suspected.

Treatment includes continued cervical spine precautions, a neurosurgical consultation, and complete evaluation with imaging. If tracheal intubation is necessary, the head cannot be tilted; oropharyngeal intubation with in-line traction to maintain spinal column alignment or nasotracheal intubation is required (Fig. 12-7).

Case Variation 12.7.4. **The patient has priapism.**

✦ Priapism is a finding in patients with a **fresh spinal cord injury**. Other findings include loss of anal sphincter tone, loss of vasomotor tone, and bradycardia due to loss of peripheral sympathetic activity and intestinal ileus.

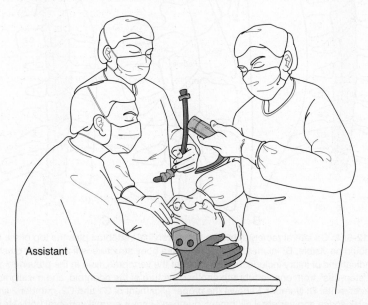

Assistant

Figure 12-7: To safely intubate a trauma patient, an assistant must maintain stability and in-line traction to prevent injury to the potentially unstable cervical spine. (From Peitzman AB, Rhodes M, Schwab CW, et al, eds. *The Trauma Manual*, 2nd ed. Philadelphia: Lippincott Williams & Wilkins; 2002:90.)

Case 12.8   Initial Assessment of Thoracic Injury

A 25-year-old man presents with a stab wound to the left chest lateral to the nipple. He is verbally complaining of pain. His vital signs are BP, 120/60 mm Hg; heart rate, 90 beats per minute; and respiratory rate, 20 breaths per minute.

◆ **Is any immediate action necessary?**

◆ It is very likely that the pleural space has been violated and that a hemopneumothorax exists. Chest tube insertion or tube thoracostomy (≥38 F catheter) should occur in the left side, fifth intercostal space.

You perform the tube thoracostomy.

◆ **What management is appropriate in the following situations?**

Case Variation 12.8.1. Immediately, 1,700 mL of blood is evacuated.

◆ The decision to perform an **emergent thoracotomy** is usually based on where the stab wound is located (e.g., close to a vital structure such as the heart or great vessels) and the initial volume of blood evacuated. Generally, if a tube thoracostomy is placed with 1,500 mL evacuated in a brief amount of time, a thoracotomy should be performed to evaluate for lung hilar injury or an injury to the heart.

Case Variation 12.8.2. The initial volume output from the chest tube is 1,000 mL, but the patient continues to have blood loss from the chest tube.

> **QUICK CUT** In thoracic injuries, the rate of blood loss is as important as the initial blood loss. Usually, a blood loss of greater than 200 mL/hr for 3 hours also requires thoracotomy to evaluate the injury.

Case Variation 12.8.3. The patient initially presents with hypotension with a BP of 80/50 mm Hg.

◆ Hypotension in this setting is most likely **secondary to blood loss in the left chest** (Fig. 12-8). Although a tension pneumothorax is a possibility, it is a less likely cause, and the rapid placement of a chest tube in the left thorax is necessary. If the hypotension does not respond quickly to insertion of a chest tube, the bleeding is extremely rapid, and urgent thoracotomy is indicated.

Case Variation 12.8.4. The injury is immediately inferior to the clavicle.

◆ A **subclavian arterial or venous injury** with a stab wound below the clavicle is a concern. If the patient is stable, it is necessary to perform an angiogram to inspect the vessels because operative evaluation of structures in this location is difficult and requires planning the approach. If the patient is not stable, urgent exploration is necessary (Fig. 12-9).

Case Variation 12.8.5. The injury is below the nipple on the left side (Fig. 12-10).

◆ Suspected injury to the diaphragm and organs inferior to the diaphragm occurs as a result of gunshot entrance wounds and stab wounds below the nipple. **Diaphragmatic injuries** may be missed on initial survey because herniation of intra-abdominal contents into the

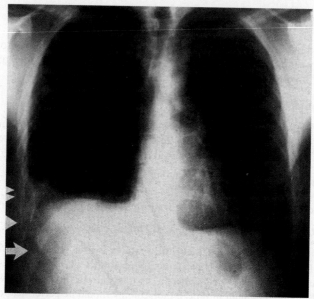

Figure 12-8: Chest radiograph demonstrating a right hemothorax (*arrow*) with multiple rib fractures. (From Greenfield LJ, Mulholland MW, Oldham KT, et al, eds. *Surgery: Scientific Principles and Practice*, 2nd ed. Philadelphia: Lippincott Williams & Wilkins; 1997:321.)

thorax may not occur in the initial period. For this reason, if suspicion of a diaphragmatic injury is high, **exploration throughout the abdomen** for related injuries, including the stomach, small bowel, colon, pancreas, and other visceral organs, is necessary. Thoracoscopy and laparoscopy are sometimes useful in this setting if the patient is stable.

Suppose the patient has a gunshot wound to the chest rather than a stab wound (see Fig. 12-10).

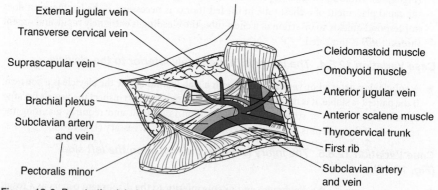

Figure 12-9: Penetrating injuries immediately below the clavicle can injure many vascular structures. (From Peitzman AB, Rhodes M, Schwab CW, et al, eds. *The Trauma Manual*, 2nd ed. Philadelphia: Lippincott Williams & Wilkins; 2002:195.)

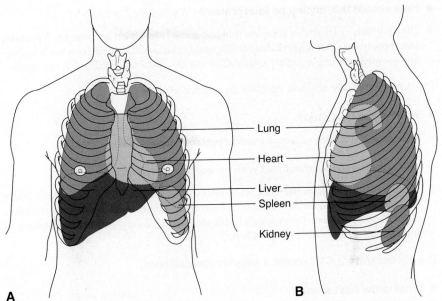

Figure 12-10: Penetrating injuries below the nipple may injure several abdominal organs. (Redrawn from Peitzman AB, Rhodes M, Schwab CW, et al, eds. *The Trauma Manual*, 2nd ed. Philadelphia: Lippincott Williams & Wilkins; 2002:195.)

◆ **How does the proposed management change?**

> **QUICK CUT** The difference in management between gunshot wounds and stab wounds relates to the unpredictable path of bullets.

Because the path of a bullet is not predictable, abdominal exploration is essential if the wound is near the abdomen. It is necessary to mark the entrance and exit wounds with a metallic marker and perform radiography to determine the current location of the bullet.

Suppose the patient has blunt trauma to the chest. You place a chest tube and find a hemopneumothorax and significant blood output.

◆ **How does the proposed management change?**

◆ The management is similar to that described for the patient with the stab wound (see Case Variation 12.8.2).

Case 12.9 Management of an Indistinct or Widened Mediastinum

A 46-year-old man who was in an automobile crash is brought to the emergency department, where he undergoes initial survey and resuscitation. On CXR, the mediastinum is wide on a portable anteroposterior film.

◆ **How should this finding be interpreted?**

◆ The possibility of a partial or complete **thoracic aortic transection is a concern**. A **portable anteroposterior CXR is unreliable** for diagnosing this condition because it tends to magnify the mediastinum. A slightly rotated CXR can also distort the mediastinal structures.

The patient is stable and has no other significant injuries.

◆ **What is the next step?**

◆ If the patient is stable and normotensive, a **posteroanterior CXR** is warranted.

◆ **What findings are associated with an aortic disruption?**

◆ A widened mediastinum has been traditionally associated with a thoracic aortic injury (Fig. 12-11). However, the most reliable findings are an indistinct aortic knob or descending aorta; they are associated with a high incidence of aortic injury. In addition, a variety of findings may also be present (Table 12-4).

The posteroanterior CXR shows a widened mediastinum.

◆ **What is the next step?**

◆ The accepted methods of establishing this diagnosis are aortic angiography (Fig. 12-12) (the "gold standard") and dynamic computed tomography angiography (CTA) scanning of the chest, which has become the most common modality to study the aorta.

A partially transected aorta is apparent on CTA (Fig. 12-13).

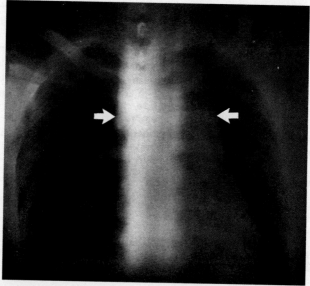

Figure 12-11: Chest radiograph in a patient with an aortic disruption showing loss of the aortic knob and a left apical pleural cap (*). Other findings include left pleural effusion and a widened mediastinum (*arrows*). (From Greenfield LJ, Mulholland MW, Oldham KT, et al, eds. *Surgery: Scientific Principles and Practice*, 2nd ed. Philadelphia: Lippincott Williams & Wilkins; 1997:327.)

Table 12-4: Radiographic Findings in Aortic Transection*

Obliteration of aortic knob

Deviation of trachea to right

Pleural cap, which is pleural fluid at top of lung cupola, suggestive of hematoma

Obliteration of aortic–pulmonary window

Deviation of esophagus to right

Depression of left mainstem bronchus or elevation of right mainstem bronchus

*An aortic transection may also be present with a normal chest radiograph or any one of these findings.

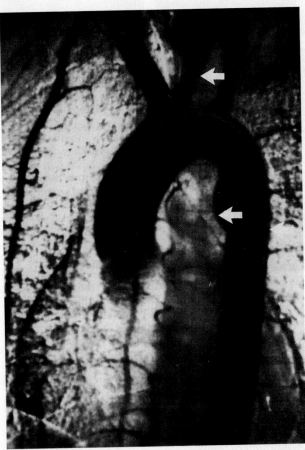

Figure 12-12: Thoracic aortogram showing a traumatic aortic aneurysm (*arrows*). (From Greenfield LJ, Mulholland MW, Oldham KT, et al, eds. *Surgery: Scientific Principles and Practice*, 2nd ed. Philadelphia: Lippincott Williams & Wilkins; 1997:369.)

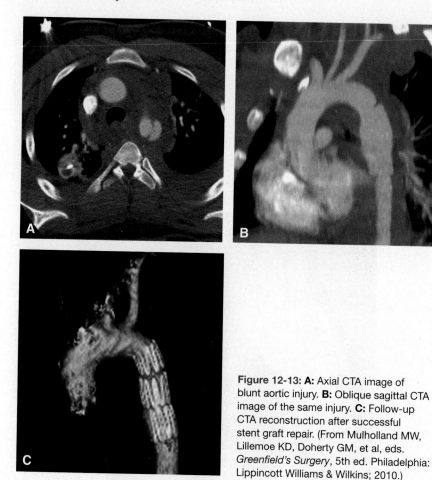

Figure 12-13: A: Axial CTA image of blunt aortic injury. **B:** Oblique sagittal CTA image of the same injury. **C:** Follow-up CTA reconstruction after successful stent graft repair. (From Mulholland MW, Lillemoe KD, Doherty GM, et al, eds. *Greenfield's Surgery*, 5th ed. Philadelphia: Lippincott Williams & Wilkins; 2010.)

◆ **What is the next step?**

◆ The grade of the injury is determined (Table 12-5). Grade I injuries and some grade II injuries are observed and treated medically. Grade III and grade IV injuries are treated surgically, most commonly with an endovascular repair if technically feasible or an open repair if an endovascular repair cannot be performed.

Table 12-5: Description of Injury

I	Intimal tear or intramural hematoma
II	Small pseudoaneurysm (<50% of the aortic circumference)
III	Large pseudoaneurysm (>50% of the aortic circumference)
IV	Rupture or transection

| Case 12.10 | Initial Abdominal Assessment Based on Mechanism of Injury |

A pedestrian, a 40-year-old man, who was struck by an automobile sustained blunt trauma. When he is brought to the emergency department, he is awake and alert, with a patent airway. Initial assessment reveals adequate ventilation and a BP of 120/80 mm Hg. You are responsible for evaluating his abdomen and making management decisions.

◆ **How does the mechanism of injury influence the approach to the patient?**

◆ Trauma patients require careful abdominal evaluation when obvious injury to the abdomen is present; the mechanism of injury is associated with a **high risk of injury or a limited reserve to tolerate injury** (Table 12-6). Injury by a mechanism described in Table 12-6 warrants further abdominal imaging.

On questioning, you discover that the patient was struck by an automobile traveling at a speed of 25 mph. Physical examination reveals no abdominal distention and minimal pain on palpation. Vital signs are stable and unchanged from admission.

◆ **Is additional abdominal evaluation necessary, or is simple observation sufficient?**

◆ Based on the previously described mechanism of injury, most trauma surgeons would further evaluate this patient with a focused assessment with sonography for trauma (FAST) despite the fact that no other findings are present.

Suppose the patient has a gunshot wound instead of blunt trauma.

Table 12-6: Injuries that Require Further Evaluation Based Solely on the Mechanism of Injury

Unprotected trauma
Pedestrians hit by motorized vehicles
Motorcycle crashes
Bicycle crashes
Assaults with objects
High-energy trauma
Motor vehicle crashes with the following:
No restraints
Substantial deformities
Known high speeds
Death at the scene
Substantial vehicular damage
Falls >15 ft
Minor trauma in patients with limited reserve to tolerate injury
Elderly patients
Patients with chronic debilitating diseases
Immunosuppressed patients

◆ **How would the decision about management change?**

◆ Gunshot wounds to the abdomen have an 80%–90% rate of intra-abdominal injuries; therefore, aggressive exploration after gunshot wounds is usually performed. If there is uncertainty whether the bullet entered the abdomen, a CT scan can help determine if there is intra-abdominal penetration and whether selective management can be attempted.

Case 12.11 Initial Assessment of Abdominal Injury

A 28-year-old man, who has been in an automobile crash, has undergone an initial trauma survey and is being resuscitated. Ventilation is good. You are responsible for evaluating the patient's abdomen.

◆ **What are the options for evaluation?**

◆ Several options allow further evaluation.

 QUICK CUT Exploration of the abdomen is justified in patients with obvious, penetrating injuries such as gunshot wounds or deep penetrating lacerations, as well as in unstable patients with a rapidly expanding (distending) abdomen or severe abdominal pain.

However, pre-emptive abdominal exploration is difficult to justify in most cases. Other options include diagnostic peritoneal lavage (DPL) and noninvasive imaging of the abdomen, which entails exploring the abdomen initially with images rather than with surgery. Commonly used methods include CT with contrast and FAST (Figs. 12-14 and 12-15).

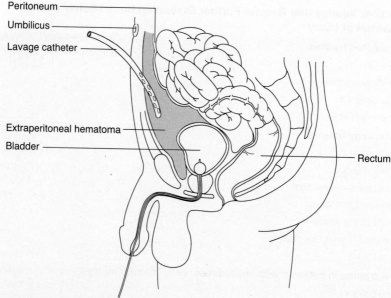

Figure 12-14: Diagnostic peritoneal lavage is performed by inserting a lavage catheter into the peritoneal cavity and testing the effluent for blood or intestinal contents. (From Greenfield LJ, Mulholland MW, Oldham KT, et al, eds. *Surgery: Scientific Principles and Practice*, 2nd ed. Philadelphia: Lippincott Williams & Wilkins; 1997:355.)

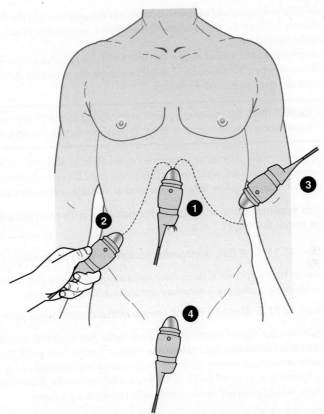

Figure 12-15: Evaluation of the abdominal contents for traumatic injuries can be performed using FAST. This technique is particularly useful for detecting blood and pericardial effusion. Evaluation for fluid in: *1*, the pericardial space; *2*, Hepatorenal space; *3*, Perisplenic; *4*, Pevis. (From Peitzman AB, Rhodes M, Schwab CW, et al, eds. *The Trauma Manual*, 2nd ed. Philadelphia: Lippincott Williams & Wilkins; 2002:239.)

 QUICK CUT DPL is most useful in situations in which the diagnosis of abdominal injury is not clear and hemodynamic instability is present.

The advantages of DPL are the rapidity of performance, low cost, and low false-negative rate (1%–2%). However, **DPL may miss injuries to retroperitoneal structures such as the duodenum and pancreas** if there is no communication between the injury and the peritoneal cavity.

In DPL, a small midline incision is made, and the peritoneum is opened. The urinary bladder must be emptied prior to this test to avoid injury to the bladder. If 10 mL or more of gross blood is encountered on opening the peritoneum, the test is positive, and the abdomen is closed.

A **positive DPL is an indication for exploration**. DPL is also positive if 100,000/mL or more RBCs are present in the lavage fluid. The appearance of vegetable matter or bile on opening the peritoneum is significant; these findings are other indications for exploration. If no blood is encountered, 1,000 mL of saline is placed into the abdomen for lavage and then removed for analysis.

Indications for FAST are similar to indications for DPL. FAST has become much more common place than a DPL due to improved technique and its less invasive nature. To perform FAST, it is necessary to complete an ultrasound examination of the four quadrants of the abdomen to check for the presence of fluid. Fluid, presumably blood, indicates the presence of an injured organ.

The interpretation of FAST is similar to DPL; FAST also provides a yes-or-no answer to the question of injury. However, FAST is rather nonspecific regarding the organ injured. It is also used to detect a pericardial effusion.

QUICK CUT CT scanning is used in stable patients with unclear abdominal injuries or a mechanism of injury that warrants further investigation.

CT scanning requires that patients be transported to the CT suite and given IV and oral contrast dye before the actual scan, which means being away from the resuscitation unit and more sophisticated care. **This procedure should be avoided in unstable or severely injured patients.**

✦ **What is the appropriate management for patients with the following additional initial findings?**

Case Variation 12.11.1. ***A flat, nontender abdomen with no evidence of injury***

✦ Observation may be sufficient if there is no mechanism of injury that warrants further evaluation. Abdominal imaging is necessary if there is such a mechanism.

Case Variation 12.11.2. ***Complaints of severe diffuse abdominal pain***

✦ Severe pain, which is a sign of significant irritation to the peritoneum from blood or intestinal contents, is an **indication for exploration** without further tests particularly with any hemodynamic changes. In centers with FAST ultrasound examination or CT scanners in the trauma receiving unit, either FAST or CT is a useful method for determining whether fluid is present in the peritoneal cavity, which would confirm an injury.

Case Variation 12.11.3. ***A tire mark across the abdomen***

✦ This finding indicates a **severe direct trauma** to the abdomen, which should make the physician very suspicious for an abdominal injury.

Case Variation 12.11.4. ***Coma on admission***

✦ It is not possible to perform a useful physical examination of the abdomen in a comatose patient. Abdominal imaging with one of the previously discussed methods (e.g., DPL, CT, FAST) is necessary.

Case Variation 12.11.5. ***A CXR that shows the stomach in the left chest (Fig. 12-16)***

✦ This patient has a **ruptured diaphragm**, which should be repaired in the operating room. Prior to surgery, the rapid evaluation of other major nonabdominal injuries is necessary.

Case Variation 12.11.6. ***A CXR that shows free air in the abdomen***

✦ The patient has a **perforated viscus.** The treatment is similar to that used in Case Variation 12.11.5.

Case Variation 12.11.7. ***Development of hypotension, with no obvious cause of blood loss***

✦ This patient is a **good candidate for FAST or DPL** for diagnosis of an abdominal injury. If either procedure is positive, the patient should urgently proceed to the operating room.

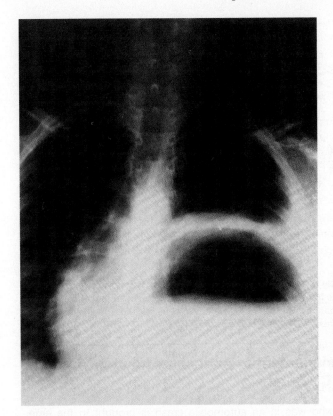

Figure 12-16: Radiograph of a diaphragmatic hernia. (From Greenfield LJ, Mulholland MW, Oldham KT, et al, eds. *Surgery: Scientific Principles and Practice*, 2nd ed. Philadelphia: Lippincott Williams & Wilkins; 1997:337.)

It is always important to perform an initial survey to assess other serious injuries. **A CT scan is inappropriate because the patient is unstable.** It is very dangerous to transport an unstable patient to CT scan where direct access to care for the patient is denied or limited.

Case Variation 12.11.8. Development of hypotension and a distending abdomen

◆ This patient most likely has a **major abdominal injury** and should proceed to the operating room rapidly.

Case Variation 12.11.9. Development of hypotension and an obviously fractured pelvis

◆ **A major vascular injury from the fractured pelvis** should be a concern. One approach involves rapid assessment of the abdomen for fluid with FAST. If significant fluid is present, the patient requires abdominal exploration first. If no fluid is present, then pelvic bleeding is the major issue. Management entails stabilizing the pelvis with a binder, and moving the patient to the angiography suite and performing a **pelvic angiogram**. Most angiography suites have well-equipped invasive monitoring and resuscitation capability, allowing for care of severely injured patients. Typically, **significant bleeding from a branch of the internal iliac artery is evident, which is controlled by embolization.** Reduction and external fixation of the fractured pelvis is also an important aspect in the control of bleeding in certain types of pelvic fractures (Fig. 12-17).

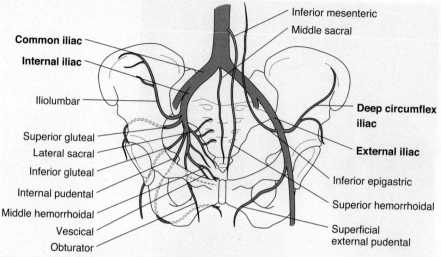

Figure 12-17: Arterial supply to the pelvis. These pelvic arteries and associated veins bleed profusely with certain pelvic fractures that disrupt the continuity. The treatment of choice is embolization. (From Peitzman AB, Rhodes M, Schwab CW, et al, eds. *The Trauma Manual*, 2nd ed. Philadelphia: Lippincott Williams & Wilkins; 2002:311.)

Case 12.12   Management of Abdominal Injuries Visible on CT Scan

A 52-year-old woman who was in an automobile crash is brought to the emergency department. After the initial survey and resuscitation, the patient is stable. No abdominal injury is obvious, but you decide to perform a CT scan of the abdomen based on the mechanism of injury.

◆ **What is the appropriate management of the following CT findings?**

Case Variation 12.12.1. Splenic laceration with fluid adjacent to the injury (Fig. 12-18)

◆ This patient has a ruptured spleen with a localized hematoma. Unstable patients should go to the operating room. Different approaches may be useful in stable patients such as this one. All approaches have the following principle in common: **Preserve the spleen if possible** to avoid postsplenectomy sepsis. Most surgeons also agree with the following statement: **Avoid blood transfusions if patients can be safely managed without them.** The management of splenic injury represents a balance between these two principles.

A splenic injury in an unstable patient should be explored. In stable patients, splenic injuries are graded with CT by the extent of injury (Table 12-7). For most grade III and lesser injuries, observation is safe and appropriate with a 90% success rate. If the CT scan demonstrates a blush or the patient has a high-grade injury with concern for active bleeding, then angiogram and embolization is highly successful in stopping the bleeding. If the spleen continues to bleed, surgery is required with a splenectomy or splenorrhaphy to control bleeding. The patient must be stable enough to transport to and undergo angiography. Infarction is rarely a problem when embolizing a portion of the spleen because of the rich collateral blood

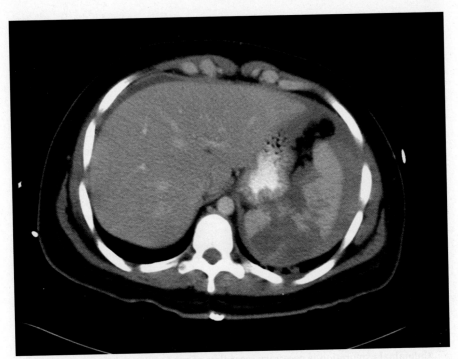

Figure 12-18: CT scan of splenic laceration.

Table 12-7: Grades of Splenic Injury

	Grade	Description of Injury
I	Hematoma	Subcapsular, nonexpanding, <10% surface area
	Laceration	Capsular tear, nonbleeding, <1 cm parenchymal depth
II	Hematoma	Subcapsular, nonexpanding, 10%–50% surface area Intraparenchymal, nonexpanding, <2 cm in diameter
	Laceration	Capsular tear, active bleeding; 1–3 cm parenchymal depth, which does not involve trabecular vessel
III	Hematoma	Subcapsular, >50% surface area or expanding; ruptured subcapsular hematoma >2 cm or expanding; intraparenchymal hematoma >2 cm or expanding
	Laceration	>3 cm parenchymal depth or involving trabecular vessels
IV	Hematoma	Ruptured intraparenchymal hematoma with active bleeding
	Laceration	Laceration involving segmental or hilar vessels producing major devascularization (>25% of spleen)
V	Laceration	Completely shattered spleen
	Vascular	Hilar vascular injury, which devascularizes spleen; hematoma >2 cm and expanding

From Wilson RF, ed. *Handbook of Trauma: Pitfalls and Pearls*. Philadelphia: Lippincott Williams & Wilkins; 1999:361.

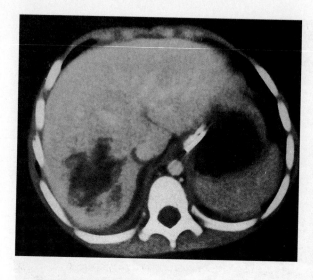

Figure 12-19: CT scan demonstrating a hepatic hematoma secondary to blunt trauma. (From Greenfield LJ, Mulholland MW, Oldham KT, et al, eds. *Surgery: Scientific Principles and Practice*, 2nd ed. Philadelphia: Lippincott Williams & Wilkins; 1997:383.)

supply from the short gastric vessels. Any patient who has had a splenectomy should receive immunization with vaccines for diplococcus, meningococcus, and *Haemophilus*.

Case Variation 12.12.2.   Liver laceration

◆ This patient has a liver injury (Fig. 12-19). CT is used to grade liver injuries (Table 12-8). **Abdominal exploration is necessary regardless of grade in unstable patients, particularly in those with grade IV, V, and VI injuries.** In stable patients, attempted observation is standard practice. Angiographic embolization is used for extravasation noted on CT scan. The risk of serious bleeding is related to the grade (see Table 12-8).

Table 12-8: Grades of Liver Injury

	Grade	Description of Injury
I	Hematoma	Subcapsular, nonexpanding, <10% surface area
	Laceration	Capsular tear, nonbleeding, <1 cm parenchymal depth
II	Hematoma	Subcapsular, nonexpanding, 10%–50% surface area Intraparenchymal, nonexpanding, <2 cm in diameter
	Laceration	Capsular tear, active bleeding; 1–3 cm parenchymal depth, <10 cm
III	Hematoma	Subcapsular, >50% surface area or expanding Ruptured subcapsular hematoma with active bleeding Intraparenchymal hematoma >2 cm or expanding
	Laceration	>3 cm parenchymal depth
IV	Hematoma	Ruptured intraparenchymal hematoma with active bleeding
	Laceration	Parenchymal disruption involving 25%–50% of hepatic lobe
V	Laceration	Parenchymal disruption involving >58% of hepatic lobe
	Vascular	Juxtahepatic venous injuries (i.e., retrohepatic vena cava/major hepatic veins)
VI	Vascular	Hepatic avulsion

From Wilson RF, ed. *Handbook of Trauma: Pitfalls and Pearls.* Philadelphia: Lippincott Williams & Wilkins; 1999:342.

> **Deep Thoughts**
>
> Because of the portal venous system and the high flow through the hepatic veins, which communicate directly to the inferior vena cava coursing behind the liver, patients can bleed very rapidly from these venous systems. Angiography will not control venous bleeding.

Case Variation 12.12.3. Injury to the mesentery

◆ Injuries at the root of the mesentery require injury forces that are significantly large. These forces **may also tear or rupture the bowel.** Leaking bowel is obviously a serious injury that requires operative intervention. It is **particularly difficult to detect these injuries on CT.** Therefore, they must be suspected based on either mechanism or associated injuries seen on CT scan. Free fluid on CT scan in the absence of a solid organ injury is suspicious for an injury to the intestine.

Case Variation 12.12.4. Rupture of the left kidney and an associated retroperitoneal hematoma around the kidney

◆ **In unstable patients, kidney ruptures require operative intervention,** although most patients are stable with isolated kidney fractures. In the setting of urgent operative intervention, it is important to **document the presence of two functioning kidneys** before removing the injured kidney. A single IV pyelogram obtained in the resuscitation area or operating room can determine this. **In stable patients,** the injury can be assigned a grade. **Angiography** is useful for the study of high-grade disruptions or intimal tears to examine for major vascular injuries. Some vascular injuries warrant planned operative repair. A large injury to the urinary collecting system may require drainage or operative repair.

Case Variation 12.12.5. Hematoma located centrally in the area of the superior mesenteric artery

◆ Centrally located hematomas suggest major injuries to either the **upper abdominal aorta or major aortic branches or direct injury to the pancreas and duodenum** (Fig. 12-20). In unstable patients, urgent exploration is necessary. In stable patients, angiography and further assessment prior to exploration are appropriate.

Case Variation 12.12.6. Partial transection of the pancreas (Fig. 12-21)

◆ This serious injury requires exploration and evaluation of the pancreas and duodenum. Treatment of pancreatic injury depends on the location of the injury and if there is ductal disruption. Contusions and minor injuries can be treated with drainage to control leakage of pancreatic enzymes. Surgical exploration, CT scan, magnetic resonance cholangiopancreatography, and endoscopic retrograde cholangiopancreatography can be used to determine if there is a major duct injury. Major duct injuries in the body and tail of the pancreas usually require distal pancreatic resection, often including the spleen, and closure of the more proximal duct with drainage. A pancreatic head injury will require drainage. A large injury to the pancreatic head and duodenum or the ampulla of Vater may require a formal pancreaticoduodenectomy.

Case Variation 12.12.7. Hematoma of the duodenum, with no other injuries in the abdomen (Fig. 12-22)

◆ A duodenal hematoma is a common injury in children who hit their abdomen on bicycle handlebars. Typically, it is an intramural hematoma that obstructs the duodenal lumen

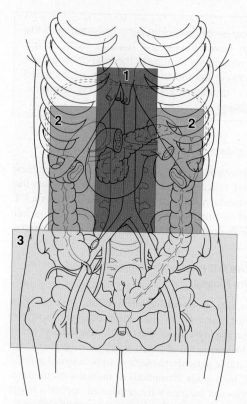

Figure 12-20: A zone *1*, or central hematoma, is a retroperitoneal hematoma that may involve injury to a major vascular structure, and it is usually surgically explored. A zone *2*, or flank hematoma, frequently is secondary to a renal parenchymal injury, and it can be observed in stable patients. A zone *3*, or pelvic hematoma, is observed in stable patients; if bleeding is present, the bleeding site is located angiographically and embolized. (From Peitzman AB, Rhodes M, Schwab CW, et al, eds. *The Trauma Manual*, 2nd ed. Philadelphia: Lippincott Williams & Wilkins; 2002:265.)

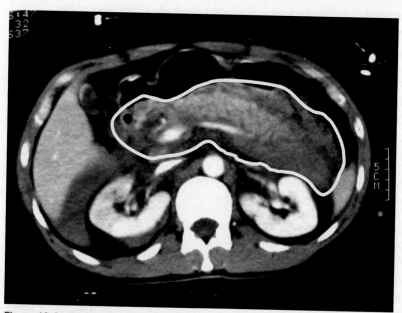

Figure 12-21: Pancreatic injury.

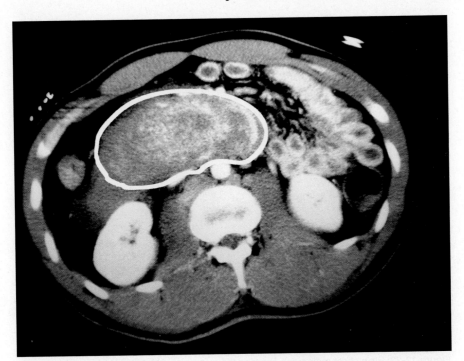

Figure 12-22: Duodenal hematoma.

and can be diagnosed on upper GI series or CT scan. If it is an isolated injury, management involves observation and no oral intake until the obstruction resolves, commonly in 5–7 days. If the hematoma persists, exploration and evacuation of hematoma is appropriate after several weeks.

Case Variation 12.12.8. *Large pelvic hematoma (see Fig. 12-20)*

◆ Pelvic fractures are associated with significant vascular injuries and pelvic hematomas.

 QUICK CUT Angiography and embolization is appropriate in patients with continued bleeding or instability.

The first step to control bleeding from a pelvic fracture is to reduce the fracture using a compressive device such as a bedsheet crisscrossed over the patient at the level of the greater trochanters or a pelvic binder. Angiograph and embolization of the bleeding arteries or the hypogastric vessels can be performed to control the bleeding. Direct surgical exploration of these patients is not likely to control bleeding. However, extraperitoneal packing where the pelvic retroperitoneum is exposed and the blood clot evacuated with packing placed against the peritoneum to tamponade the bleeding can be used to control pelvic bleeding.

Case Variation 12.12.9. *Ruptured diaphragm (Fig. 12-23)*

◆ A ruptured diaphragm requires **surgical repair**. The abdominal organs are returned to the abdomen, and the diaphragm is either primarily repaired or repaired with a prosthetic mesh.

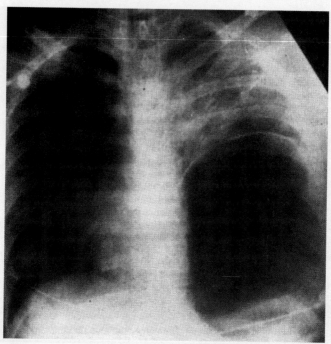

Figure 12-23: Plain chest radiograph showing the stomach herniated into the left chest in traumatic rupture of the diaphragm. (From Wilson RF, ed. *Handbook of Trauma: Pitfalls and Pearls*. Philadelphia: Lippincott Williams & Wilkins; 1999:333.)

*Case Variation 12.12.10. **Free fluid in the peritoneal cavity and no evidence of solid organ injury***

◆ Free fluid in this setting could be **blood or intestinal contents**. One should be suspicious for bowel injury and confirm it either by surgical exploration or by serial examinations and imaging.

Case 12.13   Management of Operative Findings with Abdominal Trauma

You are caring for a 47-year-old man who was in an automobile crash. The CT scan shows a small liver laceration and a grade 3 splenic laceration. The patient's vital signs continue to be stable, and no other major injuries are present. You chose treatment with close observation. Thirty minutes later, the patient deteriorates, becoming hypotensive and combative.

◆ **What is the next step?**

◆ Management of trauma patients is based on **continual assessment** of the clinical condition. Most patients with significant injuries have a dynamic course, with sometimes rapid and unexpected changes. Nonoperative management has failed in this case, and urgent surgical abdominal exploration is warranted.

On entering the peritoneum, there is a moderate amount of blood.

◆ **What should the basic steps in the operative plan be?**

 QUICK CUT The initial step is to stop the bleeding as quickly as possible by packing all four quadrants of the abdomen with gauze packs.

◆ Injuries are "attacked" in the order of their severity, with more severe injuries receiving priority. After removing one pack, the surgeon quickly assesses the area and attempts hemostasis. This is repeated in all four quadrants. Liver injuries are commonly treated by packing the laceration to achieve control rather than attempting to suture vessels.

It is possible to control the bleeding by packing the liver laceration and repairing the splenic injury.

◆ **What is the next step?**

◆ After the bleeding has been controlled, it is necessary to **inspect the remainder of the abdominal contents and repair the injuries.** Primary repair is appropriate for simple injuries, such as small bowel and stomach injuries. However, many injuries are complex and require involved procedures, including duodenal and pancreatic injuries. Primary repair of low-risk colonic injuries without a colostomy is safe. Patients with multiple injuries, hypotension, major bleeding, pancreatic injury, or significant treatment delay with peritoneal contamination are considered to be at high risk for complications, so management with resection and colostomy is usually necessary. Careful inspection of the duodenal and pancreatic areas is essential for detection of injuries.

None of the previously listed injuries are present, but a retroperitoneal hematoma is found.

◆ **What is the appropriate management?**

◆ Retroperitoneal hematomas are classified into three groups (Table 12-9; see Fig. 12-20). Management depends on the location of the hematoma and the stability of the patient.

Table 12-9: Classification of Retroperitoneal Hematomas (see Fig. 12-19 on page 388 for description)

Type	Management
Zone 1 (central hematomas)	**Usually abdominal exploration** because major injuries to the great vessels, pancreas, and duodenum might otherwise be overlooked (patients with blunt abdominal trauma). Preoperative angiogram is useful based on clinical presentation when appropriate.
Zone 2 (usually involve kidney)	**No exploration is warranted, unless hematoma is expanding. Exploration is typically appropriate** in unstable patients or in those with **penetrating trauma** to exclude major vascular injuries. With exploration, proximal arterial control of the kidney as the first step is desirable, if possible. Knowledge of presence of contralateral functional kidney is also necessary.
Zone 3 (pelvic hematomas)	**No exploration is warranted in blunt trauma. Exploration is typically appropriate** in patients with **penetrating trauma** to exclude major vascular injuries. **Angiographic embolization and pelvic fracture reduction** are appropriate, especially in unstable patients after other sources of hemorrhage have been evaluated.

Patients with **penetrating trauma** typically have zones 1, 2, and 3 hematomas **explored** to exclude major vascular injuries.

Case 12.14 Initial Neurologic Injury Assessment and Management

An 18-year-old man appears to have sustained an isolated major closed head injury in a motorcycle accident.

✦ **What is involved in the initial evaluation?**

✦ Evaluation of head trauma must always begin with a **primary survey**: ABCs. Once an adequate airway is established and the patient is adequately ventilated, vital signs can be obtained. If vital signs are stable and initial assessment reveals no other injuries requiring immediate attention, evaluation of the patient's neurologic status should take place.

The patient has stable vital signs and a head injury but evidence of no other injury.

✦ **What is involved in the assessment of the severity of the neurologic injury?**

 QUICK CUT A rapid neurologic examination and assessment of pupillary responses and other cranial nerve functions, peripheral motor and sensory function, and any deficits or focal findings, along with level of consciousness, is appropriate.

✦ It is also necessary to examine the head for evidence of direct trauma, such as a depressed skull fracture or scalp laceration. If available, the patient's state of consciousness at the scene of the accident is useful.

✦ **What signs might be present with a basal skull fracture?**

✦ A basal skull fracture is a fracture at the base of the skull where it connects to the spine. Fractures at this location may cause loss of consciousness, sinus fractures, and local hemorrhage. Blood in this location can migrate to sites visible to the surgeon, such as the ear, mastoid bone, and orbits.

✦ **How is level of consciousness assessed?**

✦ The Glasgow Coma Scale provides a quantitative measure of a patient's level of consciousness (see Table 12-2).

On examination, the patient responds to verbal stimuli, moves all extremities normally, and has intact sensation and no focal findings.

✦ **What is his Glasgow Coma Scale score?**

✦ In this example, the patient opens his eyes spontaneously (4 points), responds to verbal stimuli (5 points), and moves all extremities spontaneously (6 points). The Glasgow Coma Scale score is 15 (see Table 12-2).

✦ **What is the next step?**

✦ It is necessary to take a more complete history and perform a neurologic assessment to confirm that there are no other findings. Some physicians would observe a patient who has suffered a brief loss of consciousness (under 5 minutes) for a period of time (several hours). Other surgeons would perform a CT scan because of the loss of consciousness. Neurologic change warrants a CT scan of the head. Otherwise, the patient can be sent home if someone is there to continue the observation.

A normal CT scan virtually eliminates the possibility of a serious head injury and makes discharge from the hospital very safe. The decision to admit a patient should be based on the length of unconsciousness, the reliability of the individual, and the existence of symptoms such as nausea and vomiting. If a patient is neurologically intact, has no symptoms, has a normal head CT scan, and has a reliable home situation, the risk of a subsequent neurologic event is very low.

Case 12.15 Other Neurologic Problems

You are evaluating a 38-year-old man in the emergency department. He has an isolated head injury and loss of consciousness.

◆ **What therapeutic measures warrant consideration during the evaluation?**

◆ The possibility that a **severe head injury will cause edema of the brain, increasing the intracranial pressure (ICP) and decreasing the cerebral perfusion pressure**, should be a concern. Decreasing perfusion leads to further ischemia, edema, and eventual brain herniation and death if left untreated.

 QUICK CUT Initial management should include neurosurgical consultation and maintenance of good pulmonary ventilation and tissue perfusion.

Maneuvers that may lessen the amount of brain edema when the patient is first seen include elevation of the head to 30 degrees. Mannitol is also useful because it dehydrates the brain within 15–20 minutes, leading to decreased ICP. Mannitol administration should be slow because rapid infusion can cause asystole. It is crucial to maintain perfusion and mean arterial pressure (MAP) with appropriate resuscitation and vasopressors as needed. Cerebral perfusion pressure (CPP) is MAP − ICP. To maximize CPP, the clinician must support MAP and minimize ICP.

Deep Thoughts The best way to minimize secondary injury to the brain after a trauma is to support the perfusion to the brain by maintaining MAP with adequate fluid support and circulation support. Too much fluid can lead to brain edema, but inadequate fluid resuscitation leads to a decrease in CPP.

Once a CT scan and a neurologic evaluation have been performed, many neurosurgeons recommend maintaining the patient in a normocarbic state (stopping the hyperventilation). Routine hyperventilation is no longer practiced and may worsen the neurologic outcome. **In general, hyperventilation is currently reserved if the patient has apparent signs of impending brain herniation such as the development of a blown pupil or lateralizing signs.**

◆ **How should the following different situations be managed?**

Case Variation 12.15.1. Glasgow Coma Scale score of 3

◆ The patient is considered comatose (Glasgow Coma Scale score <8) (see Table 12-2). Endotracheal intubation is necessary, and a neurosurgery consult is warranted. To minimize the risk of cerebral edema, it is necessary to elevate the head of the bed 30 degrees and limit fluid volume. Hyposmolar fluids should not be used because they lead to increased cerebral edema in this severe injury.

QUICK CUT Unequal pupils or a lateralizing motor deficit suggest a large focal lesion.

An immediate head CT is necessary, and the patient may require emergent operation to evacuate the lesion. This patient may have a focal injury that needs surgery, but he could also have diffuse axonal injury, which occurs in 45% of coma-producing head injuries. Diffuse axonal injury is caused by microscopic injury that is distributed throughout the brain. An affected patient may remain deeply comatose with decorticate or decerebrate posturing. This condition is associated with a high mortality that is not improved by surgery.

Case Variation 12.15.2. Glasgow Coma Scale score of 10 and a dilated right pupil that sluggishly reacts to light

◆ This is a sign of development of a **space-occupying central nervous system lesion**. An immediate CT scan is necessary, and a neurosurgical consult is warranted. The typical signs and symptoms of epidural hematoma include a loss of consciousness followed by a lucid interval, a second loss of consciousness, and a dilated and fixed pupil on the same side as the lesion. Temporal lobe intracerebral hematoma can also exhibit the same signs and symptoms because it also arises from tentorial herniation. Emergent evacuation of the hematoma is required in either case.

Case Variation 12.15.3. Blood behind the tympanic membrane

◆ Blood behind the tympanic membrane indicates a **basal skull fracture**, as do ecchymosis in the mastoid region (Battle sign) or around the eyes (raccoon eyes). The patient may also have cerebrospinal fluid (CSF) leaking from the ear (otorrhea) or the nose (rhinorrhea). A skull fracture may be evidence of an underlying intracranial hematoma.

Patients with skull fractures may require admission for observation. A neurosurgical consult is warranted. Most surgeons do not place these patients on prophylactic antibiotics, but when a CSF leak is present, some do. If the patient requires a nasogastric (NG) tube or a nasotracheal tube for ventilation, physicians should take extreme caution to ensure that the tube does not perforate fractured skull bones, particularly the cribriform plate, and enter the brain. Safer alternatives are an orogastric tube and an endotracheal tube.

Case Variation 12.15.4. Sodium level of 125 mEq/L

◆ Brain injury can lead to syndrome of inappropriate antidiuretic hormone (SIADH), which is thought to be in direct response to stimulation of hypothalamic osmoreceptors. This produces a syndrome characterized by hyponatremia, concentrated urine, elevated urine sodium concentration, and a normal or mildly expanded volume of extracellular fluid. The extracellular hypotonicity leads to intracellular edema, which may cause severe cerebral edema. When hyponatremia is acute in onset, it leads to restlessness, irritability, confusion, and eventually convulsions or coma. Treatment is **water restriction**. If symptoms are severe, 3% sodium chloride solution, 200–300 mL, given over 3–4 hours, is appropriate.

QUICK CUT It is important not to correct the hyponatremia too rapidly because this may lead to central pontine myelinolysis. The general recommendation is to correct half the sodium deficit over 24 hours.

Case Variation 12.15.5. Sodium level of 160 mEq/L

◆ Just as head trauma can lead to SIADH, severe head trauma has also been associated with diabetes insipidus. This is caused by failure of release of antidiuretic hormone, resulting in polyuria, polydipsia, and excessive thirst (if the patient is conscious). If the thirst mechanisms are restricted either by unconsciousness or inadequate access to water, dehydration may develop, leading to symptoms of weakness, fever, psychic disturbances, and death. Clinically, rising serum osmolality and serum sodium concentration, which can exceed 175 mmol/L, occurs. Diabetes insipidus can be diagnosed by measuring urine osmolality after dehydration and after administration of antidiuretic hormone. Treatment is either subcutaneous **vasopressin** or desmopressin (synthetic vasopressin, also called ddAVP) and administration of **free water**.

Case 12.16 Management of Continuing Hemorrhage

A 23-year-old man has sustained a liver injury in a motor vehicle accident. The injury is a large stellate fracture in the dome of the right lobe, which can be controlled only by packing the injury and closing the abdomen. You plan to re-explore the patient the next day.

◆ **What is the appropriate management for the following postoperative conditions?**

Case Variation 12.16.1. Temperature of 95°F

◆ Studies have shown that hypothermia is a predictor of poor outcome in trauma patients.

 QUICK CUT Hypothermia leads to coagulopathy from platelet dysfunction and prolongation of the prothrombin time (PT) and partial thromboplastin time (PTT).

It is important to rewarm the patient with blankets, heating pads, or heating lamps. In this case, it is difficult to determine whether coagulopathy is secondary to liver dysfunction, massive transfusion, or hypothermia. Once the patient is rewarmed, it is possible to discover the existence of other causes. If the coagulopathy is not corrected by normalization of the temperature, the treatment is administration of fresh frozen plasma to restore coagulation factors.

Case Variation 12.16.2. Platelet count of 30,000/mm³

◆ A decline in platelet number to 30,000/mm³ may result from inadequate replacement of circulating platelets, and it worsens the overall coagulopathy. Decreased platelets can also result from disseminated intravascular coagulation (DIC) from a transfusion reaction or sepsis, which may result from lysis of blood products. Due to the severity of injury and the risk of ongoing bleeding, platelet transfusions to keep the platelet count above 60,000/mm³ are necessary.

Case Variation 12.16.3. Metabolic acidosis

◆ Metabolic acidosis may result from **hypothermia or hypovolemia and subsequent tissue hypoperfusion**. Both conditions require correction.

Case Variation 12.16.4. Development of abdominal distention and oliguria

◆ Abdominal distention and oliguria may indicate **continued hemorrhage** from the liver and accumulation of intra-abdominal fluid and blood. The oliguria may be caused by decreased renal blood flow resulting from a tense abdominal compartment, so-called abdominal compartment syndrome. Affected patients may also have difficulty with ventilation due to increased inspiratory pressures required because of elevated diaphragms. In either case, a hematocrit can confirm continued hemorrhage, in which case emergent exploration in the operating room is necessary.

Case 12.17   Management of Postoperative Problems in Trauma Patients

A 25-year-old man ruptures his spleen in a motorcycle accident. The injury requires splenectomy, with an estimated blood loss (EBL) of 500 mL in the operating room. He is now in the recovery room.

◆ **What is the appropriate evaluation and management in terms of fluids and electrolytes?**

◆ It is appropriate to both review the patient's operative blood loss and fluid replacement in the operating room and assess whether he has received adequate replacement. Any deficits should be corrected. Blood losses should be replaced with packed RBCs milliliter for milliliter or with 0.9 normal saline (3 mL saline per milliliter blood loss). At that point, if his urine output is adequate (0.5–1 mL/kg/hr), his vital signs are stable, and he does not appear to be hemorrhaging, maintenance fluid replacement is appropriate.

Suppose the patient has multiple additional injuries such as a lung contusion and a fractured femur in addition to the spleen injury.

◆ **How should the management plan be modified?**

◆ Because of the multiple injuries, the body has sustained greater stress and will mount a greater inflammatory response. Additional fluid loss into the third space will necessitate greater fluid replacement. However, physicians should avoid overaggressive volume administration in the setting of a pulmonary contusion in which the damaged lung is more susceptible to edema.

You replace his fluid losses to an appropriate level, and since then, he has been stable during your frequent visits. You see him 48 hours postoperatively and there is a change. His BP is 105/60 mm Hg, and his urine output has been 10 mL/hr over the past 4 hours.

◆ **What is the next step in his evaluation and management?**

◆ This patient most likely has large third-space losses due to the multiple injuries, and he is most likely again hypovolemic. A fluid challenge with 1–2 L of normal saline or lactated Ringer solution is necessary.

You give him a fluid bolus of 2 L and see no response in urine output or BP.

◆ **What is the next step?**

◆ If the patient does not respond to a 2-L bolus, measurement of his **CVP** is necessary to determine if hydration is adequate. CVP provides an index of the preload of the right ventricle. If the CVP is decreased, this indicates hypovolemia, and additional volume replacement is appropriate.

The patient's CVP is 10 cm H₂O, and he remains oliguric and hypotensive.

◆ **What is the next step?**

◆ The patient appears to be adequately hydrated as measured by the CVP and yet is still not responding to the fluid challenge. One explanation is a low cardiac output from an abnormally functioning heart. A second, more likely, explanation is that the CVP is not a correct reflection of the left heart filling pressures; the patient is still volume-depleted with decreased preload, resulting in a low cardiac output.

There are limitations to the use of CVP alone. One is the assumption that right ventricular function parallels left ventricular function, which is usually true in normal individuals but not necessarily true in sick patients. Decreased preload to the left ventricle and decreased cardiac output may be present despite a normal CVP. A **pulmonary artery catheter** permits measurement of the cardiac output; right atrial, pulmonary artery, and pulmonary capillary wedge pressure (PCWP); and systemic vascular resistance (SVR). These measurements allow you to assess ventricular function and guide the administration of fluids or cardiac medications designed to enhance pump function. An echocardiogram looking at cardiac function and vena caval filling can give information about the intravascular volume status as well. If the left ventricle is not filled or the vena cava collapses on expiration, then the patient is still hypovolemic. At this point, placement of a pulmonary artery catheter to determine filling pressures to both sides of the heart is appropriate.

Your resident asks you to describe a Swan-Ganz catheter and the method for its insertion.

◆ **How do you respond?**

◆ The Swan-Ganz catheter allows measurement of CVP and pulmonary artery pressure (Fig. 12-24). When the balloon near the tip is inflated, the catheter tip measures a pulmonary artery occlusion pressure, or **PCWP**, which correlates closely with left atrial pressure ultimately measuring left ventricular end diastolic pressure. The PCWP can be interpreted in the left atrium similarly to the CVP in the right atrium. If the **PCWP is low, hypovolemia** and decreased left heart preload are present. If the PCWP is high (in the range of 20–25 mm Hg), pulmonary edema and fluid overload, caused by either left heart failure or overhydration, are present.

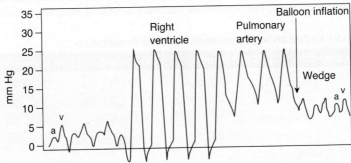

Figure 12-24: Pressure tracing seen while inserting a Swan-Ganz catheter. (From Sabiston DC, ed. *Davis-Christopher Textbook of Surgery*, 13th ed. Philadelphia: WB Saunders; 1986:71.)

The Swan-Ganz catheter also has a highly sensitive temperature probe near its top, which allows for the performance of cardiac output measurements. More sophisticated catheters that can measure the venous blood oxygen saturation in the pulmonary artery are available.

The catheter is inserted through a central venous access line, and the balloon is inflated, which tends to drag the catheter in the direction of blood flow through the heart. During passage through the line, the location of the catheter can be determined by monitoring the pressure readings at the catheter tip. When the catheter is in the right ventricle, arrhythmias are common and should be managed by either advancing or withdrawing the catheter.

◆ **What is the normal SVR, and what conditions change this value?**

◆ The normal SVR should be 800–1,400 dynes-sec/cm^5. SVR elevation may occur in cardiogenic shock, hypovolemic shock, hypertension, or with administration of vasoconstrictors. SVR reduction may occur in septic shock, neurogenic shock, or with administration of vasodilators (Table 12-10).

You measure the patient's PCWP and cardiac output (see Table 12-10).

◆ **What is the correct interpretation of the results and the proper management of the patient in example 1 (see Table 12-10)?**

◆ In example 1, the PCWP is low, indicating hypovolemia, which results in decreased venous return, eventually lowering cardiac output. The low cardiac output stimulates increased SVR by vasoconstriction. The value of 2.5 is low enough to suggest that the tissues are not being adequately perfused, and more volume is needed. Treatment involves restoration of circulatory volume.

The patient has the hemodynamic findings presented in example 1 (see Table 12-10). On the basis of these data, he is hypovolemic, and the administration of IV fluids until his PCWP reaches 15 mm Hg appears to be appropriate. He initially responds with an improvement in BP. However, over the next 24 hours, he again becomes oliguric and hypotensive. Measurement of hemodynamic parameters yields the values presented in example 3 (see Table 12-10).

◆ **What is the correct interpretation of the findings in example 3 (see Table 12-10)?**

◆ In example 3, the patient is in a **hyperdynamic state** because the cardiac output is high; this finding is characteristic of high-output septic shock. SVR falls and cardiac output increases for two reasons: (1) the left ventricle has little resistance against which to pump and (2) an adequate preload is restored.

The sequence described here is not atypical of sepsis. Early sepsis causes fluid sequestration (third-space losses) and vasodilation that result in hypovolemia and decreased cardiac

Table 12-10: Calculation of Systemic Vascular Resistance

Example (see text)	PCWP (mm Hg)	CO (L/min)	SVR (dynes-sec/cm^5)
1	3	2.5	2,000
2	20	2.0	2,400
3	15	9.5	300
4	20	15.0	300

SVR = (MAP − CVP)/CO × 80.
PCWP, pulmonary capillary wedge pressure; CO, cardiac output (L/min); SVR, systemic vascular resistance; MAP, mean arterial pressure; CVP, central venous pressure.

preload, leading to an early decrease in cardiac output. Once the fluid deficit is replaced, the low-SVR, high–cardiac output picture appears.

◆ **What management is appropriate?**

◆ Treatment includes **antibiotics and elimination of the infectious source**. In the surgical patient, elimination of the septic site often means careful examination of the patient and abdominal imaging to locate a septic site. If an abscess is present, it should be drained surgically or percutaneously. Many patients improve as a result of this treatment if it is implemented expeditiously. If this is not performed, the patient may progress to late sepsis and a septic shock characterized by decreased cardiac output and continued decreased SVR. Mortality is greatly increased in patients who progress to hypodynamic septic shock. Resuscitation should continue and a vasoconstrictor such as nor-epinephrine may be necessary if vasodilation prevents organ perfusion despite adequate volume resuscitation.

Suppose your patient had the findings in example 2.

◆ **What is the correct interpretation of the results and management of the patient in example 2 (see Table 12-10)?**

◆ In example 2, the patient may be suffering from cardiogenic shock, in which the CVP or PCWP is increased and the cardiac output is severely decreased. The SVR is increased due to an outpouring of sympathetic impulses. In this situation, the CXR would most likely reveal pulmonary edema. This type of shock does not respond to IV fluids. The etiology of heart failure may be due to a traumatic injury to the myocardium or due to pre-existing myocardial disease. To care for the patient appropriately, it is necessary to determine the exact cause of the problem.

Suppose your patient has a spinal cord injury at the C5 level.

◆ **What are the expected hemodynamic parameters?**

◆ Hypotension secondary to spinal cord injury is termed **neurogenic shock**. Impairment of the sympathetic nervous system leads to systemic vasodilation and decreased contractile force of the heart. The diagnosis is usually made in a hypotensive trauma patient with a normal or slow pulse and evidence for a spinal cord injury. Pulmonary artery catheter measurements typically demonstrate a low SVR, a low PCWP, and a low cardiac output due to decreased cardiac preload and contractility. Treatment is adequate replacement of intravascular volume. The addition of vasoconstrictors such as dopamine, phenylephrine, or norepinephrine to increase the SVR and cardiac drugs to increase the heart rate may be necessary.

Case 12.18   Traumatic Arteriovenous Fistula

A 25-year-old man presents to the emergency department with acute shortness of breath, which has progressed over the past several months. His past history is significant for a stab wound to the left groin area 5 years ago, which was treated with observation. He has no other illnesses. On physical examination, he has a BP of 120/80 mm Hg, a heart rate of 125 beats per minute, bilateral rales, and jugular venous distention. Cardiac examination reveals a systolic ejection murmur and an S_3 gallop.

◆ **Could the patient's stab wound from 5 years ago possibly cause his current problem?**

◆ The patient could have an undiagnosed traumatic arteriovenous fistula from the injury. At the time of injury, the fistula was small, but over time, it has enlarged and become hemodynamically significant. **High-output cardiac failure** is now present.

◆ **How is confirmation of this diagnosis obtained?**

◆ On physical examination, the patient would most likely have a **palpable thrill and audible bruit over the fistula**. Occlusion of the fistula with direct pressure leads to an expected significant drop in heart rate as a result of the rise in peripheral resistance. A drop of 10 beats per minute or more is thought to be significant and is termed **Branham sign**. A duplex study or angiogram could also confirm the diagnosis.

The patient has a significant arteriovenous fistula causing cardiac failure.

◆ **What is the next step?**

◆ Surgical repair of the fistula is necessary, but until the patient's cardiac status improves, repair should not be undertaken. A cardiologist should be consulted, and the patient's cardiac status optimized. The best intraoperative management probably is a pulmonary artery catheter.

A pulmonary artery catheter is inserted.

◆ **What values would you expect to find?**

◆ The expected values are presented in example 4 (Table 12-11).

The patient undergoes repair of the fistula.

◆ **How do you repair the fistula?**

◆ It is necessary to control the artery and vein proximal and distal to the fistula, disconnect the connection, and repair the vessels. Typically, the artery is very dilated, thin-walled, and difficult to handle. Clamping the artery should result in a rapid improvement in hemodynamics.

Table 12-11: Normal Cardiovascular Pressures

Location	Pressure (mm Hg systolic/mm Hg diastolic)
Right atrium	0–6
Right ventricle	20–30/0–6
Pulmonary artery	20–30/6–12
Pulmonary artery mean	12–18
PCWP	6–12
Left atrium	4–12
Left ventricle	100–140/5–14
Arteries	100–140/60–80
Mean arterial pressure = 75–100 mm Hg	
Cardiac output = 4–8 L/min	
SVR = 800–1,400 dynes-sec/cm^5	

PCWP, pulmonary capillary wedge pressure; SVR, systemic vascular resistance.

◆ **Do hemodynamically significant fistulae in surgical patients occur in any other situations?**

◆ This condition commonly occurs in two other situations. The first situation involves patients with chronic renal failure who are on hemodialysis with one or more **arteriovenous fistulas for dialysis access**. Significantly high blood flow rates (3–6 L/min) may occur and be hemodynamically significant, especially in the presence of the anemia of renal failure. The second situation involves patients with **an abdominal aortic aneurysm that ruptures into the inferior vena cava**. This creates a large fistula over a very brief period of time that results in rapid decompensation of the patient and pulmonary edema. Hemorrhage into the surrounding tissues usually does not occur.

Case 12.19 Management of Continuing Pulmonary Problems

A 30-year-old woman is hit by an automobile while she is a pedestrian. She sustains multiple bilateral rib fractures, a right pneumothorax, and multiple severe soft tissue contusions. Her airway is patent, and she is ventilating adequately. You perform a right tube thoracostomy (insert a chest tube).

◆ **What is the correct interpretation and management of the following situations?**

Case Variation 12.19.1. Severe rib pain

◆ The patient's rib pain is most likely secondary to **rib fractures** and the presence of a thoracostomy tube. It is important to administer adequate analgesics to prevent excessive splinting, which leads to atelectasis, hypoxia, and increased risk of pneumonia.

Case Variation 12.19.2. Pulse oximetry of 90% and a respiratory rate of 28 breaths per minute

◆ At this time, the patient is exhibiting **moderate respiratory distress**, and reassessment of airway patency is essential. Examination of the patient's chest and breathing, looking for symmetry of respiratory movement, is necessary, along with auscultation of the chest. It is important to send an arterial blood gas (ABG) to determine the patient's ventilatory status as well as oxygenation. Placement on oxygen to increase the arterial oxygen saturation to more than 95% is also appropriate. The patient should have a CXR to confirm the position of the chest tube and complete expansion of the lung.

   One possible source of the patient's hypoxemia is a persistent pneumothorax related to a problem (leak or kink) in the tube thoracostomy system. It is necessary to assess if the Pleurovac chamber is bubbling correctly and is connected to wall suction. Other causes of hypoxia are chest splinting from pain, atelectasis, and pulmonary contusion.

After giving the patient a dose of morphine, her arterial oxygen saturation drops from 92% to 85% and her respiratory rate drops from 32 to 10 breaths per minute with shallow breaths. An ABG indicates that the Pco_2 is 55 mm Hg. Inspection and palpation of the chest wall indicates a large, painful anterior area that does not move and expand with inspiration in the normal expansion direction but instead depresses.

◆ **What is the diagnosis and management?**

◆ The patient has two problems, **hypoventilation related to oversedation** and most likely a **flail chest**, which occurs when multiple rib fractures leave a segment of chest wall unstable (Fig. 12-25). This causes paradoxical movement of the chest wall. The examiner may also

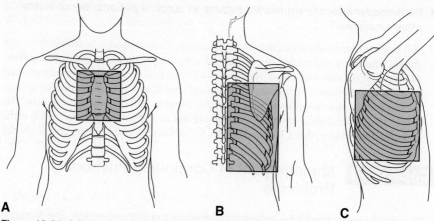

Figure 12-25: A flail chest causes a mobile segment of chest wall that moves paradoxically with respiration. **A:** Anterior view. **B:** Posterior view. **C:** Lateral view. (From Campbell DR. Trauma to the chest wall, lung and major airways. *Curr Probl Surg.* 1998:726.)

feel crepitus overlying the ribs, and there is often severe injury to the underlying lung, which contributes to the hypoxia.

Treatment includes adequate ventilation, administration of oxygen, and careful fluid balance to avoid pulmonary edema. The patient is not ventilating adequately with narcotic treatment, and several management options are appropriate. One possibility is **intubation**. A second option is regional anesthesia with a **thoracic epidural catheter** for relief of rib pain. Typically, bupivacaine, a local anesthetic, and morphine are infused into the epidural space to relieve pain and improve respiratory dynamics. If it is effective, the narcotic can be eliminated; it can cause sedation and other undesirable neurologic effects in older patients and patients who have the catheter at a high thoracic level. Epidural anesthesia can be especially helpful in the elderly because it may avoid mechanical ventilation, which leads to a high likelihood of pneumonia and other complications. A third option is **patient-controlled analgesia**, which lowers the peak narcotic levels and perhaps improves the risk–benefit ratio.

This patient's current ventilatory state requires urgent intubation and mechanical ventilation. More careful observation might have avoided intubation.

Case Variation 12.19.3. *Chest injury requiring a chest tube*

◆ You are managing a patient similar to the one described in Case Variation 12.19.2 who has a chest injury requiring a chest tube. Pulse oximetry is 86% on 4 L of nasal oxygen, and the respiratory rate is 40 breaths per minute.

◆ **What management is appropriate?**

◆ This patient has severe respiratory distress and requires immediate treatment with **emergent intubation** to avoid respiratory arrest. She cannot maintain a respiratory rate of 40 breaths per minute for very long.

Case 12.20 Management of Respiratory Distress

The woman described in Case 12.19 develops further respiratory distress and requires intubation and mechanical ventilation. On CXR, bilateral hilar infiltrates and an infiltrate over the area of the flail chest are apparent. The fractional concentration of oxygen in inspired gas (FIO_2) is 40%, arterial oxygen saturation is 85%, and ABGs reveal a PCO_2 of 54 mm Hg.

◆ **How should the following conditions be interpreted and managed?**

Case Variation 12.20.1. PCO_2 of 55 mm Hg

◆ The patient is **underventilated**. It is necessary to correct this condition by increasing the ventilatory rate or volume. This may also improve her hypoxia. Her CXR indicates a lung contusion and the probability of acute respiratory distress syndrome (ARDS) suggested by the hilar infiltrates.

Case Variation 12.20.2. PCO_2 of 25 mm Hg

◆ The **ventilatory rate is excessive.** By bringing the PCO_2 closer to 40 mm Hg, it is possible to decrease the rate. You will still have to reassess her oxygenation.

Case Variation 12.20.3. You increase her FIO_2 to 60%, which fails to increase the patient's oxygenation above 56 mm Hg.

◆ This could signify **worsening ARDS, a mucous plug, or possible malposition of the endotracheal tube.** It is necessary to repeat the CXR to determine placement of the endotracheal tube. If the CXR shows massive atelectasis on one side, it could mean significant underventilation of that lung due to tube misplacement or occlusion of the tube by a mucous plug. Treatment entails repositioning or suctioning the tube. If suctioning does not resolve the problem, bronchoscopy should be performed to remove mucous plugs, obtain sputum samples, and open occluded airways. Bronchoscopy should always be performed cautiously in hypoxic patients because of the risk of worsening the hypoxia and causing cardiac arrest. It is appropriate to continue to increase the FIO_2 to bring the PO_2 above 60 mm Hg. To accomplish this, the addition of positive end-expiratory pressure (PEEP) to the ventilator may be necessary. PEEP maintains a constant baseline pressure on the airway, which recruits more alveoli to remain patent and available for gas exchange.

Case Variation 12.20.4. You increase her FIO_2 to 80%, which still does not improve oxygenation.

◆ At this point, it is necessary to bring the FIO_2 up to 100% until the cause of the hypoxia is determined. PEEP should be added to the ventilator and started at 10 cm H_2O. An arterial line should be placed both to monitor BP and to allow frequent blood gas measurements. A CXR should be obtained to help determine the cause of the hypoxia.

The addition of PEEP for adequate oxygenation is necessary.

◆ **She is now on PEEP. How would you manage the following situations?**

Case Variation 12.20.5. When you add 10 cm H_2O PEEP, it results in a decline in BP from 120/80 mm Hg to 90/60 mm Hg.

 QUICK CUT The addition of 10 cm H_2O of PEEP causes the cardiac output to drop by impairing venous return to the heart.

◆ A pulmonary artery catheter may be necessary to monitor the patient's cardiac output and preload. This allows the physician to counterbalance the negative cardiovascular effects of PEEP by altering preload and cardiac function.

Case Variation 12.20.6. When you add 10 cm H₂O PEEP, it results in a decline in the patient's urine output, which remains at 10 mL/hr.

◆ Likewise, the high level of PEEP is causing the cardiac output to drop, decreasing perfusion to the renal parenchyma and resulting in oliguria. The treatment is the same as in Case Variation 12.20.5.

The patient's oxygenation and hemodynamics stabilize with 10 cm H_2O PEEP. During evening rounds, the intensive care unit (ICU) nurse urgently calls you because the patient has suddenly become extremely hypoxic and hypotensive and cannot be ventilated.

◆ **What intervention is appropriate?**

◆ With hypoxia, hypotension, and difficulty ventilating, it is necessary to determine if the patient has a **tension pneumothorax**. This is an *emergent* diagnosis. First, place the patient on 100% oxygen and attempt to bag the patient by hand. Listen to the lungs on both sides to determine whether breath sounds are present. If you cannot hear breath sounds on one side, it is necessary to perform a needle thoracostomy with an angiocatheter in the second intercostal space in the midclavicular line. If you hear a rush of air and note improvement in the patient's vital signs, your action has most likely solved the problem. In either event, you should place a thoracostomy tube in the fifth intercostal space in the midaxillary line and then obtain an upright CXR.

Case 12.21   Stab Wound to the Neck

A 25-year-old man is brought to the emergency department with a stab wound to the neck. He has no other apparent injuries.

◆ **What are the initial management steps?**

◆ The initial step is evaluation of the airway. With neck injuries, the chance of airway problems, including direct injury such as a transection of the trachea in the neck, is significant. Injuries to other structures can also cause airway compromise by compression and distortion of the airway such as might occur with an expanding hematoma, placing pressure on the pliable trachea. If airway injury is indicated, early elective intubation is preferable to emergent intubation or tracheostomy. If there is active hemorrhage from the wound, a quick assessment of the injury and application of direct digital pressure to control the bleeding is also appropriate.

The patient is able to talk normally. Assessment of the airway indicates that it is patent and that ventilation is good. There are no other injuries apparent elsewhere on his body. His vital signs are stable, with a normal BP and a heart rate of 80 beats per minute.

◆ **What is the next step in the evaluation of the patient's neck?**

◆ It is necessary to perform a careful examination of the neck to determine what structures are injured as identified by palpation (Table 12-12). In addition, you should ascertain whether a hematoma is present and, if so, whether it is expanding and threatening the airway.

Examination indicates that the injury, which is in the anterior triangle of the neck at the level of the thyroid cartilage, penetrates the platysma. There is a 4-cm–diameter hematoma that appears to be enlarging in size. A small amount of blood is leaking from the wound. The patient's vital signs remain stable.

Table 12-12: Important Structures to Examine in a Stab Wound to the Neck

Airway structures: tenderness, mobility, distortion or displacement, air in soft tissues, bubbling from wound, voice quality (e.g., hoarseness)

Vascular structures: evidence of active or recent bleeding, stable or expanding hematoma

Salivary glands: proximity of injury to major or minor salivary glands

Esophagus: pain or difficulty on swallowing, saliva in wound

Nervous system: neurologic deficits

Lungs: breath sounds in the cupola of lung, chest radiograph

Muscular structures: degree of platysma penetration, position in relation to sternocleidomastoid muscle (anterior or posterior)

◆ **What is the next step?**

◆ Exploration of the neck is necessary because the patient has evidence of a vascular injury in zone II (Fig. 12-26). During intubation, examination of the vocal cords is warranted to determine whether an injury has occurred.

Exploration indicates an injury to the internal jugular vein, which is repaired.

◆ **What other features of the neck should be examined?**

◆ The surgeon should follow the path of the knife and examine all nearby structures. It is necessary to explore the carotid artery and vagus nerve. In addition, the trachea and esophagus may also warrant exploration if the stab path is in proximity with these structures.

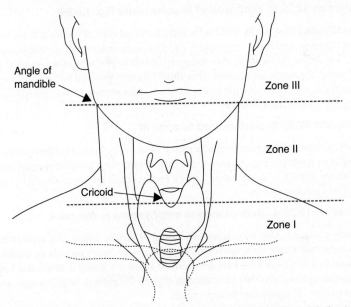

Figure 12-26: The neck can be divided into three zones. In stable patients, injuries to zones I and III are often managed by assessment, with preoperative angiography to ascertain vascular injury due to exposure of certain areas. (From Peitzman AB, Rhodes M, Schwab CW, et al, eds. *The Trauma Manual*, 2nd ed. Philadelphia: Lippincott Williams & Wilkins; 2002:192.)

You complete the exploration and close the wound. The patient returns to the floor. That evening, the nurse calls you to see the patient because there is some blood on the dressing. On examination, you note a 3-cm–diameter hematoma beneath the incision that was not present at the end of the procedure. The patient tells you that he feels fine but says that he feels a tightness in his neck and is having some trouble taking deep breaths.

◆ **What is the next step?**

◆ Airway compromise from a postoperative neck hematoma should be a concern. This situation requires urgent intervention. The removal of several sutures from the neck incision and release of the hematoma should relieve the pressure on the trachea and improve the patient's breathing. If not, then urgent intubation is necessary. Either way, he should return to the operating room for control of the airway and evacuation of the hematoma and hemostasis.

Case 12.22 Other Injuries to the Neck

You are caring for a 51-year-old woman with a traumatic injury to the neck.

◆ **How do the following findings influence decision making?**

Case Variation 12.22.1. Gunshot wound to the neck, with a BP of 80/60 mm Hg

◆ A patient who is hypotensive should go directly to the operating room for resuscitation and simultaneous exploration of the neck wound. In addition, gunshot wounds are more likely to have significant associated injuries due to the blast effect of the projectile.

Case Variation 12.22.2. Stab wound to zone I (see Fig. 12-26)

◆ Injuries to zone 1 may involve structures such as the subclavian vessels that are technically difficult to expose and repair surgically. If patients are hemodynamically stable, a preoperative CTA to define the location of an injury and to allow planning of the surgical approach is very useful. If patients are unstable, they should directly proceed to the operating room. It is necessary to remember that the thoracic outlet is part of zone I. Thus, injuries to the lung and brachial plexus can also occur.

Case Variation 12.22.3. Stab wound to zone III

◆ The management of this injury is similar to that of an injury in zone I; a preoperative CTA is very useful in stable patients. Injuries to the carotid artery are possible; surgical control and repair is very difficult in that location, and an endovascular approach should be considered for isolated vascular injuries.

Case Variation 12.22.4. Subcutaneous emphysema in the neck

◆ This finding suggests that there is an esophageal or airway injury, and exploration of the neck is indicated. Other findings associated with airway injury include air bubbling from the wound and an obvious tracheal deformity. If an airway injury is suspected, but there is no firm evidence and no other indication to explore the patient, bronchoscopy and laryngoscopy to rule out injury may be appropriate.

Case Variation 12.22.5. Difficulty swallowing

◆ This suggests an injury to the esophagus. This would be managed similarly to the injury in Case Variation 12.22.4, with use of esophagoscopy or a swallow study to rule out injury if there is no other clear indication for surgery.

Case Variation 12.22.6. Hoarseness

◆ Hoarseness could represent an airway injury similar to other airway injuries but could also indicate direct laryngeal trauma, laryngeal dislocation, or injury to the recurrent laryngeal nerve. Direct laryngoscopy and bronchoscopy is necessary, and surgical exploration and possible trachesotomy is indicated depending on the endoscopy findings.

Case Variation 12.22.7. Hemiparesis

◆ A carotid artery injury or thrombosis should be a concern. The patient should have a CTA or angiogram. It is necessary to define the injury and base the treatment on the specific findings in consultation with a vascular surgeon or neurosurgeon.

Case Variation 12.22.8. Blunt trauma to the neck

◆ Marked extension of the neck or direct blunt trauma may result in intimal disruptions and dissection of the carotid artery, which can produce carotid thrombosis and neurologic deficits. Management of asymptomatic carotid injuries and thromboses usually involves anticoagulation. The management of symptomatic carotid occlusions is controversial. Some surgeons would attempt thrombectomy if a thrombosis is less than several hours old and is associated with significant neurologic deficits. Other surgeons would recommend anticoagulation alone.

  Whether to repair a carotid injury or thrombosis is a decision that should be made in consultation with an experienced surgeon; these injuries often involve the carotid artery where it enters the base of the skull. This makes the surgical exposure very difficult and increases the complexity of the procedure.

Case Variation 12.22.9. Zone II stab wound with no symptoms, no other physical findings, and stable vital signs

◆ Management varies. Routine exploration on the patient's neck was common, now diagnostic evaluation using a CTA is usually the initial approach. Selective exploration or diagnostic evaluation with bronchoscopy and esophagoscopy is based on the clinical exam and CT findings.

Case 12.23 ┃ Burn

A 22-year-old man who is brought to the emergency department with extensive burns is conscious and breathing. History reveals that he was trapped in his house trailer when it caught fire. He has no other known medical problems.

◆ **What are the first steps in evaluation and management?**

◆ Initially, the basic principles of trauma management as assessment of ABCs. Most burn patients do not die as a result of the burn but from later complications. It is necessary to remove the clothes and stop any further burn injury. Cooling injured areas is appropriate, but prolonged cooling can cause core hypothermia. The patient should be placed on clean sheets.

 QUICK CUT In the initial assessment of the airway, determine whether an airway burn is likely. Suggestive factors are carbonaceous sputum, facial burn, facial or nasal hair burns, hoarseness, low oxygen saturation, or dyspnea.

Burns that occur in closed spaces are more likely to be associated with airway burns.

Table 12-13: Description of the Types of Burns

First-degree burns

- Microscopic destruction of **superficial layer of epidermis** (erythema of skin, as seen in sunburn)
- Of little clinical significance because water barrier of skin remains undisturbed
- Pain is usually chief symptom; it usually resolves within 48–72 hours.
- Damaged epithelium peels off in small scales after 5–10 days, leaving no scar.

Second-degree burns

- Damage extends **through epidermis into dermis**.
- Referred to as **partial-thickness burns** because epithelial regeneration can occur
- Blisters may be present; when burns are superficial, blisters heal within 10–14 days if not infected.
- May occur in more severe form, which burns more deeply into dermis; a layer of white, nonviable dermis is seen. **Deep second-degree burns** can easily develop into third-degree burns without proper burn management to prevent surface infection.

Third-degree burns

- Involve **full thickness of skin down to subcutaneous tissue**
- Total, irreversible destruction of all skin, dermal appendages, and epithelial elements
- Characterized by white, waxy appearance; lack of sensation; lack of capillary refill; and leathery texture
- Require skin grafting for repair
- Deep second- and third-degree burns are equally significant physiologically, and coverage may be estimated by the "rule of nines" (see Table 12-13).

◆ **What is involved in assessment of the patient's burns?**

◆ This assessment is most easily performed in three steps.

1. Determine the **depth of burn** (Table 12-13).
2. Identify the **type of burn**. Common types include flame burns, contact burns with a hot object, scald burns with a hot liquid, and steam burns.
3. Determine the **percentage body surface area (BSA) burned** (Table 12-14). The area of a burn wound is expressed as a percent of the total BSA.

The **"rule of 9's"** is the most common way of estimating the BSA burn. Using this rule, different body parts account for certain percentages, and the sum of these values represents the total area burned. Note that this rule is not used in children because their heads take up a larger percentage of their BSA. Separate burn charts are available for children to determine percentage BSA burn. It is possible to obtain another good estimate of the BSA by measuring the size of the burn using the size of the patient's hand as representative of 1% of the BSA.

◆ **Under what conditions would it be necessary to transfer the patient to a burn center?**

◆ Several reasons for transfer are generally accepted (Table 12-15).
The estimated weight of the man is 70 kg, and he appears to have suffered deep second- and third-degree flame burns over 30% of his BSA.

Table 12-14: "Rule of Nines" Used to Determine Percent of Surface Area Burned in Adults

Anatomic Area	% Body Surface
Head	9
Right upper extremity	9
Left upper extremity	9
Right lower extremity	18
Left lower extremity	18
Anterior trunk	18
Posterior trunk	18
Neck	1

◆ **How is the amount of fluid replacement estimated?**

◆ The overall strategy of burn resuscitation aims **to return plasma volume to normal and sustain adequate perfusion of tissues.** Evidence supports the need for both crystalloid and colloid solutions. The Parkland formula has been adopted in many burn centers to provide specific replacement guidelines; it can be used to calculate the volume of solution necessary in the first 24 hours after the burn.

◆ Total volume of lactated Ringer solution = % BSA burned × weight (kg) × 4 mL/kg where BSA = body surface area.

One-half of the solution is given over the first 8 hours, and the second half is given over the next 16 hours. **In the next 24 hours,** it is also necessary to give D_5W to replace evaporative water loss and maintain serum sodium at 140 mEq/L and administer 0.5 mL 5% albumin or fresh frozen plasma / percentage BSA burned over 8 hours to maintain colloid oncotic pressure.

Crystalloid solutions are used to expand depleted plasma and extracellular volumes as soon as possible, which helps return cardiac output to normal. **Colloid is not given in the first 24 hours** because the capillaries are "leaky," and most of the fluid will leak into the extracellular space very quickly. **Colloid is most effective for returning intravascular/ plasma volume to normal without adding edema.**

Table 12-15: Indications for Transfer to a Burn Center

Full-thickness burn >5% BSA

Partial-thickness burn >20% BSA

Age younger than 5 or older than 50 years

Burns of face, hands, feet, genitalia, perineum, or over major joints

Inhalation injury

Circumferential burns of the chest or extremities

Chemical or electrical burns

Burned children without qualified pediatric specialists

BSA, body surface area.

◆ **What is the appropriate management in the following situations?**

Case Variation 12.23.1. Need for topical treatment of burns

◆ It is important to provide an aseptic environment for topical wound care in burn patients to prevent infections. Although superficial burns do not require topical antibiotics, deeper wounds do. **Silver sulfadiazine**, mafenide, and povidone-iodine ointment are some of the topical antibiotics available for use. Occlusive dressings are used to minimize exposure to air, increase the rate of epithelialization, and decrease pain. It is necessary to change the dressings at least twice daily to inhibit bacterial growth. Third-degree burns may also require regular debridement of necrotic tissue until a biologic dressing, preferably a split-thickness skin graft of the patient's own skin, is in place.

Prophylactic systemic antibiotics are not used because they select for resistant organisms. They should be used only for clearly documented infections. The most common infections are *Staphylococcus aureus*, *Pseudomonas*, *Streptococcus*, and *Candida*.

Case Variation 12.23.2. Dark urine that is positive for blood

◆ Microscopic analysis of the urine is necessary. If no RBCs are seen, the patient has **myoglobinuria** and is at risk for **acute tubular necrosis** if this condition goes unrecognized and inadequately treated. **Fluids** should be administered to ensure urine output two to three times normal. **Alkalinization** of the urine and osmotic diuretics (e.g., mannitol) may also be used in severe cases.

If RBCs are present in the urine, the workup should include investigation into traumatic causes of hematuria. In addition, electrical injuries can cause hemolysis.

Case Variation 12.23.3. Carbonaceous sputum and hoarseness

◆ It is essential that these signs of **inhalation injury** not be overlooked because they are indications of laryngeal edema and pulmonary injury. Other signs of inhalation injury include singed facial hair, carbon particles in the oropharynx, and a history of being burned in a closed space. Some institutions perform laryngoscopy at presentation to determine the need for intubation. The threshold for intubation should be low.

Deep Thoughts It is always better to intubate a patient too early rather than too late.

Carbon monoxide poisoning should be a consideration in every patient suspected of having inhalation injury. Levels of carboxyhemoglobin of more than 5% in nonsmokers or more than 10% in smokers indicate carbon monoxide poisoning. If this has occurred, 100% oxygen should be administered until the carboxyhemoglobin level returns to normal and symptoms resolve. Hyperbaric oxygen chambers are also used to rapidly remove carbon monoxide from the blood.

Case Variation 12.23.4. Methemoglobinemia

◆ Methemoglobin is hemoglobin with the iron oxidized to the ferric (Fe^{3+}) form rather than the normal, reduced ferrous (Fe^{2+}) state. The ferric form is unable to bind or transport oxygen. Enclosed-space fires can cause a buildup of this product, which results in a shift of the oxyhemoglobin dissociation curve to the left.

Symptoms of methemoglobinemia range from a chocolate-brown appearance of the blood and central cyanosis of the trunk and proximal extremities to generalized seizures, coma, and cardiac arrhythmias. **Pulse oximetry is unreliable as a measure of oxygen saturation** because it cannot differentiate between methemoglobin and hemoglobin. Instead, ABG readings should be taken. If the patient is asymptomatic, supplemental oxygen is sufficient as treatment; methemoglobin will reduce to normal hemoglobin in 24–72 hours. Specific therapy for methemoglobinemia is administration of IV methylene blue (1–2 mg/kg). In extreme cases, if massive hemolysis occurs, hyperbaric oxygen therapy or exchange transfusion may be necessary.

Case Variation 12.23.5. Early deterioration of ABCs with CO_2 retention

◆ With early deterioration of ABG readings and CO_2 retention, **airway obstruction is likely.** This condition warrants prompt endotracheal intubation and mechanical ventilatory support. Added positive pressure helps prevent atelectasis and closure of lung units distal to the swollen airways.

Case Variation 12.23.6. Circumferential third-degree burn of the thorax

◆ Circumferential burns rapidly become thick and contracted, limiting motion and blood flow. In the chest, this may seriously impair ventilation, whereas in the extremities, it may create ischemia and necrosis of the muscles. An **escharotomy** helps avoid this problem (Fig. 12-27).

Case Variation 12.23.7. Electrical burn

◆ Electrical burns appear benign on the surface but may be associated with large amounts of **interior damage to muscles, nerves, and vessels**. Examination for entrance and exit sites is necessary. Evaluation with an ECG and cardiac enzymes is appropriate to rule out suspected cardiac injury. Necrotic muscle results in myoglobinuria, which can cause acute renal failure. Maintaining high urine output and alkalinizing the urine can prevent such renal failure.

Case 12.24 Total Parenteral Nutrition

A 50-year-old man who was in an automobile crash undergoes exploration for abdominal injury. He has a significant contusion to his bowel with intramural hematomas and several areas of perforation. The bowel is repaired but is very edematous. Postoperatively, you decide that enteral feeding is not safe and that TPN is appropriate during the postoperative period.

◆ **What is the initial step in determining the nutritional requirements for this patient?**

◆ Nutrients may be given by TPN when the GI tract is unavailable or not functioning. TPN provides calories, amino acids, electrolytes, vitamins, trace minerals, and fatty acids through a central venous catheter. For every patient who requires TPN, it is necessary to determine the nutritional status.

QUICK CUT "Nondepleted" patients (those with a good nutritional status) are in a minor catabolic state. Depleted patients were malnourished before surgery. Hypermetabolic patients are in a severely stressed catabolic state (i.e., due to trauma, burn, sepsis, cancer).

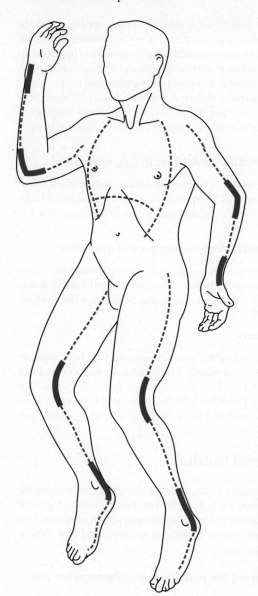

Figure 12-27: Preferred sites for escharotomy. Third-degree burns can cause immobility and contraction of muscular compartments and the chest. Escharotomy may be necessary if vascular or ventilatory compromise is present. (From Martin RR, Becker WK, Cioff WG, et al. In: Peitzman AB, Rhodes M, Schwab CW, et al, eds. *The Trauma Manual*, 2nd ed. Philadelphia: Lippincott Williams & Wilkins; 2002.)

◆ Requirements for both protein and energy vary according to the patient's nutritional state. The protein requirements of patients who are considered **nondepleted** are approximately 1.0 g/kg/day, with total daily calories of 20% above **basal energy expenditure**. The protein and calorie requirements of **depleted** patients are in an intermediate zone. The protein requirements of **hypermetabolic** patients may be 2.0–2.5 g/kg/day, with total daily calories of 50%–100% above basal energy expenditure.

This patient appears to be in a nondepleted condition, in a minor catabolic state.

Table 12-16: Estimate of Daily Baseline Metabolic Needs

Weir formula for determination of **resting energy expenditure (REE)** (kcal/min)*

$3.9(VO_2) + 1.1(VCO_2) - 2.2$(urine nitrogen [g/min]) where VO_2 is the oxygen production and VCO_2 is the carbon dioxide output.

Harris-Benedict equation for determination of **basal energy expenditure (BEE)** (kcal/24 hr)†

Males

$66 + (13.7 \times$ weight [kg]) + $(5 \times$ height [cm]) $- (6.7 \times$ age [years])

Females

$665 + (9.6 \times$ weight [kg]) + $(1.8 \times$ height [cm]) $- (4.7 \times$ age [years])

*Requires metabolic cart to measure.
†Estimate based on age, weight, height, and gender. BEE can be estimated as approximately 1,400–1,800 kcal/day (30 kcal/kg/day) for baseline needs (as much as 3,000 kcal/day in severely stressed patients).

◆ **What is the estimated daily energy expenditure?**

◆ A patient's daily energy expenditure can be measured by a variety of methods. The most accurate is indirect calorimetry, which involves calculation of the production of O_2 (VO_2) and CO_2 (VCO_2) from the timed volumetric collection of expired O_2, CO_2, and urinary nitrogen (Table 12-16). Because indirect calorimetry requires measurements of gas volumes using sophisticated equipment (metabolic cart), it is not often performed.

If you assume this patient was well-nourished prior to surgery and is the standard 70-kg male, his daily baseline caloric needs are about 30 kcal/kg/day $\times$ 70 kg = 2,100 kcal/day.

◆ **Given this caloric estimate, how would you choose the type of TPN solution?**

◆ Protein should not serve as a calorie source when a determination of the type of TPN is made. Instead, protein is needed to replace the amino acids that are constantly being recycled in the body. Calories are derived from a mixed-energy substrate system, with approximately 70% of calories supplied as dextrose and 30% of calories supplied as fat (Table 12-17).

In this patient, a standard TPN formula, which is a 50% dextrose solution with 4.25% amino acids, could be given (see Table 12-17; Table 12-18). Fat is usually given as a 10% or 20% emulsion, separate from the TPN bag. A single infusion of 500 mL is usually given over 10–12 hours. Serum triglyceride levels must be monitored to avoid high levels. If hypertriglyceridemia occurs, the amount of lipid administered must be reduced.

To determine the calories in 1 L of standard TPN solution, see Table 12-18. If 1,000 mL of $D_{50}W$ and 500 mL of fat emulsion is given over a 24-hour period, the total nonprotein calories infused is 1,700 + 550 = 2,250 kcal.

◆ **How is the daily nitrogen requirement determined?**

◆ A patient who is critically ill and on TPN should have a positive nitrogen balance as a goal, particularly with a body weight that is 10% or more below the ideal level. Nitrogen balance is defined as nitrogen intake minus nitrogen excretion. Nitrogen intake in a patient on TPN is calculated from the contents of the solution. The protein in TPN is typically 4.25%, which means there are 4.25 g of protein per liter. To calculate the nitrogen content of the same liter of TPN solution described in Table 12-17, use the formula grams nitrogen = grams protein ÷ 6.25. This calculation yields 4.25 g protein ÷ 6.25 = 0.68 g nitrogen per liter of TPN.

Table 12-17: Composition of a Standard Central Venous Solution

Basic Requirements for Standard Total Parenteral Nutrition	
Fat	9 kcal/g
Carbohydrate	3.4 kcal/g
Protein	4 kcal/g
Volume	
10% amino acid solution	500 mL
50% dextrose solution	500 mL
Fat emulsion	—
Electrolytes	~50 mL
Total volume	~1,050 mL
Composition	
Amino acids	50 g
Dextrose	250 g
Total potassium	8.0 g (50 ÷ 6.25)
Dextrose kcal	840 kcal (250 g × 3.4 kcal/g)
mOsm/L	~2,000

Electrolytes Added to TPN Solutions	Usual Concentration (mEq/L)	Range of Concentrations (mEq/L)
Sodium	60	0–150
Potassium	40	0–80
Acetate	50	50–150
Chloride	50	0–150
Phosphate	15	0–30
Calcium*	4.5	0–20
Magnesium	5	5–15

*Calcium is generally added as calcium gluconate or calcium chloride. One ampule of calcium gluconate = 1 g of calcium = 4.5 mEq.

Table 12-18: Calculation of Calories in Standard Total Parenteral Nutrition Solution in Adults

$D_{50}W$ contains 500 g/L of glucose.

500 g × 3.4 kcal/g = 1,700 kcal/L

A 10% fat emulsion represents 1.1 kcal/mL of fat. Therefore, 500 mL contains 550 kcal.

A 4.25% amino acid solution contains 4.25 g/100 mL of amino acids or 42.5 g/L.

42.5 g × 4 kcal/g = 170 kcal (not to be used for caloric calculation)

Nitrogen excretion can be partially measured and partly estimated. Up to 90% of nitrogen excretion is in the form of urea in the urine. Stool losses of nitrogen are approximately 1 g/24 hours in patients who are eating and much less in patients who are on nothing by mouth (NPO) feeding. A 24-hour urine collection and urea measurement allow the majority of urinary nitrogen excretion to be measured. To convert grams of urea to grams of protein, it is necessary to multiply the urea by 0.50. An additional 15% of protein is lost in the urine from nonurea compounds, including creatinine and ammonia.

Once the nitrogen balance has been determined, it is appropriate to adjust the standard TPN solution infusion rate to maintain a positive balance.

QUICK CUT The more severe the injury, the more severe the catabolic state and the higher the amino acid requirement.

The response to starvation in normal individuals is to use ketones for energy, which spares protein from being metabolized. During starvation, the overall metabolic rate also falls. In severe injury, the adaptation to ketone metabolism does not occur, and thus protein is used as a source for gluconeogenesis (Table 12-19). This creates a significant catabolic state. In addition, the resting metabolic state increases with severe injury, which also increases the need for energy and thus increases the catabolic state. The metabolic rate alters in response to various diseases (Fig. 12-28).

◆ **What other molecules are also in TPN solution?**

◆ The standard composition of TPN solutions is shown in Table 12-17.

The patient has been on TPN for 2 weeks and still cannot tolerate enteral feeding.

◆ **What is the appropriate evaluation and management for the following TPN-related problems?**

Case Variation 12.24.1. Fever

◆ A temperature spike greater than 101°F may indicate an **infected catheter**, among other causes. Patients should undergo complete evaluation for all possible sources of infection. The physician should examine the catheter site for erythema, tenderness, or purulence and obtain cultures both peripherally and directly from the catheter. If cultures are positive or fever persists, it is necessary to select a new catheter site and initiate antibiotics.

Case Variation 12.24.2. Metabolic coma

◆ **Hyperglycemic, hyperosmolar, nonketotic coma** is a common cause of coma in patients on TPN. This condition is **secondary to dehydration following excessive diuresis due to hyperglycemia.** This situation warrants discontinuation of TPN, administration of insulin, and very close monitoring of glucose and electrolytes.

Table 12-19: Daily Amino Acid Requirement for a 70-kg Man

Condition	Amino Acids Needed (g/kg/day)	Catabolic State
Uncomplicated postoperative course	1.0–1.5	Mild
Mild to moderate sepsis or injury	1.5–2.0	Moderate
Severe sepsis or burn	2.0–3.0	Severe

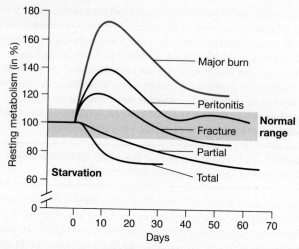

Figure 12-28: Metabolic response to surgical stress and starvation. Major burns represent the largest metabolic requirement encountered by humans. (From Wilson RF, ed. *Handbook of Trauma: Pitfalls and Pearls.* Philadelphia: Lippincott Williams & Wilkins; 1999:578. After Long CL, Schaffel N. Metabolic response to injury and illness: estimation of energy and protein needs from indirect calorimetry and nitrogen balance. *JPEN J Parenter Enteral Nutr.* 1979;3:425.)

Case Variation 12.24.3. *Elevated bilirubin and liver enzymes*

◆ Liver function tests become abnormal in as many as 30% of patients on TPN. During the first 2 weeks, transaminases rise, and a gradual increase in alkaline phosphatase occurs. Rising enzyme levels normally respond to a modest reduction in the rate of infusion. Failure of the serum enzymes to plateau or return to normal within 7–14 days should suggest another etiology. Fatty liver and structural liver damage can be induced by TPN. Prolonged TPN can cause cirrhosis, but this usually occurs over years of TPN.

Case Variation 12.24.4. *Dry, scaly skin*

◆ This condition is indicative of free fatty acid deficiency. Administration of lipids should correct the problem.

Chapter 13

Congenital Anomalies

Clint D. Cappiello, Eric D. Strauch, Bruce E. Jarrell

Key Thoughts

1. Bilious emesis in a newborn is malrotation and midgut volvulus until proven otherwise. If the patient has peritonitis or free air, this is done in the operating room. If the patient's abdominal exam is benign, then an upper gastrointestinal series (UGI) should be emergently obtained.

2. In patients with congenital diaphragmatic hernia (CDH), ventilation with the lowest possible pressure to both lungs is crucial. High ventilator pressure results in barotrauma, which can be lethal in a patient with pulmonary hypoplasia.

3. Morbidity and mortality associated with esophageal atresia and tracheoesophageal fistula (TEF) is usually related to comorbidities such as prematurity and complex congenital cardiac disease.

4. The high mortality in patients with an omphalocele is usually related to chromosomal abnormalities and complex congenital cardiac disease. There has been a significant reduction in patients born with omphalocele partially due to termination of the pregnancy in these fetuses with nonsurvivable or high mortality conditions.

5. The mortality in patients with gastroschisis is related to intestinal injury from the gastroschisis resulting in sepsis or short gut syndrome.

6. When evaluating a neonate with a bowel obstruction, it is helpful to determine if the obstruction is proximal in the GI tract or in the distal small intestine or colon. The differential diagnosis is different and the approach is different. Proximal obstructions are best diagnosed with abdominal x-ray (AXR) and UGI evaluation and usually require surgical intervention. Distal obstructions are best diagnosed with a lower gastrointestinal (LGI) study and in the case of meconium ileus and meconium plug, can be treated with an LGI.

7. Idiopathic ileocolic intussusception in children is different than small bowel intussusception in several ways. The colon is involved; there usually is no lead point; and the intussusception can be reduced with an air or contrast enema with surgery reserved for failure of nonoperative management.

8. Pyloric stenosis results in a hypokalemic, hypochloremic metabolic alkalosis because of emesis and volume loss. Although acid is lost from vomiting, the alkalosis is perpetuated by sodium retention to maintain intravascular volume by exchanging potassium and hydrogen ions in the kidney. The key to correcting the hypokalemic, hypochloremic metabolic alkalosis is sodium and volume repletion.

Case 13.1 Acute Respiratory Distress

A newborn full-term infant presents with acute respiratory distress. The patient was significantly tachypneic with a respiratory rate of 90 breaths per minute and oxygen saturations at 70% on blow by oxygen. The physical exam showed no breath sounds on the left hemithorax, the heart sounds are shifted to the right, and a scaphoid abdomen. The patient was emergently intubated and placed on the ventilator. A chest x-ray (CXR) (Fig. 13-1) was obtained.

◆ **What is the most likely diagnosis?**

◆ The differential diagnosis includes CDH, congenital pulmonary airway malformation (CPAM) (sometimes called congenital cystic adenoid malformation), bronchopulmonary sequestration (BPS), bronchopulmonary foregut malformation, bronchogenic cysts, enteric cysts, and teratoma. This CXR is consistent with a CDH.

◆ **What is the initial management?**

◆ Initial management includes the following:

1. Intubation and support with gentle low-pressure, high-frequency ventilation
2. Nasogastric (NG) decompression to prevent gastric and intestinal decompression
3. Arterial line
4. Measurement of oxygen saturations proximal and distal to the ductus arteriosus
5. Echocardiogram to look for any congenital cardiac anomalies and pulmonary hypertension

◆ **What would you do if the patient improves with this therapy?**

◆ If the patient can be adequately oxygenated, ventilated, with good perfusion to the tissues without acidosis, then the patient is observed and stabilized for several days or more until the CDH is repaired. Rushing the baby to the operating room can result in life-threatening

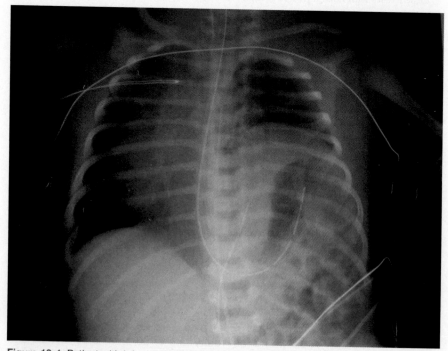

Figure 13-1: Patient with left-sided CDH. Intestines and stomach with the NG tube in place in the left hemithorax. (Photo courtesy of Dr. Eric D. Strauch.)

pulmonary hypertension and persistent fetal circulation. This results in shunting unoxygenated blood from the right-sided circulation to the left-sided circulation created more hypoxia and acidosis resulting in more pulmonary hypertension and a vicious circle is created.

◆ **What treatment can be used for pulmonary hypertension?**

◆ Acidosis causes pulmonary vasculature to constrict, which decreases blood flow to the lung and increases the right-to-left shunt. So maintaining perfusion and adequate ventilation to prevent acidosis is crucial. Pressors may be used to support the systemic pressure to minimize right-to-left shunt. For persistent hypoxemia and hypercarbia, high-frequency oscillatory ventilation (HFOV) is used. Inhaled nitric oxide (NO), a potent pulmonary vasodilator, can improve hypoxemia by treating pulmonary hypertension.

◆ **What intervention can be done if conventional therapy for pulmonary hypertension fails?**

◆ If acidosis with hypoxemia persists despite maximal support, extracorporeal membrane oxygenation (ECMO) should be considered. ECMO requires anticoagulation and has risk of bleeding particularly intracranial hemorrhage.

◆ **How is the CDH repaired?**

◆ Operative management is based on the following principles:

The herniated contents are reduced surgically back into the abdomen with a subcostal incision or thoracotomy. Recently, a thoracoscopic approach has been successful, although the recurrence rate is higher than for open repairs. The hernia defect is repaired either primarily or with a prosthetic patch. The infant's acid–base balance and respiratory function are monitored carefully and aggressive support using pressors, HFOV, NO, and ECMO are continued as needed.

The loss of abdominal domain can make primary repair difficult. A silo or abdominal patch is placed to prevent intra-abdominal compartment syndrome if needed.

◆ **What is the prognosis of patients with CDH?**

◆ Survival rates are 60%–90% because of improved perioperative and operative management strategies. The lungs are almost always hypoplastic when a diaphragmatic hernia is present. Pulmonary function approaches normal as survivors reach adulthood. Studies have shown that CDH survivors develop appropriate exercise tolerance even if pulmonary function tests indicate some level of impairment.

Case 13.2   Respiratory Distress with Oral Intake

A newborn full-term infant without respiratory distress at birth presents with acute respiratory distress and choking during the first feed. The patient was significantly tachypneic with a respiratory rate of 70 breaths per minute immediately after the feed attempt. The physical exam reveals coarse breath sounds bilaterally. The patient improved after a coughing episode.

◆ **What is the initial management for this patient?**

◆ Attempt placement of an NG tube and obtain a CXR and AXR (Fig. 13-2). The patient has an esophageal atresia (proximal pouch) with a distal TEF, which is the most common type of esophageal atresia; it occurs in about 86% of patients.

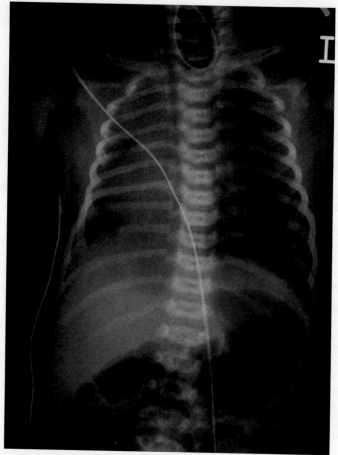

Figure 13-2: Esophageal atresia with distal TEF. Note the curled NG tube in the proximal esophageal pouch that cannot be passed further distally into the esophagus because of the proximal esophageal atresia. The air in the GI system is indicative of a distal TEF. (Photo courtesy of Dr. Eric D. Strauch.)

◆ **What other diagnostic evaluation is necessary for this patient?**

◆ The diagnosis of esophageal atresia is made by the inability to pass an NG tube into the stomach. The type of esophageal atresia is determined by the presence of gas in the GI tract. If the patient has air distally, in the GI tract, the patient must have a distal fistula, where the distal esophagus communicates with the trachea.

Types include the following (Fig. 13-3):

1. **Pure esophageal atresia** (proximal and distal blind pouches) without a fistula occurs in 7% of patients.
2. **Esophageal atresia with a proximal TEF** (the least common type) occurs in 0.5% of patients.
3. **Esophageal atresia** (proximal pouch) **with a distal TEF** is the most common type; it occurs in 86% of patients.

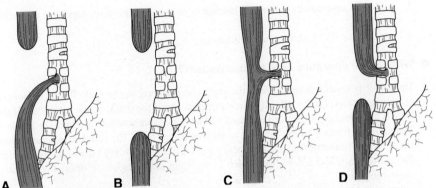

Figure 13-3: Types of esophageal atresia. (From Jarrell BE. *NMS Surgery*, 6th ed. Baltimore: Lippincott Williams & Wilkins; 2015.)

4. **TEF without atresia** (the N-type fistula) occurs in 5% of patients. It differs in its presentation in that patients tend to present at an older age with recurrent pneumonia.
5. **A proximal and distal TEF** occurs in 1.5% of patients.

Associated congenital anomalies occur in approximately 50%–70% in infants with esophageal atresia, oftentimes with multiple organ systems involved. Evaluation for the VACTERL association, a well-recognized anomaly complex, involves vertebral anomalies, anal defects, cardiac anomalies, tracheoesophageal atresia and fistula, and renal and limb dysplasia is necessary.

Cardiovascular anomalies are the most common; among these, ventricular septal defects and tetralogy of Fallot are most frequently encountered. An echocardiogram is necessary preoperatively to evaluate for the presence of any cardiac abnormalities, which, if present, can affect anesthesia and surgical care. A renal ultrasound and voiding cystoureterogram should be performed to evaluate for renal anomalies, but this does not have to be done in advance of surgical care. A complete physical examination can evaluate for the presence of any anal or limb malformations.

QUICK CUT The VACTERL association, a well-recognized anomaly complex, involves vertebral anomalies, anal defects, cardiac anomalies, tracheoesophageal fistula, and renal and limb dysplasia.

The complex may be fully or partially demonstrated; that is, one or any combination of lesions may occur.

TEF is also associated with other genetic syndromes include Down syndrome, DiGeorge sequence, and trisomy 18.

◆ **What is the preoperative care for this patient?**

◆ Preoperative management includes the following:

1. Decompression of the proximal pouch by means of a sump tube (Replogle tube) with low continuous suction is required.
2. An upright position is maintained to help prevent aspiration of refluxed gastric contents through the TEF into the lungs.

3. Acid reduction usually with an H_2 blocker to minimize pulmonary damage if aspiration occurs

4. Intravenous (IV) hydration and antibiotics

◆ **What is the operative care for this patient?**

✦ The repair is usually done through the right chest as long as the aorta lies in its normal anatomic position on the left side. Some surgeons repair the defect thoracoscopically if the baby is large and physiologically normal. Otherwise, a thoracotomy is done. The fistula is ligated at the trachea taking care not to narrow the trachea. The distal esophagus is then anastomosed to the proximal esophageal pouch. Usually, a feeding tube is placed through the anastomosis, and a drain can be left in the right pleural space to drain any potential anastomotic leak.

◆ **What would be the next step if saliva comes from the chest drain?**

✦ An anastomotic leak has occurred. This can be due to excessive tension on the anastomosis and ischemia of the esophageal ends; 95% of leaks close spontaneously with adequate drainage by a pleural tube and nutritional support. If the leak persists and is large, an anastomotic disruption has occurred and the anastomosis must be redone or a cervical esophagostomy must be performed.

◆ **How would you proceed if the baby has emesis of formula during each feed?**

✦ The patient may have gastroesophageal reflux, which is the most common complication following TEF repair reported in approximately 40%–70% of patients. Anastomotic stricture may also present in this fashion and is a common early complication following TEF repair.

◆ **How would you differentiate an anastomotic stricture from reflux?**

✦ A UGI can diagnose a stricture. Strictures are usually treated with serial dilations and acid reduction as they are exacerbated by gastroesophageal reflux disease.

Case 13.3 Bilious Emesis

A newborn full-term baby presents with bilious emesis. On physical examination, the baby's abdomen is mildly distended.

◆ **What is the initial diagnostic test?**

✦ Obtain an AXR. If the AXR shows a complete intestinal obstruction, or extraluminal or free air, the baby is taken to the operating room for a laparotomy.

◆ **What is the next diagnostic test?**

✦ Bilious emesis particularly in a newborn is the early warning sign for intestinal malrotation and volvulus. The patient may have a midgut volvulus, where the midgut from the third portion of the duodenum to the distal transverse colon twists around the superior mesenteric vessels. Midgut volvulus results in ischemia and potential death of the midgut in as soon as 6 hours. Therefore, this diagnosis must be made immediately to save the child. If the baby has peritonitis or is sick, then an emergent laparotomy is done. If the baby is stable, then a UGI study is performed (Fig. 13-4). The AXR in a baby with malrotation is usually

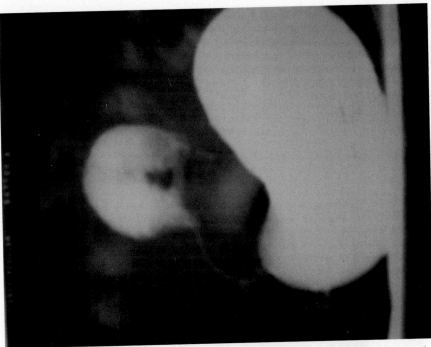

Figure 13-4: A UGI on a patient with malrotation and a midgut volvulus. The contrast abruptly stops at the third portion of the duodenum with a bird's beak appearance consistent with a midgut volvulus. (Photo courtesy of Dr. Eric D. Strauch.)

normal unless there is a volvulus with ischemic or dead intestine. Once the diagnosis of midgut malrotation is made, the baby is taken emergently to the operating room to detort the intestine and do a Ladd procedure.

◆ **What is the Ladd procedure?**

◆ This procedure consists of releasing the adhesive bands and mobilizing the duodenum. The goal is to broaden the mesentery of the intestine as much as possible and to separate the duodenum and ascending colon. Also, the appendix is removed, as it will lie in the left upper quadrant making the diagnosis of acute appendicitis difficult.

◆ **If the baby does not have malrotation, what is the diagnosis?**

◆ There are other causes of intestinal obstructions in the newborn. The baby may have duodenal atresia, which usually presents with bilious emesis. Duodenal atresia can be suspected on prenatal ultrasound if a dilated stomach and duodenum is seen.

Case Variation 13.3.1 Duodenal atresia

◆ **How is the diagnosis of duodenal atresia made?**

◆ Abdominal radiographs show the classic **double bubble sign** (Fig. 13-5), which involves air in the stomach and a proximally dilated duodenum. Paucity of distal gas suggests complete obstruction.

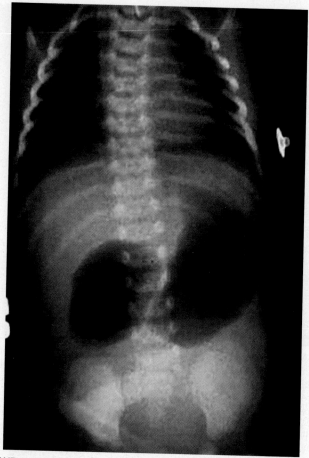

Figure 13-5: AXR showing the double bubble sign. The stomach and proximal duodenum are dilated and filled with air and there is no distal gas. This is indicative of a duodenal atresia. (Photo courtesy of Dr. Eric D. Strauch.)

◆ **How is duodenal atresia managed?**

◆ Preoperative management includes:

1. Gastric decompression and fluid resuscitation are performed as needed.
2. Preoperative antibiotics are administered.
3. Associated anomalies

Trisomy 21 occurs in 30% of infants with duodenal malformations.

Cardiac lesions are present in many infants (~25%). An echocardiogram should be done before surgery.

An annular pancreas may be present (~25%), with the pancreas forming a ring around the duodenum. This anomaly is due to failure of the ventral pancreatic bud to completely rotate dorsally. Although the annular pancreas may cause extrinsic compression, an underlying web or stenosis is the true cause of the obstruction.

◆ **How is duodenal atresia treated?**

◆ Operative repair is performed by bypassing the obstruction using a duodenoduodenostomy. If a web is present, the duodenum is opened at the site of obstruction, the web is excised, and the duodenum is closed transversely. Care must be taken to identify the ampulla of Vater because it is also located on the mesenteric side of the web.

    If an annular pancreas is present, the repair is the same and the pancreas is left untouched and the obstruction bypassed with a duodenoduodenostomy. In no circumstance is the pancreas divided since duct structures run in this tissue and if transected will result in a persistent pancreatic leak.

Case Variation 13.3.2.

◆ **What if the obstruction is in the more distal small intestine?**

◆ The AXR shows dilated small intestine with no distal gas caused by a jejunal obstruction usually from a jejunal atresia (Fig. 13-6). Jejunal, ileal, and colonic atresias are caused by in utero vascular accidents that result in ischemia of a segment of bowel, with consequent stenosis (5%) or atresia (95%). Jejunoileal atresias are evenly split between the jejunum and ileum, with the colon uncommonly affected. The severity of the lesion is related to the size of the vascular arcade that was affected in utero. Repair is undertaken when the baby is stable. Other anomalies are uncommon, but there is an increased risk (10%) of cystic fibrosis. A thorough abdominal examination for multiple atresias is performed.

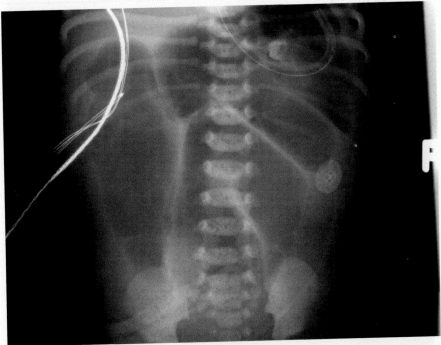

Figure 13-6: AXR in a newborn that shows significant dilation of the small intestine with no distal air indicative of a jejunal atresia. (Photo courtesy of Dr. Eric D. Strauch.)

◆ **What further studies should be done if there is an obstruction in the small intestine?**

◆ **Contrast studies** can be helpful in both diagnosis and management. If the obstruction is in the proximal jejunum, then a contrast study adds little. If the obstruction is in the distal small bowel or colon, then a contrast study is more useful. A contrast enema will reveal colonic lesions and perhaps distal ileal lesions. A microcolon suggests the atresia developed early in gestation. Hirschsprung disease, meconium ileus, and other congenital disorders may also be ruled out, making diagnosis of the atresia more certain.

◆ **How is an intestinal atresia surgically corrected?**

◆ The current **procedure of choice** is an end-to-end intestinal anastomosis. This procedure may be difficult to accomplish because of the marked size disparity of the bowel (Fig. 13-7) so a tapering of the dilated proximal bowel can be performed.

Case Variation 13.3.3.

◆ **What if the obstruction is in the distal ileum or colon?**

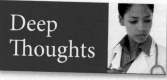

Deep Thoughts

When taking care of a neonate with an intestinal obstruction, the first decision to be made is whether the obstruction is proximal or distal. The differential diagnosis and approach is different for a proximal versus a distal obstruction.

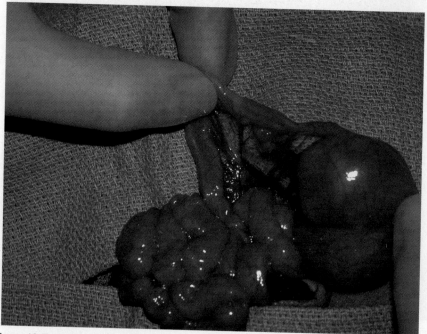

Figure 13-7: Jejunal atresia with a significant size disparity between the intestine proximal to the atresia and intestine distal to the atresia. (Photo courtesy of Dr. Eric D. Strauch.)

◆ If the baby has a distal intestinal obstruction, the differential diagnosis includes the following:

1. Ileal atresia
2. Colonic atresia
3. Meconium ileus
4. Meconium plug
5. Hirschsprung disease
6. Imperforate anus
7. Ileus

 QUICK CUT Imperforate anus should be diagnosed by physical exam and not a contrast enema.

An LGI series can help determine the diagnosis.

An ileal or colonic atresia is treated like a more proximal jejunal atresia with an end-to-end intestinal anastomosis.

◆ **What if the LGI shows inspissated meconium in the terminal ileum (Fig. 13-8)?**

◆ The treatment for meconium ileus is to attempt to washout the inspissated meconium with enema of water-soluble contrast, *N*-acetylcysteine, or saline. If washouts are unsuccessful, then surgical evacuation of the inspissated meconium is done with or without an ileostomy.

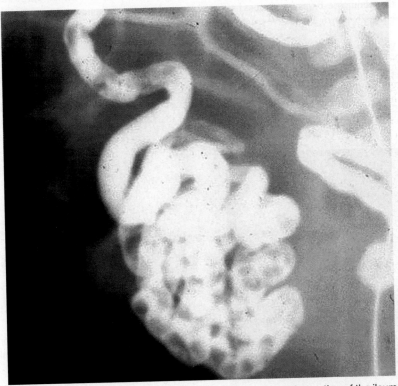

Figure 13-8: Inspissated meconium in the terminal ileum causing obstruction of the ileum secondary to meconium ileus. (Photo courtesy of Dr. Eric D. Strauch.)

Case Variation 13.3.4.

♦ **What if the LGI shows inspissated meconium in the colon?**

♦ The patient has meconium plug syndrome, where the colon is obstructed by inspissated meconium in the colon. This can be treated with colonic irrigation with saline to wash-out the inspissated meconium. Meconium plug syndrome is associated with Hirschsprung disease, cystic fibrosis, and maternal diabetes. An evaluation for Hirschsprung disease and cystic fibrosis should be performed.

Case Variation 13.3.5.

♦ **What if the LGI shows a transition zone (Fig. 13-9)?**

♦ Hirschsprung disease is caused by the congenital absence of ganglion cells in the myenteric and submucosal plexus in the intestine. As a result, the affected segment of the bowel (aganglionic segment) is unable to relax and allow effective peristalsis to occur acting as a functional obstruction. Hirschsprung disease usually involves the rectum and extends prox-imally at varying lengths most commonly involving the rectosigmoid region. Newborns with Hirschsprung disease classically present with a history of delayed passage of meco-nium and abdominal distention. An LGI will show a transition zone where the colon is more dilated than the distal rectum.

♦ **How is Hirschsprung disease diagnosed?**

♦ If the LGI shows a transition zone, then a suction rectal biopsy is performed which includes the submucosa. Biopsy specimens have an absence of parasympathetic ganglion cells and pres-ence of hypertrophied nerve trunks in the bowel wall when Hirschsprung disease is present.

♦ **What is the treatment for Hirschsprung disease?**

♦ There are a variety of different operative approaches for Hirschsprung disease. A primary pull-through procedure (one-stage) is the preferred approach in Hirschsprung patients; however, some infants require an initial diverting colostomy (two-stage procedure) prior to their definitive operation due to enterocolitis or marked dilation of proximal normal colon.

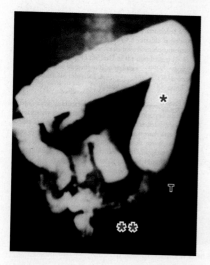

Figure 13-9: Colonic aganglionosis (Hirschsprung disease). *T*, transition zone; *, normal proximal colon; **, aganglionic spastic bowel. (From Dudek RW, ed. *BRS Embryology*, 5th ed. Baltimore: Lippincott Williams & Wilkins; 2010.)

Although different operative procedures are available for the definitive repair, all have three goals in common:

1. Resect the involved aganglionic intestine.
2. Re-establishment of a functional GI tract by bringing normal ganglionic bowel to the anus.
3. Preserve sphincter function.

 QUICK CUT Hirschsprung disease can also present later in life with potentially lethal enterocolitis.

Enterocolitis is the initial clinical presentation of a small percentage of children with Hirschsprung disease. Patients present with profuse diarrhea, abdominal distention, and fever. Enterocolitis develops due to intestinal stasis proximal to the aganglionic segment of bowel resulting in bacterial overgrowth and translocation. Treatment includes serial rectal irrigations and IV antibiotics. If the patient does not improve with medical therapy, an emergent colostomy may be required.

Case 13.4 Imperforate Anus

A newborn full term baby presents with mild abdominal distention. The nurse is unable to take a rectal temperature.

◆ **What if the patient does not have a normal anal opening?**

◆ Abnormal termination of the anorectum has a clinical spectrum that ranges from a fistulous opening in the perineal area or a rectourethral fistula to a completely blind ending of the rectum or common cloaca where the urethra, vagina, and rectum open into a common channel.

Although many classifications have been proposed for an imperforate anus, the simplest division is on the basis of sex and the relationship to the levator ani:

1. **Infralevator (low) type:** The rectum passes through the puborectalis sling usually with a fistula to the perineum.
2. **Intermediate:** This type is more common in girls, resulting in a rectovestibular fistula.
3. **Supralevator (high) type:** The rectum does not pass through the puborectalis sling. This type is more common in boys, resulting in a rectourethral fistula or a common cloaca (common opening for the rectum, vagina, and urethra in girls).

Associated anomalies are common in patients with an imperforate anus, and this congenital defect is associated with the VACTERL syndrome; 50%–60% of patients with an anorectal malformation will have an abnormality of another system. Therefore, a VACTERL workup with an echocardiogram, renal ultrasound, spine films and spinal ultrasound, passage of an NG tube, and a thorough physical exam should be performed.

Diagnosis of an imperforate anus appears easy; however, determination of the extent of the lesion is critical for management.

◆ **What is the next step if the patient has a perineal fistula?**

◆ The first step is a thorough examination of the perineum and, in girls, the introitus. If a fistula is found in the perineal area, dilation of the fistula is performed and an elective anoplasty done usually without a colostomy.

◆ **What is the next step if the patient has a fistula within the vestibule?**

◈ The patient has a vestibular fistula, which is inside the labia majora but outside the labia minora (therefore, it is not a fistula to the vagina but shares a common wall with the vagina). Some surgeons will perform a colostomy before repair and others will repair without a colostomy. If the repair breaks down or an infection occurs, then a colostomy will be done to prevent further stool drainage onto the repair to allow for healing.

◆ **What is the next step if the patient has no visible fistula?**

◈ Radiographic evaluation should be performed around 12–24 hours after birth; otherwise, the rectum may appear higher than it actually is. Additionally, this allows for additional studies to rule out other malformations. If no external fistula is identified, the surgeon must determine whether the rectum has traversed the puborectalis sling. Using ultrasound or an invertogram (a radiograph with the infant inverted and the perineum marked), the surgeon can identify the extent of the rectum by visualizing the distal extent of the intraluminal air. If the rectum is close to the skin, then surgery without a colostomy can be done. If a high lesion is found, then the boys will have a fistula to the urinary tract, usually the urethra.

    If the girls do not have a fistula, they usually have a common channel or cloaca, where the urethra, rectum, and vagina all open into the same channel.

◆ **How is a high lesion treated?**

◈ The treatment for the supralevator type of imperforate anus is, first, the formation of a colostomy, followed by the formation of a neorectum and anus. The posterior sagittal anorectoplasty (PSARP or Peña procedure) has been used for reconstruction of all levels of imperforate anus. The goal is to bring the rectum down to the perineum within the sphincter complex to try and maximize continence. Laparoscopy can be used to mobilize the intra-abdominal rectum from the rectourethral or rectovestibular fistula.

    All patients will need to have their neoanus dilated to prevent strictures.

Case 13.5   Vomiting in a 2-Week-Old

◆ **The patient is a 2-week-old with nonbilious projectile vomiting?**

◈ **Infantile hypertrophic pyloric stenosis (IHPS)** is a common cause of gastric outlet obstruction in infants due to hypertrophy of the muscular layer of the pylorus classically causing nonbilious forceful projectile vomiting.

    It is a male-predominant disease with a male-to-female ratio of 4:1. The offspring of a female with a history of pyloric stenosis have a 10-fold greater chance of developing pyloric stenosis, whereas offspring of a male with a history of pyloric stenosis have a fourfold greater chance of developing pyloric stenosis. Environmental factors associated with IHPS include breast feeding, seasonal variability, and erythromycin exposure.

◆ **How is the diagnosis of pyloric stenosis made?**

◈ Palpation of the enlarged pylorus, also termed "the olive," in the midepigastrium can be diagnostic for pyloric stenosis. Patience and persistence on physical exam with the infant supine and legs bent to relax the abdominal wall muscles is essential to palpating the enlarged pylorus.

    Complete evacuation of the stomach by an NG tube may aid in finding the mass.

    Ultrasound is the standard initial imaging technique to assist in diagnosing IHPS but does not supplant a thorough physical exam for diagnosis. A positive study confirming the diagnosis of pyloric stenosis is defined as a pyloric channel length of 16 mm or greater and a pyloric muscle thickness of 4 mm or greater.

UGI is helpful for diagnosing IHPS when ultrasound results are equivocal (Fig. 13-10). Findings include an elongated pyloric channel with a "string" sign or "railroad track" sign (one or two thin barium tracts, respectively, through the pylorus). Gastric emptying of contrast is slowed.

◆ How is pyloric stenosis treated?

◆ Preoperatively, correction of the hypokalemic, hypochloremic metabolic alkalosis is essential prior to anesthesia and surgical correction of pyloric stenosis with a goal of decreasing the serum bicarbonate level to less than 30 mEq/L. Optimal resuscitation is achieved through IV administration of normal saline boluses and 5% dextrose in 0.45 normal saline containing 20 mEq of potassium chloride at 1.5–2 times the normal maintenance rate. The alkalosis is corrected through sodium repletion and volume resuscitation. Thus, when the alkalosis is resolved, sodium and volume repletion is complete.

 QUICK CUT Surgery should not be done until the electrolytes are normal.

The surgical procedure of choice is the Ramstedt pyloromyotomy. This procedure involves an incision of the serosa down the length of the enlarged pylorus to the depth of the mucosa. A complete myotomy is demonstrated through bulging of the submucosa through the divided hypertrophied muscle. An intraoperative leak test is performed to rule out any perforation. Pyloromyotomy may be done through an open or laparoscopic approach. Studies have demonstrated equal efficacy and complication rates; therefore, most centers are performing

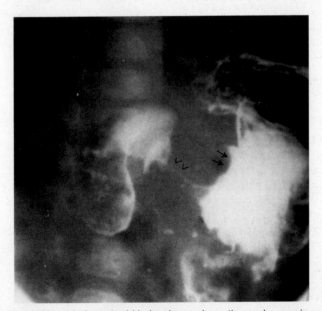

Figure 13-10: The UGI in this 6-week-old baby shows elongation and narrowing of the pyloric channel (*arrowheads*). On the stomach side, notice the rounded indentation (*arrows*) caused by the very hypertrophied pyloric muscle. This is called the shoulder sign. Together, this combination of signs is diagnostic for pyloric stenosis. (From Erkonen WE, Smith WL, eds. *Radiology 101*, 3rd ed. Philadelphia: Lippincott Williams & Wilkins; 2009.)

the procedure laparoscopically. The complication rate is very low and includes a perforation of the pylorus or an incomplete myotomy; both occur about 1% of the time.

Feeds are advanced as tolerated postoperatively.

Case 13.6 Abdominal Wall Defects

A newborn baby is born with an abdominal defect and intestine outside the abdominal wall.

◆ **What is the most important initial physical finding?**

◆ Is the intestine covered? If herniated abdominal contents are covered, then the defect is an omphalocele. An omphalocele is a central abdominal wall defect located at the umbilicus ranging from 2 to 12 cm (giant omphaloceles).

Most omphaloceles are lateral fold defects that always occur at the umbilicus and are covered with a sac (Fig. 13-11). A sac covering the extruding visceral contents is always present. If the omphalocele has ruptured, a sac remnant will be visible. The sac usually contains the liver, midgut, and frequently other organs such as the stomach, colon, spleen, and gonads.

 QUICK CUT Approximately 50%–60% of infants with an omphalocele have one or more associated anomalies.

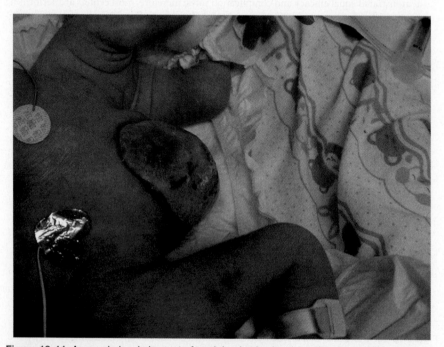

Figure 13-11: An omphalocele in a set of conjoined twins involving the shared abdominal wall of the twins. The sac has been treated with topical antibiotic and now has thickened and developed an eschar. The intact sac helps prevent heat and fluid loss and protects the abdominal contents from infection and desiccation. (Photo courtesy of Dr. Eric D. Strauch.)

◆ **What is the initial treatment for a neonate with an omphalocele?**

◆ As long as the sac is intact, there is no emergent need for operative intervention. NG decompression, IV fluid resuscitation, and broad-spectrum antibiotics are instituted. An evaluation for associated anomalies is done, particularly an echocardiogram to look for congenital cardiac anomalies and a renal ultrasound for renal anomalies. A genetic evaluation should be performed to look for chromosomal abnormalities.

◆ **How is the omphalocele defect treated?**

◆ **Operative management** in omphaloceles can vary greatly depending on both the size of the defect and whether the sac is intact or ruptured. The choice of procedures includes primary closure; staged repair; or, for an unruptured omphalocele, initial nonoperative management.

    Primary repair can prove to be problematic with larger omphaloceles due to the size of the defect, visceroabdominal disproportion, and the presence of other congenital anomalies and medical comorbidities. If primary repair is attempted, monitoring for intra-abdominal hypertension is essential because the growth of the abdominal cavity is governed by the presence of the abdominal contents. If the contents are outside the abdomen, the abdominal cavity may not have developed adequate space for the herniated contents and putting these contents back in under too much pressure may result in abdominal compartment syndrome.

    Staged repair includes the following:

1. Silastic sheeting or preconstructed silo bags can be used to stage the repair. By keeping tension on the prosthetic sac through routine bedside reductions, the Silastic sheet stretches the abdominal wall enough to accommodate the herniated viscera.
2. A prosthetic material such as a biologic or prosthetic mesh can be used to close the defect.
3. As with a staged repair of gastroschisis, closure is usually accomplished within 10 days.
4. An alternative method of treatment is to cover the defect with skin flaps, leaving the resultant ventral hernia to be repaired later on. Excess tension with this method of closure may also result in abdominal compartment syndrome.

    Nonoperative management is an alternative in patients with associated pulmonary hypoplasia and cardiac anomalies that may not tolerate reduction of a silo. Initial nonoperative management acts as a bridge to delayed closure when the infant is more stable. The sac is coated with silver sulfadiazine or a silver-impregnated sterile dressing. An eschar forms with subsequent coverage by granulation tissue; the resultant ventral hernia can be repaired later.

    The risks associated with this method are rupture of the sac, requiring subsequent repair in an infected area; sepsis; and prolonged hospitalization.

◆ **What if the defect has no sac?**

◆ Then the defect is a **gastroschisis**, which is an opening in the abdominal wall, immediately adjacent to the right of the umbilicus, which is located in the normal position. During fetal development, the abdominal wall is completely formed, but the peritoneal cavity is underdeveloped because of the protruding viscera, which usually consist of the small intestine, the stomach, and the colon.

    The intestine is edematous, semirigid, leathery, and matted together as a result of chemical peritonitis (Fig. 13-12).

    Associated anomalies and syndromes are rare, and intestinal atresia is the most frequent (10% of cases) anomaly.

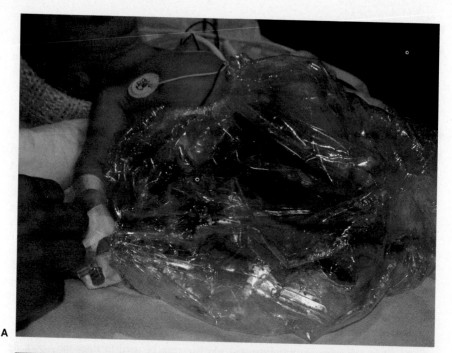

A

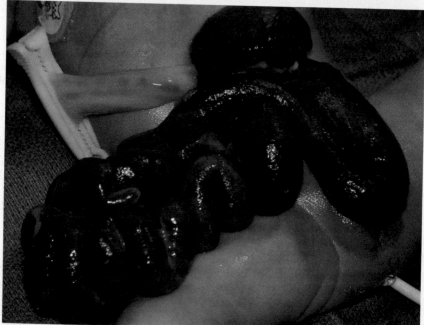

B

Figure 13-12: Gastroschisis. **A:** The baby is placed in a sterile bag to the nipples to cover the exposed GI contents to prevent heat and fluid loss and protect against infection. **B:** The inflamed intestine before closure of the gastroschisis defect. (Photos courtesy of Dr. Eric D. Strauch.)

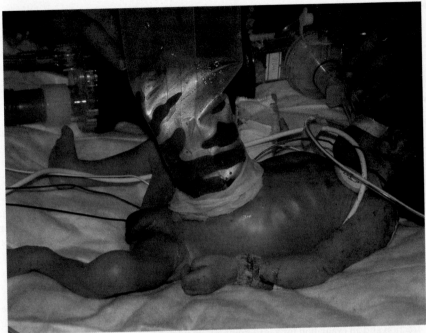

Figure 13-13: A neonate with gastroschisis without enough abdominal domain to allow primary closure and a silo covering the exposed GI contents. (Photo courtesy of Dr. Eric D. Strauch.)

◆ **How is gastroschisis treated?**

◆ Closure is emergent, as there is no covering over the GI tract to prevent heat and fluid losses. Primary closure involves decompressing the GI tract and stretching the abdominal wall over the defect.

◆ **What happens if the closure is too tight?**

◆ Abdominal compartment syndrome will occur resulting in impairment of ventilation and blood supply, abdominal wall and abdominal contents, and venous congestion of the lower extremities. To avoid this complication, it is better to cover the exposed organs temporarily with prosthetic materials. Preconstructed silicon ventral wall defect silo bags are now available for staged closure with the herniated contents reduced 1–2 times a day. Reduction can now usually be completed by days 5–7, thus minimizing the risk of infection (Fig. 13-13).

Case 13.7 Abdominal Pain in a 1-Year-Old

A 1-year-old otherwise healthy male patient presents with a 12-hour history of intermittent fussiness, decreased appetite, lethargy, and attacks of crying every 20 minutes while drawing his knees up to his chest. His abdomen is not distended and has no signs of peritonitis.

◆ **What is the most likely diagnosis?**

◆ The intermittent abdominal pain, lethargy, and drawing the knees up to the chest are classic for idiopathic ileocolic or colocolonic intussusception.

◆ **What age does idiopathic intussusception usually occur?**

◆ Idiopathic intussusception usually occurs in children age 6 months–3 years and involves the colon. It differs from small bowel intussusceptions which are usually related to a lead point, which is an intraluminal mass that is the instigator for the intussusception, involve only the small bowel, and usually occur in older patients.

◆ **What is the next step?**

◆ The next step would be AXRs looking for extraluminal or free air and signs of a bowel obstruction. If the AXRs do not show any extraluminal air, then an ultrasound is done looking for a target sign indicative of an intussusception.

◆ **How is an idiopathic intussusception treated?**

◆ After placement of an IV and resuscitation, the intussusception is treated by reduction. Most patients can have their intussusception reduced with an air contrast enema under fluoroscopy. Air is insufflated into the rectum and colon up to 120 cm pressure in an attempt to completely reduce the intussusception.

◆ **What if the intussusception cannot be reduced by air contrast enema?**

◆ The patient is taken to surgery for surgical reduction of the intussusception. This can be done laparoscopically or via an open technique. The intussusception is reduced by gentle traction and an evaluation for a lead point (5% incidence) is performed.

◆ **What do you tell the parents?**

◆ There is a recurrence rate of about 7% after reduction of an intussusception.

◆ **What if the intussusception cannot be surgically reduced?**

◆ Surgical resection of the affected intestine is required if reduction fails because the intusscepted intestine is too edematous to reduce or is already necrotic. Usually, it is safe to perform a primary anastomosis; an ostomy is reserved only for children who are unstable.

Index

Page numbers followed by *f* and *t* indicate figures and tables, respectively.

A

AAA. *See* Abdominal aortic aneurysm
ABCDE assessment, 361*t*
ABCD rule, 299
Abdomen, acute, 144–172
  differential diagnosis of, 145–147
  evaluation of, 147–148
  gastric cancer and, 158–159
  GERD and, 148–150
  hiatal hernia and, 150–151
  key thoughts on, 144–145
  peptic ulcer disease and, 151–161
  perforated ulcer and, 159–161
Abdominal aortic aneurysm (AAA), 124–129
  aneurysms associated with, 125
  bruit with, 221
  drawing of, 125*f*
  imaging of, 125, 125*f*
  postoperative care in, 126–127
  postoperative complications in, 128–129
  repair of, 126–127, 126*f*
  ruptured, 127–129, 128*t*, 403
Abdominal bruit, 129, 221
Abdominal compartment syndrome, 398
Abdominal distention, posttraumatic, 398
Abdominal pain, crampy
  colorectal cancer and, 249, 251–252
  inflammatory bowel disease and, 223–230
  small bowel obstruction and, 211–223
Abdominal pain, epigastric, 146–161
  differential diagnosis of, 146–147
  evaluation of, 147–148
  gastric cancer and, 158–159
  GERD and, 148–150
  hiatal hernia and, 150–151
  pancreatitis and, 195–201
  peptic ulcer disease and, 151–161
  perforated ulcer and, 159–161
Abdominal pain, LLQ, diverticulitis and, 261–266
Abdominal pain, postprandial
  mesenteric ischemia and, 129–130
Abdominal pain, RLQ
  appendicitis and, 230–237, 231*f*
  bladder outlet obstruction and, 232
  carcinoid tumor and, 235–237

  gastroenteritis and, 232
  pelvic abscess and, 237
  urinary tract infection and, 231–232
Abdominal pain, RUQ
  acute cholangitis and, 184–185
  acute cholecystitis and, 177–179
  differential diagnosis of, 174–175
  gallbladder empyema and, 180–182
  gallstone pancreatitis and, 180
  gallstones and, 174–177
  liver abscess and, 208–209
  palpable (inflamed) gallbladder and, 182–184
Abdominal trauma, 381–393
  blunt, 381
  computed tomography in, 382, 384–392, 387*f*–388*f*, 390*f*–391*f*
  continual assessment in, 392
  diagnostic peritoneal lavage in, 382–383, 382*f*
  focused sonography in, 381, 382–385, 383*f*
  hypotension in, 384–385
  initial assessment of, 381–385
  mechanism of injury, 381–382, 381*t*
  operative findings in, management of, 392–393
  penetrating, 375–376, 377*f*, 381–382
  surgical exploration in, 382, 384, 392–393
Abdominal ultrasound, postoperative, 186–187
Abdominal wall defects, 434–437
Abdominoperineal resection, 252–259, 308–309
  alternatives to, 257–258
  anatomy and, 253*f*
  in female patients, 258
  level of lesion from anal verge and, 254–257
  principle of, 253
  risks and complications of, 252–253
  techniques in, 253, 254*f*, 257, 257*f*
Abscesses
  amebic, 203, 209
  breast, 357, 358*f*
  colectomy and, 251
  hepatic, 203, 208–209, 208*f*
  intra-abdominal, diverticulitis and, 264–266
  pancreatic, 198, 198*f*

Abscesses (*continued*)
  pelvic
    appendicitis and, 235, 236*f*, 237, 238*f*
    postoperative, 251
  perianal, 276–277
  pilonidal, 277
  pyogenic, 209
  stitch, 39
ACC. *See* American College of Cardiology
Achalasia, 82–83
  barium swallow in, 82, 83*f*
  esophagomyotomy for, 83, 84*f*
Acidosis
  lactic, 371
  metabolic
    ischemic bowel and, 220
    small bowel obstruction and, 215
    trauma and, 397
Acral lentiginous lesions, 308
Acute abdomen. *See* Abdomen, acute
Acute respiratory distress syndrome (ARDS)
  adult (traumatic), 405–406
  infant, 419–424
    congenital diaphragmatic hernia and,
      419–421
    esophageal atresia and, 421–424
Acute suppurative thyroiditis, 294
Acute tubular necrosis, 412
Adenocarcinoma(s)
  duodenal, 194
  esophageal, 83–85
  gallbladder, 194–195, 194*f*
  lung, 52–56, 55*f*
  pancreatic
    ampullary, 194
    biopsy of, 189–190
    head of pancreas, 187–192
    imaging of, 188–189, 188*f*–189*f*
    palliative surgery for, 192, 193*f*
    resection of, 191, 192*f*, 194
  rectal, 252–254
  small bowel, 236–237
Adenoma(s)
  bronchial, 64–65
  hepatic, 201–206
  parathyroid, 288, 289*f*, 291
  thyroid, 283
Adhesions, small bowel, 213, 215*f*, 216–218
Adrenal cortical carcinoma, 298
Adrenal mass, incidental, 298, 298*f*
Advanced cardiac life support (ACLS), 35
AHA. *See* American Heart Association
Airway management
  in burn injuries, 409, 413
  in cervical spine injury, 374, 374*f*
  in neck injury, 406
  in trauma, 361–362, 394
Alcoholic cirrhosis. *See* Cirrhosis
Alkalosis, metabolic, small bowel obstruction
      and, 211
Amaurosis fugax, 103
Amebic abscess, 203, 209
American College of Cardiology (ACC), risk
      assessment tool of, 1–3, 2*t*
American Heart Association (AHA), risk
      assessment tool of, 1–3, 2*t*
American Society of Anesthesiologists (ASA),
      physical status classification of, 3, 5*t*
Amino acids, in parenteral nutrition,
      417, 417*t*
Amyloid deposits, 283
Anal carcinoma, 241, 242*f*, 260–261, 261*t*
Anal fissures, 275–276, 276*f*
Anal fistula, 276, 277*f*
Anal melanoma, 308–309
Anaplastic thyroid carcinoma, 283, 287
Anemia, preoperative care for patient with, 7
Anesthesia
  epidural, 8
  risk assessment for, 3, 5*t*
  selection of type, 3–6
Aneurysm(s)
  abdominal aortic, 124–129, 221, 403
  iliofemoral, 125
  popliteal, 125
Angina
  aortic stenosis and, 78–79
  preoperative care for patient with, 16
  unstable (preinfarction), 73–77
Angiography
  in lower GI bleeding, 270, 272
  in renal injury, 389
  in thoracic aortic dissection, 378,
      379*f*, 380*f*
Animal bites, 46
Ankle–brachial index (ABI), 17, 112–113,
      112*t*, 113*f*, 113*t*
Annular pancreas, 426–427
Anoscopy, in lower GI bleeding, 267
Antibiotics, prophylactic
  for cholecystectomy, 177
  for infective endocarditis, 23–24
  for wound infections, 45, 46*t*–48*t*
Anticoagulation therapy
  for acute arterial occlusion, 105
  for deep venous thrombosis, 133–134, 143
  GI bleeding as complication of, 142
  for pulmonary embolism, 139
Antidiuretic hormone. *See also* Vasopressin
  inappropriate secretion of, 396–397

Antrectomy
  for gastric ulcer, 156, 156*f*–157*f*
  vagotomy with, 153, 154*f*, 157
Anus, imperforate, 429, 431–432
Aortic aneurysm, abdominal, 124–129
  aneurysms associated with, 125
  bruit with, 221
  drawing of, 125*f*
  imaging of, 125, 125*f*
  postoperative care in, 126–127
  postoperative complications in, 128–129
  repair of, 126–127, 126*f*
  ruptured, 127–129, 128*t*, 403
Aortic disease, 96–97. *See also specific types*
Aortic dissection
  ischemia with, 111, 221
  thoracic, 132–133, 377–380
    angiography of, 132, 378, 379*f*, 380*f*
    grading of, 380, 380*t*
    history of, occlusion related to, 221
    radiographic findings of, 132, 378,
      378*f*, 379*t*
    types of, 132, 132*f*
Aortic stenosis, 78–79, 79*f*
Aortic valve disease, 78–79
Aortic valve replacement, 79
Aortobifemoral bypass, 120–122, 121*f*
  basic steps in, 122
  cardiovascular risk in, 122
  "trash foot" in, 122
Aortoenteric fistula, 129, 130*f*, 131*f*
Aortofemoral reconstruction, 116–118, 118*f*
Aortoiliac occlusive disease, 114–115, 120–122
  aortobifemoral bypass for, 120–122, 121*f*
  cardiac risk in reconstruction procedures
    for, 123–124, 124*f*
  management of, 120
  patterns of, 115*f*
Aphasia, 103
Apical blebs, 67–70, 71*f*
Appendicitis, 230–237
  acute gangrenous, 235
  age distribution of, 234
  corticosteroids and masking of, 234
  differential diagnosis of, 231–237, 233*f*
  fecalith with, 235
  location of pain in, 231*f*
  pelvic abscess in, 235, 236*f*, 237, 238*f*
  perforated, 234, 235
  in pregnancy, 234, 234*f*
  rectal and pelvic examinations in, 230
  retrocecal, 230–231, 233
Appendix
  carcinoid tumor of, 235–237, 236*f*
  retrocecal, 230, 230*f*

ARDS. *See* Acute respiratory distress syndrome
Arm edema, in breast cancer, 345
Arrhythmia
  head injury and, 372
  postoperative, 28–29
Arterial blood gases (ABGs), 11, 34–35
Arterial bypass grafts, 97. *See also specific
    procedures*
Arterial occlusion. *See also specific arteries*
  acute lower body (leg), 104–111
    balloon catheter embolectomy for,
      105–107, 109*f*
    common sites of, 105, 106*f*
    compartment syndrome with, 107–110
    immediate management of, 105
    limb salvage/viability in, 105, 108*t*, 109*t*
    6 P's of, 105, 107*t*
Arteriovenous fistula
  abdominal aortic aneurysm and, 403
  dialysis and, 403
  traumatic, 401–403
Arteriovenous malformations, and lower GI
    bleeding, 267–269
ASA. *See* American Society of
    Anesthesiologists
Aspirin
  for carotid artery disease, 98, 100*t*, 103
  preoperative, 6
Asymmetries, on mammography, 332
Atelectasis
  bronchial adenoma and, 64–65
  postoperative, 31, 34
Atherosclerosis, 15
  aortoiliac, 120–122
  carotid artery, 97–104
  coronary artery, 73–77
  mesenteric, 129–130
  peripheral vascular, 97–119. *See also*
    Peripheral vascular disease
Atrial fibrillation
  embolization to bowel in, 220
  preoperative care for patient with, 17
Atypical ductal hyperplasia, 337, 338*f*
Axillary vein thrombosis, 136

B
Bacterial endocarditis prophylaxis, 23–24
Balloon catheter embolectomy, 105–107, 109*f*
Balloon tamponade, of esophageal varices,
    170, 171*f*
Band ligation, of esophageal varices, 167,
    169*f*, 170
Barium enema
  in colorectal cancer, 245, 245*f*
  in diverticulitis, 262, 263*f*

Barium enema (*continued*)
  in inflammatory bowel disease, 228,
    233, 233*f*
Barium swallow
  in achalasia, 82, 83*f*
  in esophageal cancer, 83, 84*f*, 89*f*, 90–91
  in pharyngeal diverticulum, 81, 81*f*
Barlow syndrome, 77–78
Barrett esophagus, 83, 85*f*, 149–150
Basal cell carcinoma, 300
Basal energy expenditure (BEE), 414, 415*t*
Basal skull fracture, 394–395, 396
Bassini repair, 320–321, 320*f*
Biliary colic, 174
Biliary sepsis, acute, 182
Biliary stricture, 184, 185*f*
Bilious emesis, 424–431
  duodenal atresia and, 425–427
  volvulus and, 424–425
Biopsy
  breast, 334, 335*f*, 336*f*
  bronchial, 64
  esophageal, 83, 90–91
  hepatic, 204–206
  lung, 51–52, 62
  pancreatic, 189–190, 201
  pleural, 65, 67*f*
  sentinel node, 350–351, 350*f*
  skin, 300, 300*f*
  soft tissue sarcoma, 309–310, 310*f*
  thyroid, 280–283, 281*f*–282*f*, 297
BI-RADS. *See* Breast Imaging Reporting and
    Database System
Bite injuries, 46
Bladder function, abdominoperineal resection
    and, 253
Bladder outlet obstruction, 232
Bleeding ulcers, 161–165
Blindness, monocular transient, 103
Blood loss
  intraoperative, 26, 27*t*
  traumatic, 370–372, 370*t*
Blood pressure
  high. *See* Hypertension
  low. *See* Hypotension
Blood transfusion, for lower GI bleeding, 270–272
Blunt trauma
  abdominal, 381
  neck, 409
  thoracic, 377
Body surface area (BSA), in burn injuries,
    410, 411*t*
Bowel injury, 389, 392
Bowel perforation, toxic megacolon and,
    228–230

Bowel prep, 246
Bradycardia, 372
Brain edema, 395–396
Brain herniation, 395
Brain injury, traumatic, 394–397
Brain metastases, 357
Branham sign, 402
BRCA1/BRCA2 genes, 330
Breast, anatomy of, 346, 347*f*
Breast abscess, 357, 358*f*
Breast cancer, 330–359
  biopsy for, 334, 335*f*, 336*f*
  breast reconstruction in, 352, 353*f*
  diagnostic mammography for, 334, 341
  genetics of, 330
  hypercalcemia in, 291, 357
  infiltrating, 341–343, 355
  inflammatory, 343–344, 355–356
  local recurrence of, 356
  medical management of, 353–354, 354*t*
  in men, 359
  metastatic, 214, 291, 343, 355, 356–357
  new primary, 356
  pathologic findings in, 335–337, 338*f*
  in patients of advanced age and decreased
    function, 358–359
  in pregnancy, 358
  prognostic indicators in, 343–345, 343*t*
  risk factors for, 330–331, 331*t*
  screening for, 330–334
    benefits and effectiveness of, 331
    evaluation of abnormality in, 332–334
    false-negative results in, 332
    radiation exposure in, 332
    recommendations on, 330, 330*t*
  sentinel node biopsy in, 350, 350*f*
  sequelae of, 356–357
  stage I and II, treatment of, 350–352
  stage III and IV, treatment of, 355
  staging of, 341–343, 342*t*
  surgical management of, 345–352,
    348*f*–349*f*, 351*f*
Breast cysts, 345
Breast disorders, 329–359. *See also specific*
    disorders
  key thoughts on, 329–330
  in men, 359
  in pregnancy and peripartum period, 357–358
Breast edema, 343–344, 355–356
Breast enlargement, in men, 359
Breast Imaging Reporting and Database
    System (BI-RADS), 332–334, 332*t*
Breast masses
  with cellulitis and edema, 355–356
  fixation to chest wall, 345

mammography of, 332–334
in men, 359
palpable, management of, 337–340
subareolar, 345
in younger women, 339–340
Breast reconstruction, 352, 353*f*
Breast retraction, 344
Breslow thickness of melanoma, 301–302,
    301*f*, 302*t*
Bronchial adenoma, 64–65
Bronchial rupture, 365, 366*f*
Bronchitis
    postoperative, 34
    preoperative, 10
Bronchoscopy, 53–54, 56, 64
Bruits
    abdominal, 129, 221
    aortic, 79
    arteriovenous fistula and, 402
    carotid, 17, 79, 98, 104
    peripheral artery, 111
Burns, 409–413
    airway management in, 409, 413
    assessment of, 410, 410*t*
    circumferential, 413
    depth and types of, 410, 410*t*
    electrical, 413
    escharotomy for, 413, 414*f*
    fluid management in, 411–412
    full-thickness, 410*t*
    partial-thickness, 410*t*
    rule of 9's in, 410, 411*t*
    superficial, 410*t*
    topical treatment of, 412
    transfer to burn center for, 410, 411*t*

C
CABG. *See* Coronary artery bypass graft
CAD. *See* Coronary artery disease
Calcified gallbladder, 174, 195
Calcium imbalance, 287–291
    breast cancer and, 291, 357
    hyperparathyroidism with, 287–291, 287*f*
    renal failure and, 291–292
    symptomatic, 287–290
    thyroid surgery and, 283–284
Calories, in parenteral nutrition, 415, 416*t*
Cancer. *See also specific types*
    adrenal cortical, 298
    breast, 330–359
    duodenal, 194
    esophageal, 83–90, 150
    gallbladder, 194–195, 194*f*
    gastric, 158–159
    liver, 202, 203–204, 206–207

lung, 52–62
pancreatic, 187–192, 194
parathyroid, 288
skin, 299–309
thyroid, 280, 283–287, 297–298
Candida infection, in burn injury, 412
Carbon monoxide poisoning, 412
Carcinoembryonic antigen (CEA), 239, 259,
    286
Carcinoid tumor
    appendiceal, 235–237, 236*f*
    small bowel, 237, 237*f*
Cardiac disease. *See* Heart disease
Cardiac output, 400, 405
Cardiac risk
    in major vascular reconstruction, 123–124,
        124*f*
    in noncardiac surgery, 1–3, 2*t*, 13–17, 14*f*
    in surgical patient with cardiac disease, 6–7,
        15–17, 22–24
Cardiac tamponade, 367–368, 369*f*
Cardiogenic shock, 401
Cardiology consultation, 7–8
Cardiomyopathy
    dilated, 80
    preoperative care for patient with, 24
Cardiopulmonary arrest, postoperative, 35
Cardiopulmonary bypass, 76, 76*f*
Cardiovascular pressures, 402, 402*t*
Carotid artery disease, 79, 97–104
    asymptomatic, 104, 104*t*
    duplex examination for, 98, 99*f*, 100*f*, 104
    embolism formation in, 97–98, 98*f*
    key thoughts on, 96
    pharmacologic therapy for, 98, 100*t*
    surgery for, 98–99. *See also* Carotid
        endarterectomy
Carotid artery injury, 409
Carotid bruit, 17, 79, 98, 104
Carotid endarterectomy, 17, 98–103
    in asymptomatic patients, 104
    basic steps in, 101, 102*f*
    indications for, 101*t*
    monitoring in, 102
    nerve injury in, 100, 101*f*
    percutaneous *versus* open, 98–99
    pharmacologic therapy *versus,* 98, 100*t*
    preoperative evaluation for, 99
    stroke risk in, 99–100
    technical perfection in, 102
Catheter-related infections, 32, 417
CDH. *See* Congenital diaphragmatic hernia
CEA. *See* Carcinoembryonic antigen
Cecal volvulus, 273, 274*f*
Celiac artery occlusion, 129–130, 221

Cellulitis
  breast (mastitis), 357–358
  breast mass with, 355–356
  postoperative, 32
  preoperative care for patient with, 9
Central hematoma, 389, 390*f*, 393*t*
Central venous catheter, 371
Central venous pressure (CVP), 398–401
Cerebral perfusion pressure, 395
Cerebrospinal fluid (CSF) leak, 396
Cervical spine injury, 372–374
  comatose patient and, 374
  intubation in, 374, 374*f*
  neurologic deficits in, 374
  precautions and immobilization in, 373
  radiographic findings in, 373, 373*f*
Chagas disease, 83
Chemoembolization, of liver metastases, 260
Chest pain
  aortic dissection and, 132–133
  empyema and, 71–73
  pneumothorax and, 67–70
  unstable angina and, 73–77
Chest radiograph
  asymptomatic abnormality seen on,
    50–52, 51*f*
  free air under diaphragm on, 159–161, 161*f*
  postoperative, 34–35
  preoperative, 3, 4*t*
  symptomatic abnormality located in hilum
    on, 56–60, 59*f*
  symptomatic abnormality seen on, 52–56, 55*f*
Chest tube drainage
  air leak in, 69–70, 365, 403
  for chest injury, 404
  for empyema, 73, 73*f*
  for hemopneumothorax, 375
  for pneumothorax, 67–69, 69*f*, 70*f*,
    364–365, 364*f*, 403
  tube placement in, 69, 71*f*, 365
CHF. *See* Congestive heart failure
Child-Turcotte-Pugh score, 18, 19*t*
Cholangiocarcinoma, 192–194, 202
Cholangitis
  acute, 184–185
  suppurative, 181–182, 183*f*
Cholecystectomy
  antibiotic prophylaxis in, 177
  for asymptomatic disease, 174
  for cancer, 195
  complications of, 177
  for gallstone (biliary) pancreatitis, 180
  laparoscopic, 177
    for acute calculous cholecystitis, 179
    for common bile duct obstruction, 179

  complications of, 185–187
  for empyema, 181, 182*f*
  for gallstone pancreatitis, 196
  for gallstones, 176–177
  for palpable (inflamed) gallbladder,
    183–184
  for polyp, 195
  postoperative care in, 177
Cholecystitis
  acute, 174
  acute calculous, 177–179
    antibiotic therapy for, 178
    laparoscopic cholecystectomy for, 179
Choledochojejunostomy, 184, 186*f*
Cholelithiasis (gallstones), 174–182
  acute cholecystitis with, 177–179
  asymptomatic, 174
  common bile obstruction in, 179
  empyema in, 180–182
  laboratory findings in, 175–176
  laparoscopic cholecystectomy for, 176–177
  laparoscopic complications in, 185–187
  Murphy sign in, 175, 175*f*
  pancreatitis with, 179, 180, 181*f*, 196
  in pregnancy, 179–180
  ultrasound of, 174, 174*f*, 175, 176*f*
Cholesterol, preoperative, 6
Chronic obstructive pulmonary disease
    (COPD), preoperative care for
    patients with, 11–12
Circumferential burns, 413
Cirrhosis
  duodenal ulcer in, 165
  esophageal varices in, 166*f*, 167–172
  gastric varices in, 166–167, 166*f*
  total parenteral nutrition and, 418
  upper GI bleeding in, 165–172
Clark levels in melanoma, 301–302,
    301*f*, 302*t*
Claudication, 111–115
  absence of femoral pulse with, 114–115
  nonoperative therapy for, 114
  surgery for, 113–114
Clean-contaminated wounds, 44–45, 44*t*, 45*t*
Clean wounds, 44–45, 44*t*, 45*t*
Clopidogrel, for carotid artery disease, 98
Closed head injury, 371–372
Closed loop bowel obstruction, 214, 215*f*,
    216–218
Clostridium perfringens, 33
Coagulation studies, preoperative, 4*t*
Coccidioidomycosis, 51
Coin lesions, 50–52
  computed tomography of, 51, 54*f*
  radiographic appearance of, 50, 51*f*

Colectomy
    for colorectal cancer, 246, 247f
        operative (pathologic) findings in, 250
        postoperative complications of, 251–252
    for diverticulitis, 263–266
    for lower GI bleeding, 271
    sigmoid, for volvulus, 273
    for ulcerative colitis, 226
Colitis
    acute, 228–230
    Crohn disease, 225
    ulcerative. See Ulcerative colitis
Collagen, in wound healing, 39, 40f, 42
Colloid nodules, thyroid, 283
Colon
    dilation and obstruction of, acute, 272–274
    dysplasia of, 226
    ischemia and necrosis of, 221–223
    polyps of, 241–244, 243f, 249
Colonic aganglionosis, 430–431, 430f
Colonic atresia, 428–429
Colonic intussusception, 437–438
Colonic pseudo-obstruction, acute, 273–274
Colon injury, in repair of abdominal aortic
        aneurysm, 128–129
Colonoscopy
    in colorectal cancer, 245, 252, 259
    in diverticulitis follow-up, 262
    in inflammatory bowel disease, 228, 232
    in lower GI bleeding, 268
    screening, for cancer, 238–239, 239t
Colorectal cancer, 238–261
    abdominal wall invasion in, 250
    abdominoperineal resection in, 252–259
    adjuvant chemotherapy for, 248
    colostomy alternatives in, 257–258
    follow-up in, 248–249
    heme-positive stool in, 244–249
    hemorrhoids versus, 240
    invasive, 244, 249
    left- and right-sided lesions in, 245, 245f,
        245t
    locations of, 244f
    metastatic, 206, 207t, 248–250, 252,
        259–261
    obstruction in, 249
    operative (pathologic) findings in, 250
    perforated, 262
    perianal fungating mass in, 241, 242f
    polyps and, 241–244, 244f, 249
    postoperative complications of, 251–252
    preoperative radiation therapy for, 257
    recurrence of, 248–249, 251–252, 259
    screening for, 238–239, 239t
    staging of, 248, 248t, 253, 255f–256f

    surgical management of, 246, 247f, 252–259
    ulcerative colitis and, 226–227
    in younger patients, 249
Colostomy, 277–278
    abdominopelvic resection and, 252–259
    alternatives to, 257–258
Coma
    metabolic, TPN and, 417
    trauma and, 395–397
Coma scale, Glasgow, 362, 362t, 394, 396
Common bile duct obstruction, 179, 184–185,
        185f, 192–193
Common femoral vein thrombosis, 133–136,
        135f
Compartment syndrome, 107–110
    abdominal, 398
    fasciotomy for, 110, 110f
Congenital anomalies, 419–438. See also
        specific anomalies
    key thoughts on, 419
Congenital diaphragmatic hernia (CDH),
        419–421
    differential diagnosis of, 420
    initial management of, 420
    prognosis of, 421
    pulmonary hypertension with, 420–421
    surgical management of, 421
Congestive heart failure (CHF)
    mesenteric ischemia in, 221, 223
    with normal coronary arteries, 80
    preoperative care for patient with history
        of, 23
Constipation
    appendicitis versus, 233
    colorectal cancer and, 249
    fecal impaction in, 214, 274
    small bowel obstruction versus, 218–219
Contaminated wounds, 44–45, 44t, 45t
Cooper ligament repair, 321, 321f, 325, 326f
COPD. See Chronic obstructive pulmonary
        disease
Core-needle biopsy, breast, 334
Coronary artery bypass graft (CABG), 74–77
    alternatives to, 75
    conduits for, 75
    effectiveness of, 74, 75f
    left internal mammary artery–left anterior
        descending artery (LIMA-LAD), 77
    minimally invasive, 77
    multiple arterial, 77
    noncardiac surgery for patient with, 16
    prophylactic, for patients undergoing
        vascular surgery, 123–124, 124f
    robot-assisted, 77
    techniques in, 76–77

Coronary artery disease (CAD), 73–77
  left main, 74
  three-vessel, 74, 74f
Corticosteroids, appendicitis masked
    by, 234
Creatinine, preoperative levels of, 3, 4t
Crohn disease
  appendicitis *versus*, 232–233, 233f
  characteristics of, 224t
  colitis in, 225
  management of, 225
  perianal disease in, 225
  small bowel obstruction in, 223–225
  stricturoplasty in, 225
  ulcerative colitis *versus,* 226
Cushing reflex, 372
CVP. *See* Central venous pressure
Cyst(s)
  breast, 345
  echinococcal, 202–203, 203f
  hepatic, 201–203
  mediastinal, 94t
  thyroid, 280
Cystic duct stump leak, 187, 187f
Cystogastrostomy, 200–201, 201f
Cystourethrogram, retrograde, 372

D

DCIS. *See* Ductal carcinoma in situ
Deep venous thrombosis (DVT), 133–143
  anatomic definition of, 133, 134f, 136
  anticoagulation for, 133–135, 143
  conditions associated with, 136, 138t
  duplex ultrasound of, 133, 135f
  long-term morbidity of, 135–136
  monitoring treatment for, 134
  physical findings in, 133
  prevention of, 136–139
  recurrence of, 135, 136f
  risk factors for, 136, 137t
  severe, 143
  upper extremity, 97, 136
  venous incompetence and, 137f
"Depleted" patients, TPN for, 414
Diabetes insipidus, 29, 397
Diabetes mellitus, preoperative care for patient
    with, 7, 9
Diagnostic peritoneal lavage, 382–383, 382f
Dialysis, arteriovenous fistula in, 403
Diaphragm, free air under, 159–161, 161f
Diaphragmatic hernia, congenital,
    419–421
Diaphragmatic injuries, 375–376, 377f, 384,
    385f, 391, 392f

Diarrhea
  acute colitis and, 228–230
  colorectal cancer and, 249
Dilated cardiomyopathy, 80
Dipyridamole–thallium scintigraphy (DTS),
    123, 124f
Direct inguinal hernia, 316–320, 317f
Dirty wounds, 44, 44t, 45t
Distal esophagitis, with GERD, 148–149
Distal popliteal obstruction, 117–118
Distal subtotal gastrectomy, 158
Diuresis, postobstructive, 29–31
Diverticula
  bleeding, 267–269, 269f
  pharyngeal, 80–82, 82f
Diverticulitis, 261–266
  abscess or perforation in, 264–266
  algorithm for, 264, 265f
  computed tomography of, 262, 262f
  fistula with, 266, 267f
  follow-up in, 262, 263f
  Hinchey classification of, 264, 264t
  initial management of, 261–262
  recurrence of, 262, 263–264
  surgical management of, 263–266
Double bubble sign, 425, 426f
Down syndrome
  duodenal atresia in, 426
  tracheoesophageal fistula in, 423
Ductal carcinoma in situ (DCIS), 335–337, 338f
Ductal hyperplasia, atypical, 337, 338f
Dukes classification, of colorectal cancer,
    248, 248f
Duodenal adenocarcinoma, 194
Duodenal atresia, 425–427
  preoperative management of, 426
  radiographic findings of, 425, 426f
  surgical management of, 427
Duodenal hematoma, 389–391, 391f
Duodenal ulcer, 152–153
  bleeding, 161–165
    hypotension with, 164–165
    suture ligation of, 164, 165f
  with clean, white base, 164
  with fresh clot adherent to liver, 164
  with fresh clot and visible artery at base,
    164
  intractable, with history of
    hyperparathyroidism, 294–297
  in patient with acute renal failure, 165
  in patient with chronic alcoholic cirrhosis, 165
  perforated, 159–161
    radiograph findings of, 159, 161f
    surgical treatment of, 161, 162f

Duodenoduodenostomy, 427
DVT. See Deep venous thrombosis
Dyspepsia
    nonulcer, 147–148
    ulcer. See Peptic ulcer disease
Dysphagia
    achalasia and, 82–83
    esophageal cancer and, 83–92
    pharyngeal diverticulum and, 80–82
Dysplastic nevi, 301
Dyspnea, postoperative, 34

E

ECG. See Electrocardiogram
Echinococcal cyst, 202–203, 203f
ECMO. See Extracorporeal membrane
        oxygenation
Ectopic hyperparathyroidism, 287f
Edema
    arm, in breast cancer, 345
    brain, 395–396
    breast, 343–344, 355–356
    laryngeal, 362
    pulmonary, postoperative, 31
Effusion
    hemmorhagic, with pneumothorax, 375,
        376f, 377
    pleural
        empyema and, 71–73, 72f
        new-onset, without heart failure, 65–66
        radiographic findings of, 65, 66f
Ejection fraction, 74, 80
Electrical burn, 413
Electrocardiogram (ECG)
    for patients undergoing vascular surgery, 123
    postoperative, 34–35
    preoperative, 3, 4t, 6–7, 15
Electrolytes. See also Fluid management
    calculation of maintenance requirements, 27
    gastrointestinal losses and, 27, 28t
    IV fluid composition of, 27, 28t
    postoperative management of, 25–29
    preoperative levels of, 3, 4t
    small bowel obstruction and, 211
Embolectomy, balloon catheter, 105–107, 109f
Embolism
    acute arterial, lower body (leg), 104–111, 106f
    carotid artery, 97–98, 98f
    computed tomography of, 139, 140f
    ophthalmic artery, 103
    pulmonary
        computed tomography of, 139, 140f
        confounding findings in, 140–141
        IVC filter for, 141–142, 142f

long-term complications of, 140
    postoperative, 34–35, 139–140
    recurrent, on anticoagulation therapy,
        141–142
    risk factors for, 136, 137t
    treatment of, 139
Embolization, to bowel, in atrial fibrillation, 220
Embolization therapy, in lower GI bleeding, 272
Emesis, bilious, 424–431
Emphysema, subcutaneous, in neck, 408
Emphysematous gallbladder, 184
Empyema
    gallbladder, 180–182
    pleural, 71–73
        drainage of, 73, 73f
        radiographic findings of, 71, 72f
Endocarditis prophylaxis, 23–24
Endocrine disorders, 279–298. See also specific
        disorders
    key thoughts on, 279
Endoscopic retrograde
        cholangiopancreatography (ERCP)
    of acute cholangitis, 184
    of cholangiocarcinoma, 192–193
    of common bile duct obstruction, 179
    of cystic duct stump leak, 187, 187f
    of pancreatic adenocarcinoma, 189, 189f
    of suppurative cholangitis, 182
Endoscopy. See specific procedures
Energy expenditure
    estimation of, 415, 415t
    and total parenteral nutrition, 414–415
Entamoeba histolytica (amebic abscess), 203, 209
Epidermoid carcinoma. See Squamous cell
        carcinoma
Epidural anesthesia, 8
Epidural catheter, thoracic, 404
Epidural hematoma, 396
Epigastric pain, acute, 146–161
    differential diagnosis of, 146–147
    evaluation of, 147–148
    gastric cancer and, 158–159
    GERD and, 148–150
    hiatal hernia and, 150–151
    pancreatitis and, 195–201
    peptic ulcer disease and, 151–161
    perforated ulcer and, 159–161
ERCP. See Endoscopic retrograde
        cholangiopancreatography
Erectile dysfunction
    abdominal aortic aneurysm and, 127
    abdominoperineal resection and, 252–253
Erosive esophagitis, 149
Escharotomy, 413, 414f

Esophageal atresia, 421–424, 422f
    congenital anomalies associated with, 423
    diagnosis of, 422–423
    initial management of, 421
    preoperative care in, 423–424
    surgical management of, 424
    types of, 422–423, 423f
Esophageal cancer, 83–92
    barium swallow in, 83, 84f
    Barrett esophagus and, 150
    cervical and upper third, 88, 89f
    endoscopic ultrasound of, 85–87, 86f, 87f
    etiology of, 83–85
    lower third, 90, 92f
    middle third, 84f, 85, 88–89
    palliative surgery for, 91–92
    staging of, 85–87, 87f, 88t
    tracheoesophageal fistula with, 90–92
    treatment of, 87–90, 88t
Esophageal disease, 80–92. See also specific types
    key thoughts on, 50
Esophageal dysplasia, 85, 149
Esophageal manometry, 148, 149f
Esophageal reflux. See Gastroesophageal
        reflux disease
Esophageal varices, 166f, 167–172
    balloon tamponade of, 170, 171f
    band ligation of, 167, 169f, 170
    drug therapy for, 170
    portosystemic shunts for, 171
    sclerotherapy for, 167
    TIPS procedure for, 170, 172
Esophagectomy, 88–90
    formal, 89, 91f
    transhiatal, 88–89, 90f
Esophagitis
    distal, with GERD, 148–149
    erosive, 149
    reflux, 83
Esophagogastrectomy, 159, 160f
Esophagogastrojejunostomy, 157
Esophagomyotomy
    for achalasia, 83, 84f
    for pharyngeal diverticulum, 82, 82f
Estimated blood loss (EBL), 26, 27t
Excisional biopsy
    of skin lesion, 300, 300f
    of soft tissue sarcoma, 309–310
Extracorporeal membrane oxygenation
        (ECMO), 421

F
Familial hypocalciuric hypercalcemia
        (FHH), 287
Fasciotomy, 110, 110f

FAST. See Focused assessment with
        sonography for trauma
Fecal impaction, 214, 274
Fecalith, 235
Fecal occult blood test (FOBT), 238
Femoral artery puncture, 110
Femoral fracture, 371, 398
Femoral hernia, 316–319, 319f
    inguinal hernia versus, 325
    repair of, 325, 326f–327f
Femoral pulse, 105, 114–115
Femoral vein thrombosis, 133–136, 135f
Femorofemoral bypass, 120
Femoropopliteal bypass, 117–118, 119f, 119t
Fever, postoperative, 31–33
Fibroadenoma, breast, 340
Fibrocystic breasts, 340
Fine-needle aspiration (FNA), of thyroid
        nodule, 280–283, 281f–282f, 297
First-degree burns, 410t
Fissures, anal, 275–276, 276f
Fistula
    aortoenteric, 129, 130f, 131f
    arteriovenous
        abdominal aortic aneurysm and, 403
        dialysis and, 403
        traumatic, 401–403
    diverticular, 266, 267f
    perineal, 431
    postoperative, 35–36, 35f, 36f
    rectourethral, 431–432
    small bowel, 35–36, 35f, 36f, 218, 225
    tracheoesophageal, 90–92, 421–424, 422f, 423f
    vestibular, 432
Fistula-in-ano, 276, 277f
Flail chest, 403–406, 404f
Flexible sigmoidoscopy, 238
Fluid management
    in burn injuries, 411–412
    calculation of maintenance requirements,
        27, 27t
    in diverticulitis, 262
    gastrointestinal losses and, 27, 28t
    in head trauma, 395
    in hypovolemic trauma, 369–379
    intraoperative, 26–27, 27t
    IV fluid composition in, 27, 28t
    in lower GI bleeding, 266–268
    in pancreatitis, 196–197
    postoperative, 25–29
        in acute renal failure, 30
        in trauma patients, 398–401
    in SIADH, 396–397
    in small bowel obstruction, 211
    in upper GI bleeding, 164

FNA. *See* Fine-needle aspiration
Focal nodular hyperplasia, 201–202, 206*f*
Focused assessment with sonography for
　　trauma (FAST), 381–385, 383*f*
Fogarty catheter embolectomy, 105–107, 109*f*
Follicular thyroid carcinoma, 285, 286
Formal esophagectomy, 89, 91*f*
Fracture(s)
　　femoral, 371, 398
　　pathologic, 356
　　pelvic, 371, 385
　　rib, 403–404
　　skull, basal, 394–395, 396
Free air in abdomen, 384
Free air in peritoneal cavity, 217
Free air under diaphragm, 159–161, 161*f*
Free fluid in peritoneal cavity, 392
Full-thickness burns, 410*t*
Functional status assessment, 3, 3*t*
Fundoplication, 148, 149, 150*f*
Fungal disease, coin lesions in, 50–51

G
Gallbladder
　　emphysematous, 184
　　palpable (inflamed), 182–184
　　porcelain or calcified, 174, 195
Gallbladder adenocarcinoma, 194–195, 194*f*
Gallbladder disease, 174–187. *See also specific*
　　types
　　key thoughts on, 173
Gallbladder empyema, 180–182
Gallbladder polyps, 195
Gallbladder removal. *See* Cholecystectomy
Gallstone pancreatitis, 179, 180, 181*f*, 196
Gallstones (cholelithiasis), 174–182
　　acute cholecystitis with, 177–179
　　asymptomatic, 174
　　common bile obstruction in, 179
　　empyema in, 180–182
　　laboratory findings in, 175–176
　　laparoscopic cholecystectomy for, 176–177
　　laparoscopic complications in, 185–187
　　Murphy sign in, 175, 175*f*
　　pancreatitis with, 179, 180, 181*f*, 196
　　in pregnancy, 179–180
　　ultrasound of, 174, 174*f*, 175, 176*f*
Gangrene, venous, 143
Gangrenous appendicitis, acute, 235
Gastrectomy
　　for gastric cancer, 158–159
　　for gastric ulcers, 156–157, 156*f*–157*f*
Gastric cancer, 158–159
　　at gastroesophageal junction, 159, 160*f*
　　infiltrating, 159

resection of, 158–159
　　staging of, 158, 158*f*
Gastric lymphoma, 172
Gastric ulcer, 155–157
　　bleeding, 165
　　drug therapy for, 155
　　evaluation of, 147–148
　　and gastric cancer, 158–159
　　at gastroesophageal junction (type IV),
　　　155*f*, 156–157, 157*f*
　　on lesser curvature (type I), 155, 155*f*
　　prepyloric (type III), 155*f*, 157
　　of stomach body (type II), 155*f*, 157
　　surgical treatment of, 156–157, 156*f*–157*f*
　　types of, 155, 155*f*
Gastric varices, 166–167, 166*f*
　　in chronic pancreatitis, 167
　　in cirrhosis, 166–167
　　portosystemic shunting for, 167, 167*f*–169*f*
　　TIPS procedure for, 167, 167*f*
Gastric volvulus, 151, 152*f*
Gastrin levels, elevated, 295
Gastrinoma, 294–297, 295*t*, 296*f*
Gastritis, upper GI bleeding in, 166–167
Gastroenteritis, abdominal RLQ pain in, 232
Gastroesophageal junction
　　gastric cancer at, 159, 160*f*
　　gastric ulcer at, 155*f*, 156–157, 157*f*
Gastroesophageal reflux disease (GERD),
　　148–150
　　Barrett esophagus with, 149–150
　　distal esophagitis with, 148–149
　　esophageal manometry in, 148, 149*f*
　　evaluation of, 146–148
　　hiatal hernia with, 150–151
　　infant, 424
　　Nissen fundoplication for, 148, 149, 150*f*
Gastrointestinal bleeding
　　anticoagulant therapy and, 142
　　lower, 266–272. *See also* Lower
　　　gastrointestinal bleeding
　　upper, 161–172. *See also* Upper
　　　gastrointestinal bleeding
Gastrointestinal disorders. *See also specific*
　　disorders
　　lower, 210–278
　　　key thoughts on, 210
　　upper, 144–172
　　　differential diagnosis of, 145–147
　　　evaluation of, 146–147
　　　key thoughts in, 144–145
Gastrointestinal fistula, postoperative, 35–36,
　　35*f*, 36*f*
Gastrointestinal fluid loss, 27, 28*t*
Gastrojejunostomy, 156–157

Gastroschisis, 435–437, 436f–437f
General anesthesia, 3–6
Genitofemoral nerve, hernia repair and, 323, 324f
GERD. See Gastroesophageal reflux disease
Germ cell tumors, 94t
Glasgow Coma Scale, 362, 362t, 394, 396
Glucose testing, preoperative, 3, 4t, 7, 9
Graham patch, 161, 162f
Granulation tissue, 41
Greater saphenous vein grafts, 75
Greenfield filter, 141–142, 142f
Groin pain, hernia and, 316–318
Growth factors, in wound healing, 42
Gunshot injuries, 375–377, 381–382, 408
Gynecomastia, 359

H
Halsted procedure (radical mastectomy), 346
Harris-Benedict equation, for energy expenditure, 415t
Hartmann procedure, 221, 222f, 229, 278
Hashimoto thyroiditis, 294
Head injury, 394–397
    closed, 371–372
    initial assessment of, 394–395
Healing. See Wound healing
Heart defects, congenital, 423
Heart disease, 73–80
    coronary artery, 73–77
    key thoughts on, 49
    preoperative care for patient with, 6–7, 15–17, 22–23
    valvular, 77–79
Heart failure
    congestive
        mesenteric ischemia in, 221, 223
        with normal coronary arteries, 80
        preoperative care for patient with history of, 23
    high-output, 402
Heart transplantation, 80
Helicobacter pylori infection, 151–161
    detection of, 147–148
    drug therapy for, 151–153, 155
    duodenal ulcer in, 152–153
    gastric cancer in, 158–159
    gastric ulcer in, 155–157
    pyloric channel ulcer in, 151–152, 152f
    surgical treatment of, 153, 153f–154f, 156–157, 156f–157f
    upper GI bleeding in, 161–165
Heller myotomy, 83
Hemangioma, hepatic, 201, 203–206, 205f

Hematocrit
    postoperative, 28–29
    preoperative, 7
Hematoma
    central, 389, 390f, 393t
    duodenal, 389–391, 391f
    epidural, 396
    neck, 406–408
    pelvic, 390f, 391, 393t
    retroperitoneal, 388f, 393, 393t
    temporal lobe, 396
Hematuria, postoperative, 30
Heme-positive stool
    anal cancer and, 260–261
    colonic polyps and, 241–244
    colorectal cancer and, 244–249, 252–259
    hemorrhoids and, 239–241
    rectal masses and, 252–259
    small bowel obstruction and, 214
Hemicolectomy
    for colorectal cancer, 246
    for lower GI bleeding, 271
Hemiparesis, 409
Hemoglobin, postoperative, 28–29
Hemopneumothorax, 375, 376f, 377
Hemoptysis, bronchial adenoma and, 64–65
Hemorrhoids, 239–241
    external, location of, 240, 240f
    internal, banding of, 240, 241f
    thrombosed, 240
Hemostasis, 38
Heparin
    for acute arterial embolism, 105
    for deep venous thrombosis, 133–134
    for pulmonary embolism, 139
Heparin-induced thrombocytopenia, 134
Hepatic abscesses, 203, 208–209, 208f
Hepatic adenoma, 201–206
Hepatic cysts, 201–203
Hepatic disease, 201–209. See also specific types
    key thoughts on, 173
    total parenteral nutrition and, 418
Hepatic failure
    complications affecting surgical plan in, 20–21
    preoperative care for patient with, 17–21
    severity of and risk assessment in, 18–19, 18t, 19t
Hepatic injury, 388–389, 388f, 388t, 392–393, 397–398
Hepatic metastases, 206, 207t, 248–250, 259–261
Hepatic resection, 206, 207f
Hepatobiliary iminodiacetic acid (HIDA) scan, 186–187, 186f

Hepatocellular carcinoma, 202, 203–204,
    206–207
Hernia(s), 316–328
  congenital diaphragmatic, 419–421
  femoral, 316–319, 319f, 325, 326f–327f
  hiatal, 150–151
  inguinal, 316–328
    complications of surgery for, 323, 324f,
        325–326
    detection and evaluation of, 318
    direct, 316–320, 317f
    groin pain with, 316–318
    indirect, 316–319, 317f
    laparoscopic repair of, 321–323, 323f
    open repair of, 320–321, 320f–322f
    pediatric, 325, 325f
    postoperative care in, 323
    sliding, 325–328, 327f
    small bowel obstruction with, 214, 215f,
        217–218, 317–319, 319f
    strangulated, 317–319, 319f
    surgical management of, 319–323
  ventral, 39, 44, 328
Hiatal hernia, 150–151
  paraesophageal (type II), 150–151,
      151f–152f
  sliding (type I), 150
HIDA. See Hepatobiliary iminodiacetic acid
      (HIDA) scan
Highly selective vagotomy (HSV), 153, 154f
Hinchey classification, of diverticulitis, 264,
      264t
Hirschsprung disease, 430–431, 430f
Histoplasmosis, 51
Hoarseness
  burns and, 412
  laryngeal edema and, 362
  neck injury and, 409
Hodgkin disease, mediastinal, 93–94
Hollenhorst plaque, 103
Horner syndrome, 62
HSV. See Highly selective vagotomy
Human bites, 46
Hürthle cells, 283
Hutchinson freckle, 307, 307f
Hypercalcemia, 287–291
  acute, medical management of, 290–291, 291t
  asymptomatic, 290
  breast cancer and, 291, 357
  familial hypocalciuric, 287
  hyperparathyroidism with, 287–291, 287f
  persistent postoperative, 288–289
  symptomatic, 287–290
Hyperdynamic state, 400–401
Hypergastrinemia, 295

Hypermetabolic patients, 414
Hyperparathyroidism, 287–297
  asymptomatic, 290
  ectopic, 287f
  history of, intractable duodenal ulcers with,
      294–297
  hypertension with, pheochromocytoma
      and, 292–293
  pathologic causes of, 288
  persistent postoperative, 288–289
  presenting symptoms of, 288t
  primary, 287–290, 287f, 290t
  secondary, 287f, 291–292
  sestamibi scan in, 288, 289f
  surgical management of, 288–290, 289f, 290t
  symptomatic, 287–290
  tertiary, 287f, 292
Hyperphosphatemia, renal failure and,
      291–292
Hypertension
  pheochromocytoma and, 292–293
  preoperative, 10
Hypertrophic scars, 40
Hyperventilation, in trauma patients, 395,
      403–404
Hypocalcemia
  renal failure and, 291–292
  thyroid surgery and, 283–284
Hypoparathyroidism, 287f
  thyroid surgery and, 283–284
Hypotension
  abdominal trauma and, 384–385
  bleeding ulcer and, 164–165
  cardiac tamponade and, 367–368
  hypovolemia and, 369–372
  lower GI bleeding and, 272
  myocardial infarction and, 369
  pancreatitis and, 196–197
  tension pneumothorax and, 365–368
  thoracic injury and, 375
  trauma and, 365–372
Hypothermia, in trauma, 397
Hypovolemia
  hypotension in, 369–372
  lower GI bleeding and, 266
  postoperative, 28–29, 398–401
Hypovolemic shock, 371

I

IBD. See Inflammatory bowel disease
Idiopathic intussusception, 437–438
Ileal atresia, 428–429
Ileal pouch–anal anastomosis, 226–228, 227t
Ileitis, terminal, 232–233
Ileorectal anastomosis, 226

Ileostomy, 226, 229, 278, 278f
Ileus
  meconium, 429, 429f
  paralytic, 218–219
Iliac artery occlusion, 116, 117f
  superficial femoral artery occlusion with,
    116–117
Iliac vein thrombosis, 136
Iliocaval thrombosis, 143
Iliofemoral aneurysm, 125
Iliohypogastric nerve, hernia repair and,
    323, 324f
Ilioinguinal nerve, hernia repair and,
    323, 324f
Imperforate anus, 429, 431–432
Incidental adrenal mass, 298, 298f
Incisional biopsy
  of skin lesion, 300, 300f
  of soft tissue sarcoma, 309–310, 310f
Indirect inguinal hernia, 316–319, 317f
Infantile hypertrophic pyloric stenosis (IHPS),
    432–434
  surgical management of, 433–434
  upper GI imaging of, 433, 433f
Infection(s)
  postoperative, 31–33, 401
  vascular graft, 129
  wound, 32–33, 37, 41–46, 251
Infective endocarditis prophylaxis, 23–24
Inferior vena cava (IVC) filter, 141–142, 142f
Inferior vena cava (IVC) thrombosis, 136
Infiltrating ductal carcinoma,
    341–343, 355
Inflammatory bowel disease (IBD), 223–230.
    See also Crohn disease; Ulcerative
      colitis
  acute colitis in, 228–230
  appendicitis versus, 232–233, 233f
  characteristics of, 224t
  toxic megacolon in, 228–230, 229f
Inflammatory breast carcinoma, 343–344,
    355–356
Inflammatory phase, of wound healing,
    38, 43f
Inflow disease, 116
Inguinal hernia, 316–328
  complications of surgery for, 323, 324f,
    325–326
  detection and evaluation of, 318
  direct, 316–320, 317f
  groin pain with, 316–318
  indirect, 316–319, 317f
  laparoscopic repair of, 321–323, 323f
  open repair of, 320–321, 320f–322f
  pediatric, 325, 325f

postoperative care in, 323
  sliding, 325–328, 327f
  small bowel obstruction with, 214, 215f,
    217–218, 317–319, 319f
  strangulated, 317–319, 319f
  surgical management of, 319–323
Inguinal region, anatomy of, 323, 324, 324f
Inhalation injury, 412
Innominate vein thrombosis, 136
Insulinoma, 297, 297t
Intermittent claudication, 111–115
Internal iliac artery injury, 385
Internal jugular vein injury, 406–408
Internal jugular vein thrombosis, 136
Internal mammary artery grafts, 75
Intestinal anastomosis, 428, 428f
Intestinal atresia
  colonic, 428–429
  duodenal, 425–427, 426f
  ileal, 428–429
  jejunal, 427–428, 427f–428f
Intestinal intussusception, 437–438
Intestinal obstruction. See Small bowel
    obstruction
Intra-abdominal abscesses, diverticulitis and,
    264–266
Intracranial pressure (ICP), 395
Intraductal papilloma (breast), 341, 342f
Intussusception, idiopathic, 437–438
Iodine-131, for thyroid carcinoma, 286
Ischemic bowel, 214, 215, 219–223, 220f
IV fluids, 27, 28t
Ivor-Lewis procedure, 89, 91f

J
Jaundice
  cholangiocarcinoma and, 192–194
  cholelithiasis (gallstones) and, 175–176
  duodenal adenocarcinoma and, 194
  evaluation of, 187
  pancreatic adenocarcinoma and, 187–192,
    194
Jejunal atresia, 427–428, 427f–428f
Jugular vein thrombosis, 136

K
Keloids, 40
Kidney disease, preoperative care for patient
    with, 21–22
Kidney failure
  dialysis-related arteriovenous fistula in, 403
  duodenal ulcer in patient with, 165
  hyperparathyroidism in, 291–292
  postoperative, 29–31
Kidney injury, 389

Kidney transplantation, surgery in patient with history of, 21–22
Klatskin tumor (cholangiocarcinoma), 192–194, 202

L

Lactic acidosis, 371
Ladd procedure, 425
Laparoscopic cholecystectomy, 177, 185–187, 196
Laparoscopic hernia repair, 321–323, 323f
Laparoscopy, pulmonary risks in, 12
Large intestine. See Colon
Laryngeal edema, 362
Laryngeal nerves, thyroid surgery and, 283–284
Laryngeal trauma, 409
Lateral femoral cutaneous nerve, hernia repair and, 323, 324f
LCIS. See Lobular carcinoma in situ
Left bundle branch block (LBBB), 16
Left internal mammary artery–left anterior descending artery (LIMA–LAD) bypass, 77
Left lower quadrant pain. See Abdominal pain, LLQ
Left main disease, 74
Lentigo maligna melanoma, 307
Leriche syndrome, 120–122
Lichtenstein repair, 321, 322f
Linitis plastica, 159
Littré hernia, 325–328
Liver abscesses, 203, 208–209, 208f
Liver adenoma, 201–206
Liver cancer, 202, 203–204, 206–207
Liver cysts, 201–203
Liver disease, 201–209. See also specific types
   key thoughts on, 173
   total parenteral nutrition and, 418
Liver failure
   complications affecting surgical plan in, 20–21
   preoperative care for patient with, 17–21
   severity of and risk assessment in, 18–19, 18t, 19t
Liver hemangioma, 201, 203–206, 205f
Liver injury, 388–389, 388f, 388t, 392–393, 397–398
Liver masses, 201–206
   cystic, 201–203
   differential diagnosis of, 201–202
   evaluation and management of, 202–206
   history and physical findings of, 202
   solid-appearing, 201–202, 203–206, 204f
Liver metastases, 206, 207t, 248–250, 259–261
Liver resection, 206, 207f

Lobular carcinoma in situ (LCIS), 337
Local anesthesia, 3–5
Lower gastrointestinal bleeding, 266–272
   angiography in, 270, 272
   blood transfusion for, 270–272
   coagulation therapy for, 268
   diverticular disease and, 267–269, 269f
   embolization for, 272
   etiology of, 267
   initial evaluation and management of, 266–267
   massive, 266–269
   massive, persistent, 269–272
   recurrence of, 268
   surgical management of, 270–272
   technetium-labeled RBC scanning in, 270, 271f
   vascular ectasias and, 267–269
   vasopressin for, 272
Lower gastrointestinal disorders, 210–278. See also specific disorders
   key thoughts on, 210
Lumpectomy, 349f, 350, 351–352, 351f, 358
"Lumpy" breasts, 340
Lung cancer, 52–62
   epidermoid (squamous cell), 54
   hilum abnormality in, 56–60, 59f
   metastatic, 59f, 60–61, 61f
   non–small cell, 54–55
   preoperative care for patient with, 11
   prognosis of, 56, 61t
   resection of, 54–60
   small cell, 54
   staging of, 54, 56, 57f–58f
Lung contusion, 398
Lung disease, 50–73. See also specific types
   key thoughts on, 49
   preoperative care for patient with, 10–12
Lung masses. See also specific types
   asymptomatic abnormality seen on chest radiography, 50–52, 51f
   key thoughts on, 49
   malignancy-simulating, 53t
   with possible metastases, 59f, 60–61, 61f
   primary, 51
   resection of, 52, 54–55, 56–60
   symptomatic abnormality seen on chest radiography, 52–56, 55f
Lung metastases, 51, 53t, 306–307, 313–316
Lymphadenectomy
   in colorectal cancer, 246
   in gastric cancer, 158–159, 237, 246
   history of, and sarcoma, 309
   in melanoma, 303–306
   in small bowel tumors, 237

Lymphadenitis, hernia and, 316
Lymph nodes
  in cancer staging. *See* Tumor–node–metastasis (TMN) staging
  palpable
    in breast cancer, 345
    in melanoma, 306
  sentinel, in breast cancer, 350–351, 350*f*
Lymphocytic thyroiditis, chronic, 283, 294
Lymphoma(s)
  gastric, 172
  mediastinal, 93–94, 94*t*
  thyroid, 283

M
MACIS scale, 286
Mallory-Weiss syndrome, 170
Mammography
  abnormalities in
    categories of, 332, 332*t*
    evaluation of, 332–334
  benefits and effectiveness of, 331
  diagnostic, 334, 339, 341
  false-negative results in, 332
  masses on, 332
  microcalcifications in, 332, 332*f*, 334
  radiation exposure in, 332
  recommendations on, 330, 330*t*
  screening, 330–334
Manometry, esophageal, 148, 149*f*
Mastectomy, 346–352, 348*f*–349*f*
  breast reconstruction after, 352, 353*f*
  lumpectomy with radiation *versus*, 351–352, 351*f*
  in men, 359
  modified radical, 346
  partial, 349*f*, 350, 351–352, 351*f*, 358
  in pregnancy, 358
  radical, 346
  simple, 346
  skin-sparing, 346
Mastitis, 357–358
McVay repair, 321, 321*f*, 325, 326*f*
Mechanical heart valves, 79
Mechanical ventilation, 404–406
Meconium ileus, 429, 429*f*
Meconium plug syndrome, 429, 430
Mediastinal masses, 93–95
  anatomic location of, 94*t*
  anterosuperior, 94*t*
  key thoughts on, 50
  middle, 94–95, 94*t*
  neurogenic, 95
  posterior, 94*t*, 95

Mediastinoscopy, 53–54, 56*f*
Mediastinum
  compartments of, 95*f*
  indistinct or widened, 377–380
Medical risks
  cardiac
    in major vascular reconstruction, 123–124, 124*f*
    in noncardiac surgery, 1–3, 2*t*, 13–17, 14*f*
    in surgical patient with cardiac disease, 6–7, 15–17, 22–24
  common, associated with routine surgery, 7–9
  in patients with kidney disease, 21–22
  in patients with liver failure, 17–21
  in patients with pulmonary symptoms/lung disease, 10–12
  in routine surgery on healthy patient, 1–6
Medullary thyroid carcinoma, 280, 283, 285–286, 297–298
Megacolon, toxic, 228–230, 229*f*
Melanoma, malignant, 299–309
  ABCD rule in, 299
  anal, 308–309
  biopsy of, 300, 300*f*
  diagnosis of, 301–306
  evaluation of lesion for, 299–301
  facial, 307–308
  family history of, 299
  histologic findings in, 302–306
  metastatic, 306–307, 309
  with palpable lymph node, 306
  small bowel obstruction in, 214, 309
  sole of foot, 308
  special problems in, 307–309
  staging of, 301–302, 301*f*, 302*t*, 303*f*, 304*t*–305*t*
  subungual, 308, 308*f*
MELD. *See* Model for End-Stage Liver Disease
MEN. *See* Multiple endocrine neoplasia
Mesenteric injury, 389
Mesenteric ischemia
  aortic dissection and, 221
  chronic, 129–130
  congestive heart failure and, 221, 223
  in older patients, 199, 219–223
  small bowel obstruction and, 215, 219–223, 220*f*
Mesenteric vessel stenosis, 221
Mesenteric volvulus, 199
Mesothelioma, 65, 66*f*
Metabolic acidosis
  ischemic bowel and, 220
  small bowel obstruction and, 215
  trauma and, 397

Metabolic alkalosis, small bowel obstruction and, 211
Metabolic coma, 417
Metabolic equivalent task (MET), 3, 3t
Metastases
    to brain, 357
    to liver, 206, 207t, 248–250, 259–261
    to lung, 51, 53t, 306–307, 313–316
    to spine, 356
Metastatic breast cancer, 214, 291, 343, 355, 356–357
Metastatic colorectal cancer, 206, 207t, 248–250, 252, 259–261
Metastatic liver cancer, 206
Metastatic lung cancer, 59f, 60–61, 61f
Metastatic melanoma, 306–307, 309
Metastatic pancreatic cancer, 190–191, 190f–191f
Metastatic soft tissue sarcoma, 313–316
Methemoglobinemia, 412–413
Metronidazole
    for perianal problems in Crohn disease, 225
    for pouchitis, 228, 278
MI. See Myocardial infarction
MIGB scan, 293, 293f
Microcalcifications, breast, 332, 332f, 334
Microinvasive follicular thyroid carcinoma, 285
Midgut volvulus, 424–425
Minimally invasive coronary artery bypass grafting (MIDCAB), 77
Mitral valve disease, 77–78
Mitral valve prolapse, 77–78
Mitral valve regurgitation, 77–78
Mitral valve repair, 78
Mitral valve replacement, 78
Mitral valve stenosis, 22–23, 78
Model for End-Stage Liver Disease (MELD), 18–19, 19t
Modified radical mastectomy, 346
Moles
    atypical, 299–301
    dysplastic, 301
Monocular transient blindness, 103
Mucosectomy, for ulcerative colitis, 226
Multiple endocrine neoplasia, 285–286
    MEN1, 295–296
    MEN2, 286, 297–298
Murphy sign, 175, 175f
Myasthenia gravis, 93
Myocardial contusion, 368
Myocardial infarction (MI)
    postoperative, 34–35
    preoperative care for patient with history of, 6–7, 15
    in trauma patient, 369

Myofibroblasts, 42
Myoglobinuria, with burn injuries, 412
Myxomatous degeneration, 77

N
Nasogastric tube, fluid and electrolyte losses from, 27, 28t
Neck emphysema, subcutaneous, 408
Neck injuries, 406–409
    blunt, 409
    gunshot wound, 408
    stab wound, 406–409
    structures to examine in, 406–407, 407t
    zones of, 407, 407f
Neck vein distention
    cardiac tamponade and, 367–369
    tension pneumothorax and, 365–369
Necrotic appendix, 234
Necrotic bowel, 215, 219–223
Necrotizing fasciitis, 33
Needle aspiration. See also Fine-needle aspiration
    for cardiac tamponade, 368
    for pneumothorax, 366
Neurogenic shock, 401
Neurogenic tumors, 95
Neurologic injury, 394–397
Neurologic risk, in surgery for peripheral vascular disease, 17
Nevi (moles)
    atypical, 299–301
    dysplastic, 301
Nipple discharge, 340–341
Nipple lesions, 345
Nipple retraction, 344
Nissen fundoplication, 148, 149, 150f
Nitrogen, in parenteral nutrition, 415–417
"Nondepleted" patients, TPN for, 413–414
Non-Hodgkin lymphoma, mediastinal, 93–94
Non–small cell lung carcinoma, 54–55
Nonsteroidal anti-inflammatory drugs (NSAIDs), preoperative, 6
Nutrition therapy, total parenteral, 413–418

O
Obese patients, preoperative care for, 7–8
Ogilvie syndrome, 273–274
Oliguria
    measurements of, 30, 30t
    PEEP and, 406
    postoperative, 28–31, 398
    trauma and, 398
Omphalocele, 434–435, 434f
Operative risks. See Medical risks
Ophthalmic artery occlusion, 103

Osteitis fibrosa cystica, 287
Outflow disease, 116
Ovarian cancer, small bowel obstruction in, 214
Oxygen saturation
 postoperative, 34
 in trauma patients, 371

P
6 P's, of arterial occlusion, 105, 107*t*
Paget disease of breast, 345
Palliation
 in esophageal cancer, 91–92
 in pancreatic cancer, 192, 193*f*
Palpable breast mass, 337–340
Palpable (inflamed) gallbladder, 182–184
Palpable lymph nodes
 in breast cancer, 345
 in melanoma, 306
Pancoast tumor, 62, 63*f*, 64*f*
Pancreas, annular, 426–427
Pancreatic abscess, 198, 198*f*
Pancreatic cancer
 ampullary adenocarcinoma, 194
 head of pancreas (adenocarcinoma),
  187–192
  biopsy of, 189–190
  imaging of, 188–189, 188*f*–189*f*
  palliative surgery for, 192, 193*f*
  resection of, 191, 192*f*
 metastatic, 190–191, 190*f*–191*f*
 prognosis of, 191–192
Pancreatic disease, 188–201. *See also specific types*
Pancreatic injury, 389, 390*f*
Pancreaticobiliary disorders, 174–201. *See also*
  specific disorders
 key thoughts on, 173
Pancreaticoduodenectomy, 191, 192*f*, 194
Pancreatic pseudocyst, 199–201
 computed tomography of, 199, 200*f*
 cystogastrostomy for, 200–201, 201*f*
Pancreatitis, 195–201
 chronic
  gastritis and gastric varices in, 167
  pancreatic cancer *versus,* 190
 computed tomography of, 196, 196*f*
 evaluation of, 146–147
 fluid resuscitation in, 196–197
 gallstone, 179, 180, 181*f*, 196
 in older patients, 199
 pancreatic pseudocyst with, 199–201
 pulmonary status in, 197–198
 Ranson prognostic signs in, 197, 197*t*
 severe necrotizing, 196–199
Papillary thyroid carcinoma, 283, 284–285, 286
Papilloma, intraductal (breast), 341, 342*f*

Paraesophageal hiatal hernia, 150–151,
  151*f*–152*f*
Paralytic ileus, 218–219
Parathyroid adenoma, 288, 289*f*, 291
Parathyroid carcinoma, 288
Parathyroidectomy, 288–292
Parathyroid glands, thyroid surgery and,
  283–284
Parathyroid hormone (PTH) imbalance,
  287–297, 287*f*. *See also*
  Hyperparathyroidism
Parenteral nutrition, total, 413–418
Partial mastectomy, 349*f*, 350, 351–352, 351*f*,
  358
Partial-thickness burns, 410*t*
Pathologic fracture, 356
Patient-controlled analgesia, 404
PCWP. *See* Pulmonary capillary wedge
  pressure
PE. *See* Pulmonary embolism
Peau d'orange, 343
Pedunculated polyps, colonic, 241–244, 243*f*
PEEP. *See* Positive end-expiratory pressure
Pelvic abscess
 appendicitis and, 235, 236*f*, 237, 238*f*
 colectomy and, 251
Pelvic examination, in appendicitis, 230
Pelvic fracture, 371, 385
Pelvic hematoma, 390*f*, 391, 393*t*
Pelvic inflammatory disease (PID), 232
Pelvic vasculature, 385, 386*f*
Penetrating trauma
 abdominal, 375–376, 377*f*, 381–382
 arteriovenous fistula with, 401–403
 neck, 406–409
 thoracic, 375–377, 376*f*, 377*f*
Peptic ulcer disease (PUD), 151–161
 drug therapy for, 151–153, 155, 162, 163*t*
 evaluation of, 146–147, 151–152
 and gastric cancer, 158–159
 perforating, 159–161
  radiograph findings of, 159, 161*f*
  surgical treatment of, 161, 162*f*
 prophylaxis in hospital setting, 162–163
 surgical treatment of, 153, 153*f*–154*f*,
  156–157, 156*f*–157*f*
 upper GI bleeding in, 161–165
Percutaneous transluminal coronary
  angioplasty (PTCA), 75
 noncardiac surgery for patient with history
  of, 16
 for patients undergoing vascular surgery,
  123–124, 124*f*
Perforated appendicitis, 234, 235
Perforated colon cancer, 262

Perforated diverticulitis, 264–266
Perforated ulcer, 159–161
  radiograph findings of, 159, 161*f*
  surgical treatment of, 161, 162*f*
Perforated viscus, 384
Perianal abscess, 276–277
Perianal mass, fungating, 241, 242*f*
Perianal problems, 225, 275–277
Pericardial tamponade, 368, 369*f*
Pericardiocentesis, 368, 369*f*
Perineal fistula, 431–432
Peripancreatic collection, 198
Peripartum period, breast problems in, 357–358
Peripheral vascular disease, 97–119
  cardiac and neurologic risk in surgery for, 13–17, 14*f*
  claudication in, 111–115
  inflow disease in, 116
  key thoughts on, 96
  outflow, 116
  toe ulceration in, 115–119
  vascular insufficiency in
    ankle–brachial index in, 112–113, 112*t*, 113*f*, 113*t*
    Doppler findings of, 112
    signs of, 111, 111*t*
Peritoneal cavity
  free air in, 217
  free fluid in, 392
Peritoneal lavage, diagnostic, 382–383, 382*f*
Pharyngeal diverticulum, 80–82, 82*f*
Pheochromocytoma, 292–293, 297
  MIBG scan of, 293, 293*f*
  surgical management of, 293
Phlebitis, suppurative, 32
Phlegmasia cerulea dolens, 143
Phosphate imbalance, renal failure and, 291–292
Phyllodes tumor, 340
PID. *See* Pelvic inflammatory disease
Pilonidal abscess, 277
Pleural abrasion, 70
Pleural biopsy, 65, 67*f*
Pleural effusion
  empyema and, 71–73, 72*f*
  new-onset, without heart failure, 65–66
  radiographic findings of, 65, 66*f*
Pleurodesis, 70
Pneumaturia, diverticulitis and, 266
Pneumonectomy, 56–60
Pneumonia
  abdominal distention in, 218–219
  postoperative, 31, 34
Pneumothorax, 362–367
  bleb excision for, 70, 71*f*
  central line insertion and, 371

chest tube drainage for, 67–69, 69*f*, 70*f*, 364–365, 364*f*, 403
  continuing pulmonary problems with, 403–404
  hemorrhagic effusion with (hemopneumothorax), 375, 376*f*, 377
  initial management of, 362–365
  pleural abrasion (pleurodesis) for, 70
  radiographic findings of, 363, 363*f*
  simple, 364
  spontaneous, 67–70
  tension, 365–368, 367*f*–368*f*
  water seal in, 68–69, 70*f*
Polycythemia, preoperative care for patient with, 7
Polycythemia vera, 221
Polyp(s)
  colonic, 241–244, 243*f*, 249
  gallbladder, 195
Polypectomy, colonic, 243
Popliteal aneurysm, 125
Popliteal obstruction, distal, 117–118
Popliteal vein thrombosis, 136
Porcelain gallbladder, 174, 195
Portosystemic shunting, 167, 167*f*–169*f*, 171
Positive end-expiratory pressure (PEEP), 405–406
Postobstructive diuresis, 29–31
Postoperative cardiopulmonary problems, 34–35
Postoperative care, 25–36
Postoperative fever, 31–33
Postoperative fistulas, 35–36, 35*f*, 36*f*
Postoperative oliguria, 28–31, 398
Postoperative pulmonary embolism, 34–35, 139–140
Postoperative tachycardia, 28–29
Pouchitis, 227–228, 278
Pre-existing conditions. *See also specific conditions*
  preoperative care for patients with, 6–24
Pregnancy
  appendicitis in, 234, 234*f*
  breast cancer in, 358
  breast problems in, 357–358
  cholelithiasis (gallstones) in, 179–180
  hemodynamic effects of, 372
Preinfarction (unstable) angina, 73–77
Premature ventricular contractions (PVCs), preoperative care for patient with, 16–17
Preoperative care, 1–24
  key thoughts on, 1
  for patients with heart disease, 6–7, 15–17, 22–24
  for patients with kidney disease, 21–22

Preoperative care (*continued*)
  for patients with liver failure, 17–21
  for patients with pre-existing conditions, 6–24
  for patients with pulmonary symptoms/ lung disease, 10–12
  for problems in patient waiting to enter operating room, 9–10
  for routine surgery in healthy patient, 1–6
Preoperative tests, 3, 4t. *See also specific tests*
Prepyloric gastric ulcer, 155f, 157
Priapism, spinal cord injury and, 374
Primary hyperparathyroidism, 287–290, 287f, 290t
Primary intention, 37–38, 38f
Proctectomy, sphincter-preserving, 257, 258f
Proctocolectomy, total, 226, 227f
Proliferative phase, of wound healing, 38, 43f
Prophylactic antibiotics
  for cholecystectomy, 177
  for infective endocarditis, 23–24
  for wound infections, 45, 46t–48t
Prosthetic heart valves, 78, 79
Psammoma bodies, 283
Pseudocyst, pancreatic, 199–201
  computed tomography of, 199, 200f
  cystogastrostomy for, 200–201, 201f
Pseudohypoparathyroidism, 287f
Pseudomonas infection
  acute suppurative thyroiditis, 294
  burn injury, 412
Pseudo-obstruction, acute colonic, 273–274
PUD. *See* Peptic ulcer disease
Pulmonary artery catheter, 30, 197, 371, 398, 402, 405
Pulmonary capillary wedge pressure (PCWP), 399–401, 402t
Pulmonary edema, postoperative, 31
Pulmonary embolism (PE)
  computed tomography of, 139, 140f
  confounding findings in, 140–141
  IVC filter for, 141–142, 142f
  long-term complications of, 140
  postoperative, 34–35, 139–140
  recurrent, on anticoagulation therapy, 141–142
  risk factors for, 136, 137t
  treatment of, 139
Pulmonary function tests, 11, 12t
Pulmonary hypertension, congenital diaphragmatic hernia and, 420–421
Pulmonary symptoms, preoperative care for patients with, 10–11
Pulsion diverticulum, 81
Pupils, in head injury, 395–396
Pyloric channel ulcer, 151–152, 152f

Pyloric stenosis, infantile hypertrophic, 432–434
  surgical management of, 433–434
  upper GI imaging of, 433, 433f
Pyloromyotomy, 433–434
Pyloroplasty, vagotomy with, 153, 153f, 157
Pyogenic abscesses, 209

R
Radical mastectomy, 346
Radiofrequency ablation, of liver metastases, 260
Ramstedt pyloromyotomy, 433–434
Ranson prognostic signs, 197, 197t
Rectal cancer, 252–259. *See also* Colorectal cancer
  abdominoperineal resection of, 252–259
  colostomy alternatives in, 257–258
  level of lesion from anal verge, 254–257
  metastatic, 252
  preoperative radiation therapy for, 257
  recurrence of, 259
  staging of, 253, 255f–256f
Rectal examination, in appendicitis, 230
Rectal prolapse, 275, 275f
Rectourethral fistula, 431–432
Recurrent laryngeal nerve, thyroid surgery and, 283–284
Red blood cell scan, in lower GI bleeding, 270, 271f
Reflux. *See* Gastroesophageal reflux disease
Reflux esophagitis, 83
Regurgitation, of undigested food, 80–82
Remodeling phase, of wound healing, 38, 43f
Renal disease, preoperative care for patient with, 21–22
Renal failure
  dialysis-related arteriovenous fistula in, 403
  duodenal ulcer in patient with, 165
  hyperparathyroidism in, 291–292
  postoperative, 29–31
Renal injury, 389
Renal transplantation, surgery in patient with history of, 21–22
Respiratory distress
  adult (traumatic), 403–406
  infant, 419–424
    congenital diaphragmatic hernia and, 419–421
    esophageal atresia and, 421–424
Resting energy expenditure (REE), 415t
Retrocecal appendicitis, 230–231, 233
Retrograde cystourethrogram, 372
Retroperitoneal hematoma, 388f, 393, 393t
Revascularization, mesenteric, 219

Rheumatic heart disease, 78
Rib fracture, 403–404
Richter hernia, 325
Right bundle branch block (RBBB), 16
Right lower quadrant pain. *See* Abdominal pain, RLQ
Right upper quadrant (RUQ) pain. *See* Abdominal pain, RUQ
Rigid abdomen, 159–161
Robot-assisted coronary bypass, 77
Roux-en-Y esophagogastrojejunostomy, 157
Rule of 9's, in burn injuries, 410, 411*t*
Ruptured abdominal aortic aneurysm, 127–128, 128*t*, 403
Ruptured bronchus, 365, 366*f*
Ruptured diaphragm, 384, 385*f*, 391, 392*f*
Ruptured kidney, 389

S
Sarcoma, soft tissue, 309–316
  biopsy of, 309–310, 310*f*
  key thoughts on, 299
  lower extremity, 309–313
  metastatic, 313–316
  pathologic features of, 310
  patient history and physical findings of, 309
  radiation therapy for, 311–313
  staging and prognosis of, 311, 312*f*–313*f*, 314*t*
  surgical management of, 311, 315*f*
Scars, 40
Scleral icterus, 249
Sclerosing adenosis, 337
Sclerotherapy, for esophageal varices, 167
Secondary hyperparathyroidism, 287*f*, 291–292
Secondary intention, 38*f*, 41
Second-degree burns, 410*t*
Seizures, brain metastases and, 357
Sentinel node biopsy, 350, 350*f*
Sessile polyps, colonic, 241–244, 243*f*
Sestamibi scan, in hyperparathyroidism, 288, 289*f*
Shock
  cardiogenic, 401
  hypovolemic, 371
  neurogenic, 401
Shouldice repair, of inguinal ligament, 321
SIADH. *See* Syndrome of inappropriate antidiuretic hormone
Sigmoid colectomy, 273
Sigmoidoscopy, flexible, 238
Sigmoid volvulus, 273, 273*f*
Silver sulfadiazine, 412
Simple mastectomy, 346

6 P's, of arterial occlusion, 105, 107*t*
Skin and soft tissue disorders, 299–316.
  See also specific disorders
  key thoughts on, 299
Skin cancer, 299–309. *See also* Melanoma, malignant
Skin graft, split-thickness, 42
Skin lesions
  biopsy of, 300, 300*f*
  evaluation of, 299–301
Skin-sparing mastectomy, 346
Skull fracture, basal, 394–395, 396
Sleeve resection (lobectomy), 56–60
Sliding hiatal hernia, 150, 151*f*
Sliding inguinal hernias, 325–328, 327*f*
Small bowel adenocarcinoma, 236–237
Small bowel carcinoid tumor, 237, 237*f*
Small bowel fistula, 218, 225
  failure to heal, 36, 36*f*
  management of, 35–36
Small bowel intussusception, 437–438
Small bowel obstruction, 211–223
  acid–base imbalances in, 211, 215
  adhesions and, 213, 215*f*, 216–218
  closed loop, 214, 215*f*, 216–218
  common causes of, 215*f*
  Crohn disease and, 223–225
  diagnosis, in complex situations, 218–219
  inguinal hernia and, 214, 215*f*, 217–218, 317–319, 319*f*
  ischemia or necrosis in, 214, 215, 219–223, 220*f*
  management of, 211–212
  melanoma and, 214, 309
  partial, 214
  proximal, 213
  radiographic findings of, 211, 212*f*, 217
  surgical indications in, 214–215, 216
  tumor-related, 214, 215*f*
Small cell lung carcinoma, 54
Small intestinal disorders, 211–223. *See also specific disorders*
Small vessel disease, 115
Smoking, as surgical risk, 10
Soft tissue disorders, 299–316. *See also specific disorders*
  key thoughts on, 299
Solitary pulmonary nodules, 50–52, 52*t*
Sphincterotomy, 276, 276*f*
Sphincter-preserving proctectomy, 257, 258*f*
Spinal anesthesia, 3–5
Spinal injury
  cervical, 372–374
  neurogenic shock in, 401
  priapism in, 374

Spinal metastases, 356
Splenectomy
  in chronic pancreatitis, 167
  in gastric cancer, 159
  postoperative management in, 398–401
  in splenic injury, 386–388
Splenic injury, 386–388, 387f, 387t, 392–393,
    398–401
Split-thickness skin graft, 42
Spontaneous pneumothorax, 67–70
Squamous cell carcinoma
  anal, 260–261, 261t
  esophageal, 83, 85, 91
  lung, 54
  skin, 300–301
Stab wounds, 375–377
  arteriovenous fistula with, 401–403
  to neck, 406–409, 407t
Staphylococcus infections
  acute suppurative thyroiditis, 294
  antibiotic prophylaxis against, 24
  burn injury, 412
  empyema, 71–73
  mastitis, 357
  vascular graft, 129
  wound, 33
Stents
  coronary, 75
  self-expanding, 110, 111f
Stereotactic breast biopsy, 334, 335f
Stitch abscess, 39
Stomas, in colostomy, 277–278
Stool, heme-positive. See Heme-positive stool
Strangulated hernia, 317–319, 319f
Streptococcus infections
  acute suppurative thyroiditis, 294
  antibiotic prophylaxis against, 24
  burn injury, 412
  empyema, 71
  mastitis, 357
  wound, 33
Stricturoplasty, in Crohn disease, 225
Stroke
  carotid artery disease and, 103–104, 104t
  preoperative care for patient with
      history of, 17
  risk in carotid endarterectomy, 99–100
Subacute thyroiditis, 294
Subclavian artery injury, 375
Subclavian vein injury, 375
Subclavian vein thrombosis, 136
Subcutaneous emphysema, in neck, 408
Subungual melanoma, 308, 308f
Sucking chest wound, 365
Superficial burns, 410t

Superficial femoral artery occlusion, 112,
    116, 117f
  aortofemoral bypass for, 116–118, 118f
  distal popliteal obstruction with, 117–118
  iliac artery occlusion with, 116–117
Superior laryngeal nerve, thyroid surgery and,
    283–284
Superior mesenteric artery occlusion,
    129–130, 131f
Superior sulcus tumor, 62, 63f, 64f
Suppurative cholangitis, 181–182, 183f
Suppurative phlebitis, 32
Suppurative thyroiditis, acute, 294
Surgical abdomen. See Abdomen, acute
Surgical Care Improvement Project (SCIP), 45
Suture knot, 39
Suture ligation, of bleeding ulcer, 164, 165f
SVR. See Systemic vascular resistance
Swallowing, neck injury and, 408
Swan-Ganz catheter, 399–400, 399f
Syncope
  aortic stenosis and, 23, 78–79
  ruptured aortic aneurysm and, 127–128
Syndrome of inappropriate antidiuretic
    hormone (SIADH), 396–397
Systemic vascular resistance (SVR),
    399–401, 400t
Systolic murmur, preoperative care for patient
    with, 23

T
Tachycardia, postoperative, 28–29
Technetium-labeled RBC scanning, in lower
    GI bleeding, 270, 271f
TEF. See Tracheoesophageal fistula
Temporal lobe hematoma, 396
Tension pneumothorax, 365–368, 367f–368f
Teratoma, mediastinal, 93
Terminal ileitis, 232–233
Tertiary hyperparathyroidism, 287f, 292
Tetralogy of Fallot, 423
Third-degree burns, 410t, 413, 414f
Third intention, 38f, 42
Thoracentesis, 65
Thoracic aortic dissection, 132–133, 377–380
  angiography of, 132, 378, 379f, 380f
  grading of, 380, 380t
  history of, occlusion related to, 221
  radiographic findings of, 132, 378, 378f, 379t
  types of, 132, 132f
Thoracic epidural catheter, 404
Thoracic trauma, 375–380
  aortic dissection in, 377–380
  blunt, 377
  initial assessment of, 375–377

penetrating, 375–377, 376f, 377f
vascular injuries in, 375, 376f
Thoracostomy, tube. *See* Chest tube drainage
Thoracotomy, emergent, 375
Three-vessel disease, 74, 74f
Thrombolysis, 107
Thymectomy, 290
Thymus tumor, 93, 94t
Thyroid adenoma, 283
Thyroid carcinoma, 283–287
    anaplastic, 283, 287
    family history of, 280
    follicular, 285, 286
    MACIS scale in, 286
    medullary, 280, 283, 285–286, 297–298
    papillary, 283, 284–285, 286
    patient history and physical findings in,
        279–280
    postoperative management of, 286–287
    surgical management of, 283–286, 285f, 298
        anatomy and, 284, 284f
        options in, 285f
        risks and complications of, 283–284
    undifferentiated, 286, 287
Thyroidectomy, 283–286, 285f, 298
Thyroiditis
    acute suppurative, 294
    chronic lymphocytic, 283, 294
    Hashimoto, 294
    subacute, 294
Thyroid lobectomy and isthmusectomy,
    284–285, 285f
Thyroid nodules, 279–287. *See also* Thyroid
    carcinoma
    colloid, 283
    cytology-based measures for, 280–283
    fine-needle aspiration of, 280–283,
        281f–282f, 297
    patient history and physical findings of,
        279–280
TIA. *See* Transient ischemic attack
TIPS. *See* Transjugular intrahepatic
    portosystemic shunt
Tissue prosthetic valves, 79
Toe ulceration, in peripheral vascular disease,
    115–119
Totally extraperitoneal repair, of hernia, 321
Total parenteral nutrition (TPN), 413–418
    amino acid requirements in, 417, 417t
    calorie calculations in, 415, 416t
    choosing solution for, 415, 416t
    complications of, 417–418
    for depleted patients, 414
    dermatologic effects of, 418
    energy expenditure in, 414–415, 415t

hepatic effects of, 418
metabolic responses in, 417, 418f
nitrogen requirement in, 415–417
for nondepleted patients, 413–414
nutritional requirements in, 413–414
standard formula for, 415, 416t
Total proctocolectomy, 226, 227f
Total thyroidectomy, 283–286, 285f, 298
Toxic megacolon, 228–230, 229f
TPN. *See* Total parenteral nutrition
Tracheoesophageal fistula (TEF), 90–92,
    421–424, 422f, 423f
Transabdominal preperitoneal repair, of
    hernia, 321, 323f
Transhiatal esophagectomy, 88–89, 90f
Transient ischemic attack (TIA), 97–104
Transjugular intrahepatic portosystemic shunt
    (TIPS), 167, 167f, 170
"Trash foot," 122
Trauma, 360–409
    abdominal, 381–393
    airway management in, 361–362
    blood and fluid loss in, 370–372, 370t
    cervical spine management in, 372–374
    continuing hemorrhage in, 397–398
    continuing pulmonary problems in, 403–406
    head (neurologic), 394–397
    hypotension in, 365–372
    key thoughts on, 360
    neck, 406–409
    postoperative problems in, 397–401
    primary survey in, 360, 361t, 394
    pulmonary management in, 362–365.
        See also Pneumothorax
    secondary survey in, 360–361
    thoracic, 375–380
Traumatic arteriovenous fistula, 401–403
Traumatic brain injury, 394–397
Truncal vagotomy and antrectomy, 153, 154f, 157
Truncal vagotomy and pyloroplasty (V&P),
    153, 153f, 157
Trypanosoma cruzi infection, 83
Tube thoracostomy. *See* Chest tube drainage
Tubular necrosis, acute, 412
Tumor–node–metastasis (TMN) staging
    of breast cancer, 341–343, 342t
    of colorectal cancer, 248, 248t
    of lung cancer, 54
    of melanoma, 301, 303f, 304t–305t
    of soft tissue sarcoma, 311, 314t

U
Ulcer(s)
    bleeding, 161–165
    duodenal, 152–153, 159–165, 294–297

Ulcer(s) (*continued*)
    gastric, 147–148, 155–159
    peptic, 146–147, 151–161
    perforating, 159–161
    prophylaxis in hospital setting, 162–163
    pyloric channel, 151–152, 152*f*
Ulcerative colitis
    acute colitis in, 228–230
    characteristics of, 224*t*
    colorectal cancer risk in, 226–227
    Crohn disease *versus*, 226
    ileal pouch–anal anastomosis for, 226–228, 227*t*
    long-standing, complications of, 226–228, 227*t*
    operative options in, 226
    postoperative follow-up in, 227
    pouchitis in, 227–228
    total proctocolectomy for, 226, 227*f*
    toxic megacolon in, 228–230, 229*f*
Undifferentiated thyroid carcinoma, 286, 287
Unstable angina, 73–77
Upper gastrointestinal bleeding, 161–172
    cirrhosis and, 166–172
    esophageal varices and, 166*f*, 167–172
    fluid resuscitation in, 164
    gastric varices and, 166–167, 166*f*
    gastritis and, 166–167
    Mallory-Weiss syndrome and, 170
    patients at higher risk for, 163, 163*t*
    peptic ulcer disease and, 161–165
    ulcer prophylaxis to prevent, 162–163
Upper gastrointestinal disorders, 144–172.
    See also specific disorders
    differential diagnosis of, 145–147
    evaluation of, 146–147
    key thoughts on, 144–145
Upper gastrointestinal endoscopy, 81, 146–147
    in gastric cancer, 158–159
    in gastric lymphoma, 172
    in GERD, 148
    in hiatal hernia, 150
    in peptic ulcer disease, 151–152
Urethral injury, 372
Urinary tract infection (UTI)
    abdominal RLQ pain in, 231–232
    postoperative, 32
    preoperative, 9
Urine analysis, in burn injuries, 412
Urine output
    normal, 29
    postoperative, 28–31
Urosepsis, 30–31
UTI. *See* Urinary tract infection

V

V&A. *See* Vagotomy and antrectomy
VACTERL association, 423, 431
Vagotomy, highly selective, 153, 154*f*
Vagotomy and antrectomy (V&A), 153, 154*f*, 157
Vagotomy and pyloroplasty (V&P), 153, 153*f*, 157
Valvular heart disease, 77–79. *See also specific types*
    endocarditis prophylaxis in, 23–24
    preoperative care for patient with, 22–24
Varices
    esophageal, 166*f*, 167–172
    gastric, 166–167, 166*f*
    portosystemic shunting for, 167, 167*f*–169*f*, 170–171
    TIPS procedure for, 167, 167*f*, 170, 172
Vascular disorders, 96–143. *See also specific types*
    cardiac and neurologic risk in surgery for, 13–17, 14*f*
    claudication in, 111–115
    key thoughts on, 96–97
Vascular ectasias, and lower GI bleeding, 267–269
Vascular graft infection, 129
Vascular injury
    in pelvic fractures, 385, 386*f*
    in stab wound to neck, 406–408
    in thoracic trauma, 375, 376*f*
Vascular reconstruction. *See also specific procedures*
    cardiac risk in, 123–124
Vasopressin
    for diabetes insipidus, 397
    for lower GI bleeding, 272
Venous disease, 133–143. *See also specific types*
    key thoughts on, 97
Venous gangrene, 143
Ventilation, mechanical, 404–406
Ventral hernia, 39, 44, 328
Ventricular septal defects, 423
Vestibular fistula, 432
Virchow triad, 136
Viscus, perforated, 384
Volvulus
    cecal, 273, 274*f*
    gastric, 151, 152*f*
    mesenteric, 199
    midgut, 424–425, 425*f*
    sigmoid, 273, 273*f*
V&P. *See* Vagotomy and pyloroplasty

W

Water seal, in chest tube drainage,
    68–69, 70*f*
Weir formula, for energy expenditure, 415*t*
Whipple procedure (pancreaticoduodenectomy),
    191, 192*f*, 194
Wound(s)
    classification of, 44–46, 44*t*, 45*t*
    clean, 44–45, 44*t*, 45*t*
    clean-contaminated, 44–45, 44*t*, 45*t*
    contaminated, 44–45, 44*t*, 45*t*
    dirty, 44, 44*t*, 45*t*
    management of, 37–40
Wound contraction, 41

Wound healing, 37–48
    complications in, 39–40
    factors delaying, 38–39, 39*t*
    phases of, 38*f*, 43*f*
    primary intention in, 37–38, 38*f*
    secondary intention in, 38*f*, 41
    strength *versus* time in, 39, 40*f*
    third intention in, 38*f*, 42
Wound infections, 32–33, 37,
    41–46, 251

Z

Zenker diverticulum, 80–82
Zollinger-Ellison syndrome, 153, 294–297